THE IRISH SWEEP

or before

For
Peter

*

THE IRISH SWEEP

A HISTORY OF THE IRISH HOSPITALS
SWEEPSTAKE
1930–87

Marie Coleman

UNIVERSITY COLLEGE DUBLIN PRESS
PREAS CHOLÁISTE OLLSCOILE BHAILE ÁTHA CLIATH

First published 2009
by University College Dublin Press
Newman House
86 St Stephen's Green
Dublin 2
Ireland
www.ucdpress.ie

© Marie Coleman 2009

ISBN 978-1-906359-40-9 hb
ISBN 978-1-906359-41-6 pb

CIP data available from the British Library

Typeset in Ireland in Adobe Caslon and Bodoni Oldstyle
by Elaine Burberry and Ryan Shiels
Printed in England on acid-free paper by
CPI Antony Rowe, Chippenham, Wilts.

Contents

—

Illustrations
vii

List of Tables
ix

Abbreviations
x

Acknowledgements
xiii

Glossary
xv

Note on the Text
xvi

INTRODUCTION
I

ONE
THE ORIGINS OF THE IRISH HOSPITALS SWEEPSTAKE
4

TWO
THE SWEEPSTAKE IN IRELAND IN THE 1930s
23

THREE
THE DEVELOPMENT OF IRISH HOSPITALS IN THE 1930s
52

FOUR

THE SWEEPSTAKE IN GREAT BRITAIN IN THE 1930s

89

FIVE

THE SWEEPSTAKE IN NORTH AMERICA IN THE 1930s

III

SIX

SURVIVAL AND RECOVERY

1939–61

144

SEVEN

DECLINE AND CLOSURE

1961–87

172

EIGHT

THE SWEEPSTAKE AND HOSPITAL DEVELOPMENT

1939–87

197

NINE

CONCLUSION

224

APPENDIX

Accounts of Sweepstake Draws

227

Notes

236

Bibliography

276

Index

287

Illustrations

—

Between pp. 176 and 177

Cover Image: The Cambridgeshire Sweepstake Draw, October 1933 © NLI, Irish Independent collection, IND_H_2798 11055

1   Joseph McGrath. Portrait by William (Liam) Belton, RHA, and Michael Brett (1969), based on an original by Leo Whelan, RHA (State Art Collection, Office of Public Works, Dublin) © Liam Belton and Michael Brett

2   Joseph McGarrity © The Digital Library, Falvey Memorial Library, Villanova University

3   Connie Neenan © The Digital Library, Falvey Memorial Library, Villanova University

4   Bernard Partridge, 'Charity begins abroad', Punch, 28 March 1934 © Punch Ltd

5   The parade of tickets counterfoils through Dublin for the Grand National Sweepstake Draw, March 1933 © NLI, Irish Independent collection, IND_H_2651 11055

6   Hospitals Trust staff mixing counterfoils for the Grand National Sweepstake Draw, March 1933 © NLI, Irish Independent collection, IND_H_2662 11055

7   The sweepstake drum decorated for the Grand National Sweepstake Draw, March 1933 © NLI, Irish Independent collection, IND_H_2652 11055

8   The parade of counterfoils through Dublin for the Grand National Sweepstake Draw, March 1935 © NLI, Irish Independent collection, IND_H_2997 11055

9   Hospitals Trust staff in themed costumes for the Grand National Sweepstake Draw, March 1935 © NLI, Irish Independent collection, IND_H_2998 11055

10 The Grand National Sweepstake Draw, March 1935 © NLI, Irish Independent collection, IND_H_3004 11055

11 1934 Derby: Grania, daughter of Cormac MacArt © Irish Hospitals' Sweepstake (also featured on the cover)

12 1935 Grand National: Granuaile (Grace O'Malley) © Irish Hospitals' Sweepstake (also featured on the cover)

13 1935 Derby: Deirdre © Irish Hospitals' Sweepstake (also featured on the cover)

14 1935 Cambridgeshire: Fionnuala, one of the children of Lir © Irish Hospitals' Sweepstake (also featured on the cover)

15 1936 Cambridgeshire: King Laoghaire's wife © Irish Hospitals' Sweepstake (also featured on the cover)

16 1937 Grand National: Brighid, Goddess of Wisdom © Irish Hospitals' Sweepstake (also featured on the cover)

List of Tables

—

1.1   Sir Patrick Dun's Hospital: financial position and number of patients treated, 1920–8

1.2   Incorporated Dental Hospital: financial position and number of patients treated, 1920–9

1.3   St Ultan's Infant Hospital: financial position and number of patients treated, 1919–29

1.4   National Maternity Hospital: admissions, attendances and operations performed, 1923–30

3.1   Total annual deficits of voluntary hospitals, 1933–9 (£)

4.1   Percentage of Irish hospitals sweepstake prizes won by British residents, 1930–4

4.2   The value of exports to Great Britain from the Irish Free State (Éire), and the estimated value of British sweepstake contributions, 1931–9

4.3   Percentage of Irish hospitals sweepstake prizes won by residents of 'Europe' [i.e. Britain], 1935–9

5.1   Geographical distribution of prizewinners, 1930–9 – percentage of prizes won

5.2   Comparison between US contributions to the Irish sweepstake and Irish exports (incl. re-exports, excl. bullion and coin) to the USA in the 1930s

6.1   Destination of prizes in selected sweepstake draws, 1940–5

8.1   Total annual deficits of voluntary hospitals, 1940–4 (£)

8.2   Fungible assets (cash, investments, and premises) of the Hospitals Trust Fund at year ended 31 December (£)

8.3   Annual figure for hospital deficits, 1946–53 (£)

8.4   Amount paid from Hospitals Trust Fund to cover deficits to the year ended 31 March, 1954–8 (£)

8.5   Expenditure of voluntary hospitals, 1947–55 (£000s)

8.6   Income of voluntary hospitals, 1947–55 (£000s)

Abbreviations

—

ANB	*American National Biography*
ATE	American Travel Exchange
BBC	British Broadcasting Corporation
BBCWA	British Broadcasting Corporation Written Archive
BBFC	British Board of Film Censors
BC	British Columbia
BHA	British Hospitals Association
BL	British Library
BLA	British Library Association
CO	Colonial Office
CSO	Central Statistics Office
CTT	Córas Tráchtála Teoranta [Irish Export Board]
DCF	Dissolved Companies Files
DD	*Dáil Debates*
DEA	Department of External Affairs
DF	Department of Finance
DFA	Department of Foreign Affairs
DH	Department of Health
DHA	Department of Home Affairs
DIB	*Dictionary of Irish Biography*
DJ	Department of Justice
DLG&PH	Department of Local Government and Public Health
DT	Department of An Taoiseach
DTT&C	Department of Transport, Tourism & Communications
DO	Dominions Office
EEC	European Economic Community
ELC	Employer–Labour Conference
FBI	Federal Bureau of Investigation
FJ	*Freeman's Journal*
FRUS	*Foreign Relations of the United States*
FVCO	Federation of Voluntary Charitable Organisations
FWUI	Federated Workers' Union of Ireland
GAA	Gaelic Athletic Association
GPO	General Post Office

G2	Irish Army, Military Intelligence Division
HLCI	Hospital Library Council of Ireland
HO	Home Office
ICTU	Irish Congress of Trade Unions
IFS	Irish Free State
IGB	Irish Glass Bottle Company
IJMS	*Irish Journal of Medical Science*
ILHM	Irish Labour History Museum
ILO	International Labour Organisation
IMA	Irish Military Archives
IRA	Irish Republican Army
IRB	Irish Republican Brotherhood
IRCA	Irish Red Cross Archives
IRCHSS	Irish Research Council for the Humanities and Social Sciences
IRCMB	*Irish Red Cross Monthly Bulletin*
Ir. Ind.	*Irish Independent*
IRN	*Irish Radio News*
Ir. Press	*Irish Press*
IRS	Internal Revenue Service
Ir. Times	*Irish Times*
ITA	Irish Tourist Association
ITGWU	Irish Transport and General Workers' Union
IWWU	Irish Women Workers' Union
LAI	Library Association of Ireland
MA	Military Archives
MEPO	Metropolitan Police Office
MP	Member of Parliament
MRCI	Medical Research Council of Ireland
NAC	National Archives of Canada
NAI	National Archives of Ireland
NARA	National Archives and Records Administration
NHS	National Health Service
NLI	National Library of Ireland
NY Times	*New York Times*
OÉL	Oireachtas Éireann Library
ÓFLA	Tomás Ó Fiaich Memorial Library and Archive
PB	Piaras Béaslaí Papers
PREM	Prime Minister's Office
PRES	Office of the Secretary to the President
RAC	Rockefeller Archive Center

RAMI	Royal Academy of Medicine in Ireland
RCBG&L	Royal Commission on Betting, Gaming and Lotteries
RCLB	Royal Commission on Lotteries and Betting
RCPI	Royal College of Physicians of Ireland
RÉ	Radio Éireann
RFA	Rockefeller Foundation Archives
RG	Record Group
RHA	Royal Hibernian Academy
RTÉ	Radio Telefís Éireann
SAI	*Statistical Abstract of Ireland*
SD	*Seanad Debates*
SIPTU	Services, Industrial, Professional and Technical Union
State DF	State Decimal Files
TB	Tuberculosis
TD	Teachta Dála [Member of the Irish Parliament]
TNA	The National Archives
UCD	University College Dublin
UCDA	University College Dublin Archives Department
UK	United Kingdom
USA	United States of America
VA	Veterans' Association
VU	Villanova University
WUI	Workers' Union of Ireland
YP	Young Philanthropists

Acknowledgements

—

The bulk of research for this book was conducted between 2001 and 2003 when I held an Irish Research Council for the Humanities and Social Sciences (IRCHSS) post-doctoral fellowship in University College Dublin. I am very grateful to the IRCHSS (especially Maurice Bric, Marc Caball and Tim Conlon) for this opportunity; since its inception the council has revolutionised research in the humanities and it is to be hoped that it will not fall victim to the current financial stringency. At UCD I benefited greatly from the advice and support of Professor Mary E. Daly.

Although the archives of Hospitals Trust are largely no longer extant, having been destroyed either when the River Dodder flooded the company's building in Ballsbridge in 1986 or when the sweepstake closed in 1987, a wealth of material on the sweepstake exists, principally in Irish government archives, and also in Britain, Canada and the USA. I wish to thank the archivists and librarians who facilitated my research in the following institutions: An Comhairle Leabharlanna (Alun Bevan); Companies Registration Office, Dublin; Irish Labour History Museum (Theresa Moriarty); Irish Military Archives; Irish Red Cross; Labour Court (Mary Aird); National Archives of Ireland (especially Brian Donnelly); National Library of Ireland; National Maternity Hospital, Dublin (Claire Grey); Royal College of Physicians of Ireland (Robert Mills); Royal College of Surgeons in Ireland, Mercer Library (Mary O'Doherty); RTÉ library sales (Stephen D'Arcy); Trinity College Dublin Library; University College Dublin Archives Department; SIPTU; Oireachtas Éireann Library (Seamus Haughey); Cardinal Tomás Ó Fiaich Memorial Library and Archive, Armagh; British Library, London; British National Archives, Kew; British Newspaper Library, Colindale; National Archives and National Library of Canada, Ottawa; Vancouver Public Library; Falvey Memorial Library, Villanova University (Bente Polites); Library of Congress, Washington DC; National Archives and Records Administration, Washington DC and New York City; Rockefeller Archive Center, Sleepy Hollow; Tamiment Library, New York University; and the libraries of the three institutions in which I worked while writing this book: University College Dublin, the National University of Ireland Galway and the Queen's University of Belfast.

Maurice Regan gave me access to the few surviving archives of Hospitals Trust, a collection of newspaper cuttings from the 1930s and 1940s, now in the National Library of Ireland. Alan Dukes, Kevin Kealy and John Slevin granted me interviews that helped fill gaps in the archival record. Ciarán Ó hÓgartaigh explained the intricacies of the Hospitals Trust Fund's accounts.

I am grateful to the following individuals and institutions for permission to reproduce the illustrations: the National Library of Ireland National Photographic Archive (*Irish Independent* collection); Punch Ltd; the Digital Library, Falvey Memorial Library, Villanova University; the State Art Collection, Office of Public Works; Mr Liam Belton RHA; and Mr Michael Brett. At UCD Press Barbara Mennell and Noelle Moran have been very enthusiastic about the project from the outset and have worked very hard on it for the past year. Máirín Garrett created another excellent index. The cost of production was offset by a grant from the Queen's University Publications Fund.

All of the following helped me out in a number of ways: Jack Anderson, Frank Bouchier-Hayes, Marion Casey, Donie Cassidy, Mike Cronin, Bernadette Cunningham, Francis Devine, Anne Dolan, Tony Farmar, Tom Feeney, Diarmaid Ferriter, Phyllis Gaffney, Brian Hanley, David Hayton, Roisín Higgins, John Horgan, Mike Huggins, Greta Jones, Liam Kennedy, James Kirwan, Marian Lyons, Joe MacAnthony, Fearghal McGarry, James McGuire, Deirdre McMahon, George Mealey, Ed Morrison, Eve Morrison, William Murphy, Caoimhe Nic Daibhéid, Mary O'Dowd, Eunan O'Halpin, Margaret Ó hÓgarthaigh, Jimmy O'Sullivan and Liam Wylie.

As always my immediate and extended family have been a great support, especially my parents, John and Rose Coleman, and my in-laws Frank, Marie, Joe, Ann, Anna-Louise and Niall Martin. Aoife Martin gave me an excuse to take maternity leave during which this book was completed. As ever, my husband Peter Martin has been a fantastic personal support as well as providing insightful professional observations on my research and writing. I dedicate this book to him.

MARIE COLEMAN
Belfast, July 2009

Glossary

—

Associated Hospitals Sweepstake Committee
A committee composed of representatives of the voluntary hospitals that originally drew up the scheme for running the sweepstakes. Chaired by Lord Powerscourt during the 1930s.

Counterfoil
The ticket stub containing the name and address of the purchaser. The portion of ticket placed in the draw.

Hospitals Commission
A body established under Public Hospitals Act (1933) to plan for future development of Irish hospitals and advise the Minister for Health on the allocation of sweepstake proceeds to participating hospitals.

Hospitals Trust
A private company established by Richard Duggan in 1930 that acquired the monopoly to promote the sweepstakes. It went into voluntary liquidation and was re-started as Hospitals Trust (1940) Ltd in 1940. Joseph McGrath served as Managing Director from 1930 to 1966.

Hospitals Trust Board
The body responsible for the money in the Hospitals Trust Board. Originally known as the National Hospital Trustees.

Hospitals Trust Fund
The fund established under Public Hospitals Act (1933) that held the hospitals' portion of the sweepstake surplus. The Hospitals Commission advised the Minister for Health on its allocation. The money was used to build and maintain voluntary and local authority hospitals and finance operating deficits of voluntary hospitals.

Voluntary Hospitals
Hospitals established in Ireland during the eighteenth and nineteenth centuries, that were under lay or religious control and were dependent on charitable endowments and contributions for their finance.

Note on the Text

—

Contemporary descriptions are used throughout. For example, the Irish state is referred to as the Irish Free State (1922–37), Éire (1938–49), and the Republic of Ireland (1949 onwards); the Departments of Justice and Foreign Affairs are referred to as Home Affairs and External Affairs during the periods when these designations were in use; and the Taoiseach (head of government) was the President of the Executive Council until 1938, and should not be confused with the President of Ireland (head of state after 1938).

Introduction

—

The Irish hospitals sweepstake funded Irish hospitals for over fifty years. It was a landmark institution in the new Irish state, attracting millions of pounds in foreign currency into Ireland to build and equip hospitals and providing employment for thousands. It also had an important impact on the development of Irish advertising and broadcasting, horse racing in Britain and Ireland, the development of indigenous Irish businesses, and the commercial sponsorship of sports.

The sweepstake was established initially to provide funds for cash-strapped voluntary hospitals in Dublin. From 1933 onwards its revenue was also used to build and equip public hospitals; most of the public hospitals in the Republic of Ireland today were built on this basis. The popular perception of the sweepstake in Ireland is that it was essential to the development of a good public hospital system, and many of the developments in Irish public health from the 1930s onwards would not have been possible without the money it generated. However, the sweepstake also had a detrimental effect on hospital financing, as charitable contributions dried up, voluntary hospitals allowed building costs and other deficits to spiral out of control in the belief that there was an endless supply of money available from the sweepstake, and successive Irish governments were relieved of responsibility for financing the state's hospital service from public funds. The principal objective of this book is to evaluate the overall impact of the sweepstake on the development of Irish hospitals in the twentieth century.

In 1930 the majority of Irish hospitals were run by voluntary charitable organisations, under either Catholic or Protestant management. Voluntary control was gradually replaced by greater state control as these hospitals began to benefit from state-controlled sweepstake funds. The voluntary hospitals fought a strong, but largely unsuccessful, battle against the encroachment of the state. Roman Catholic hospitals were particularly opposed to state control, in line with contemporary Catholic social teaching. The evolution of the role of the state is an important development in independent Ireland and this book seeks to contribute to the understanding of that process through an examination of how the health service was funded.

I

Outside the realm of public health the sweepstake was important as one of Ireland's largest employers, with a workforce of up to 4,000 women at the height of its success. The promoters made personal fortunes, much of which was reinvested in Irish industries, including the rejuvenation of Waterford Glass during the 1960s. Horse racing was linked indelibly to the sweepstakes, which were run on the major English and Irish races; sponsorship of the Irish Derby by the sweepstake turned it into the richest horse race in Europe at the time, and the promoters became leading figures in the Irish bloodstock industry. The sweepstake is best remembered today in Ireland for its sponsorship of a radio programme – *The Irish Hospitals Sweepstake Sponsored Programme* – for almost thirty years from the 1930s to the late 1950s. Advertising was crucial to its success and it was responsible for the introduction of important initiatives in Irish advertising and broadcasting, including commercial sponsorship of sporting events and the live broadcasting of horse races.

Since its closure in 1987 the underground history of the sweepstake has become more widely acknowledged. The population of Ireland was too small to generate the substantial funds needed for the Irish hospitals, so the promoters looked to the Irish diaspora, especially in Great Britain and North America, where millions of tickets were sold, generating significant foreign capital for Ireland. For much of the sweepstake's existence gambling was illegal in these countries and the promoters established an intricate system to smuggle and distribute tickets unnoticed by the legal authorities. In my research for this book, the archives of the Irish, British, American, and Canadian governments, as well as testimony by people associated with the sweepstake, has allowed me to construct a picture of how the Irish sweepstake succeeded so well in this underground activity. Another controversial aspect of the sweepstake's history that this book uncovers is the great personal wealth that accrued to the families of the three promoters, the McGraths, Duggans and Freemans. The penultimate chapter contrasts the financial comfort of the families with the shabby treatment of their workforce after the sweepstake's closure. The McGraths are no longer household names in Ireland, but for fifty years they were probably the most famous business empire in the state. Thus the story of the sweepstake is also that of the rise and fall of the first modern Irish business dynasty.

An outstanding feature of the sweepstake is the massive amount of money that it processed in the 57 years of its existence. Using the extant audited accounts of each sweepstake draw it has been possible to calculate the sums of money subscribed and the amounts expended on hospital building, administration, prizes, and taxation for the Irish state; these figures are tabulated in the Appendix.

In spite of the sweepstake's importance, there has been very little written about it. The only book published on the subject, Arthur Webb's *The Clean*

Sweep (1968), is a popular, and in places inaccurate, account of the sweepstake up to the 1960s, focusing mostly on its sensational aspects. Joe MacAnthony's controversial article 'Where the Sweep millions go' dealt in detail with the allegations of corruption, as did the Radio Telefís Éireann documentaries *The Sweep* in 1992, and Liam Wylie's more recent *If you're not in you can't win – the story of the Irish Hospitals Sweepstakes* (2003).[1] This book is, then, the first detailed account of the history of the Irish hospitals sweepstake.

In addition to telling the story of the sweepstake, this book contributes to the growing literature on Irish medical history. Ruth Barrington highlighted some of the changes to Irish health policy that resulted from the availability of sweepstake funds and Mary Daly drew attention to the friction that developed between the voluntary hospitals and the state in the 1930s, both of which issues are examined in greater detail in this book.[2] John Horgan and Greta Jones have shown how significant sweepstake funding was to Dr Noël Browne's crusade against tuberculosis in the 1950s, although the received interpretation of this subject is revised here in light of evidence from Department of Health files.[3] Individual hospital histories also provide valuable evidence of how the sweepstake was used to develop these institutions.

The overall aim of this book is to draw together these disparate aspects of the sweepstake – its social and economic importance in independent Ireland, its contribution to the development of Irish health services, and its illicit operation outside Ireland – to construct the first detailed and comprehensive history of an iconic Irish institution.

ONE

THE ORIGINS OF THE IRISH
HOSPITALS SWEEPSTAKE

—

The popularity of the public lotteries can be traced to the fifteenth century, when they were commonly used as a means of raising revenue. In sixteenth-century Britain Queen Elizabeth I resorted to this form of fund-raising to build harbours and public works, and in the seventeenth century the settlement of the Virginia colony was similarly financed. Other examples of public works in England funded through lotteries included Westminster Bridge and the British Museum. At the end of the seventeenth century the English parliament secured a virtual state monopoly on lotteries by passing legislation, which outlawed the sale of tickets in foreign lotteries and required the passing of a specific act of parliament to allow private lotteries. From that time until their prohibition in the 1820s a number of lotteries were held to raise both ordinary revenue and extraordinary loans, such as those raised during the American War of Independence and the Napoleonic wars.[1]

THE HISTORY OF LOTTERIES IN IRELAND

Lotteries were also quite popular in Ireland at this time. Lottery activity in Ireland dates from the late sixteenth century, with the first recorded Irish lottery taking place in 1621. By 1711, concern was being expressed at the number of lotteries being held, prompting an unsuccessful attempt by the Irish parliament to outlaw them. Almost two centuries before the legalisation of the hospitals sweepstake the idea of funding hospitals through lottery proceeds had gained ground. In the 1740s and 1750s Samuel Mosse conducted a variety of lotteries to provide funds for his newly established Rotunda lying-in hospital in Dublin, and in 1779 a united hospitals lottery raised £1,522 for Dublin city's St Nicholas's and St Catherine's hospitals. Systematic use of lotteries to augment government revenue in Ireland began in 1780 with the inauguration of the Irish state lottery that was to run until the Act of Union in 1801.[2]

Unlike modern lottery tickets, their early modern predecessors were not cheap. While the poorer classes were unable to participate directly in the lotteries, they often participated in illegal insurance schemes, whereby they placed smaller bets on the outcome of the lottery. The proliferation of such illegal enterprises, combined with the corruption associated with the lotteries themselves, led to their abolition under the Lotteries Act of 1823, which made it an offence, subject to a penalty of £50, to sell lottery tickets or publish proposals for a lottery. The last public lottery was held in Britain in 1826 and from that time until new legislation was enacted in 1934 public and private lotteries effectively ceased, with the exception of those permitted under the Art Union Act (1846) to finance the purchase of art works.

ILLEGAL LOTTERIES AND SWEEPSTAKES IN IRELAND IN THE 1920s

In spite of the prohibition on lotteries and other games of chance such as prize draws, the enforcers of the law traditionally turned a blind eye to small lotteries and raffles organised for charitable purposes. One of the most prominent promoters of illegal sweepstakes in Ireland in the 1910s and 1920s was the Dublin bookmaker, Richard Duggan, whose first major sweepstake was held in 1918 when he raised £1,000 for the survivors and families of victims of the torpedoed mailboat the *Leinster*.[3] The changeover of government from the Dublin Castle administration to a domestic government in southern Ireland in 1922 created legal confusion, which was exploited by Duggan and other sweepstake promoters. In the early years of independence sweepstakes and lotteries proliferated as their promoters claimed that the law was no longer clear and because the law enforcement arms of the new state had more pressing concerns than clamping down on lottery organisers.

One of the biggest sweepstakes ever organised in Ireland until that time, with a prize fund of £10,000, was Duggan's Mater Hospital sweepstake run in conjunction with the 1922 Manchester November Handicap. Although the first prize of £5,000 went to an Irishman from Derry, the distribution of the majority of the prizes outside Ireland, and especially in Britain, suggests that this was where most tickets were sold, and prefigured a pattern which emerged during the 1920s and early 1930s of an overwhelming number of tickets in Irish sweepstakes being sold outside Ireland, mostly in Britain. Second prize in Duggan's Mater sweepstake went to England, third prize to Scotland and eleven small cash prizes were won by people in England, Scotland, Wales and Canada.[4] Clearly a large number of customers successfully evaded the efforts of the British postal authorities to prevent tickets entering Britain or counterfoils being returned to Ireland.[5] Tickets, costing ten shillings each, were also reported to have been sold in South Africa, the USA, Denmark and

Egypt. To maximise the foreign market Duggan purchased lists of names of people outside Ireland likely to buy tickets. The *Irish Times* claimed that the expense of running the sweepstake amounted to £40,000, with 250 clerks, mainly female, employed to deal 'with the flood of applications for tickets'.[6] The Mater received £10,000 but Duggan's profit was never made public.[7] Another Dublin hospital, the Charitable Infirmary in Jervis Street, also organised a sweepstake, known as the 'iodine sweep' in 1925.[8] Another intrepid organiser of sweepstakes in the early 1920s was Fr John O'Nolan, of Toome, County Down, who ran sweepstakes on the 1922 Epsom Derby and the 1923 Aintree Grand National to raise funds for his parish church.[9]

Alarmed at the proliferation of sweepstakes, the government adopted a stricter policy towards them in late 1922. In addition to those organised by Duggan and Fr O'Nolan, a number of minor sweepstakes such as those for the St Andrew's Catholic Club, Peadar Cearnaigh and the Limerick Commercial Club appeared and the government decided that in future it would enforce the legal prohibition on lotteries.[10] Two sweepstakes, one organised by Duggan on behalf of Holles Street Skin and Cancer Hospital and P. L. Smyth's for Hume Street Cancer Hospital, were permitted in 1923, but no subsequent ones would be exempted from the lottery acts.[11] Applications by three Dublin hospitals – the Royal Victoria Eye and Ear, St Vincent's and the Coombe – to organise sweepstakes on the 1923 Epsom Derby and Cesarewitch to raise much-needed funds were rejected under the new policy.[12] The government was also taking note of the displeasure of British authorities at the flood of Irish sweepstake tickets into that country.[13]

Despite the government's prohibition on holding further sweepstakes, both Duggan and Smyth continued to organise them during 1923, moving the financial base of their operations to the much more liberal financial environs of Switzerland. In June Duggan ran a sweepstake on the Epsom Derby for the Meath Hospital, raising £10,000.[14] Lack of sufficient time prevented the Free State authorities prosecuting him.[15] One sanction imposed was a warrant from the Minister for Home Affairs ordering the detention of post believed to contain documents relating to the sweepstake.[16] The postal authorities agreed to detain, but not to open, such mail.[17] Another sweepstake run on the Derby for hospitals in Cork, organised by Smyth, was reported to have incurred him a loss of £30,000, largely due to the confiscation of correspondence by postal authorities. He claimed to have received only one-tenth of the letters intended for him. Nonetheless, the Cork hospitals received the £10,000 promised to them.[18] Smyth appears to have retired from the sweepstake business after this, probably because of the losses incurred.

Duggan continued to defy the government's sweepstake ban. In June 1924 he organised another sweepstake on the Epsom Derby, which raised £5,000 for the Meath Hospital.[19] Once again the organisation was based outside Ireland and in another effort to evade the strict letter of the law the competition was run as a ballot, where the ticket holder voted for past winners of the Derby in order of merit as in a parliamentary election. As such the organisers could argue that it was a game of skill rather than of chance and therefore not a lottery. This proved sufficiently confusing for the Attorney General, Hugh Kennedy, to recommend against prosecution.[20]

The legal machinery of the state finally caught up with Duggan in November 1924 when he was convicted under the Lotteries Act (1823) and fined £50 for having published a scheme and sold tickets for 'Duggan's Dublin sweep' on the Manchester November Handicap. He was also bound over to keep the peace for twelve months and gave an undertaking not to run any more sweepstakes, a promise which did not last very long.[21] Having kept his head down for a time he re-emerged in 1927 with a sweepstake on the Epsom Derby organised from Liechtenstein.[22]

The Revenue Commissioners also pursued Duggan for taxation on his sweepstake profits. He was assessed for £40,000 income tax payable on the profits from the Mater Hospital and Holles Street Skin and Cancer Hospital sweepstakes in 1922 and 1923, but contended that he should not be liable for such a payment because profits 'derived from an unlawful and criminal enterprise [i.e. sweepstakes], were not profits or gains within the meaning of the Income Tax Acts', such profits were not annual and conducting sweepstakes was not a trade or vocation. This defence was accepted initially and the assessment against him discharged by the Special Commissioners of Income Tax in 1926. The following year this decision was overturned by the High Court, but on appeal to the Supreme Court in 1928, the original decision of the Special Commissioners was upheld. Effectively, Duggan was exempt from paying income tax on sweepstakes because they were illegal and should not have been held in the first place.[23]

The large number of lotteries, draws and raffles intercepted by the post office was evidence that the government's efforts to enforce the lottery acts were ineffective. Many such competitions were innocuous when compared with the size of Duggan's sweepstakes, which the law was principally aimed at. Therefore, government policy was modified in 1925 to permit prize draws and other small lotteries where no prize exceeded £30.[24] Some groups tried to evade this restriction by offering more than one prize of £30, to which the Minister for Justice (formerly Home Affairs)[25] objected as an abuse of the concession he had granted, and which resulted in further alteration of government regulations to insist on a graduated level of prizes.[26]

In 1926 the Home Office in Britain began to put pressure on the Irish authorities to take action to stem the flood of Irish lottery tickets into Britain, drawing attention to the variety of Irish organisations peddling tickets and providing lists of persons believed to be acting as conduits for them.[27] Justice now added a further condition to its regulations governing lotteries; they would only be permitted if an undertaking was given not to sell tickets outside the Irish Free State and any post addressed to persons outside the state that was believed to contain lottery tickets would be detained.[28]

Commenting on various cases submitted by the Department of Justice to his office for advice on the likelihood of securing prosecution for breaches of the law pertaining to lotteries, the Attorney General's constant refrain was that the law in this area was unsatisfactory. In spite of the conditions it had imposed in an effort to regulate small lotteries, the department was aware of the extent to which these were violated. The prohibition on circulation of tickets outside the Free State was a particular example of the failure of lottery organisers to comply. The option of revoking the concessions and reverting to the 1923 policy of a blanket prohibition on all lotteries and sweepstakes was considered.[29] One of the biggest difficulties with the lottery acts inherited from the UK was the failure to differentiate between different types of competitions. There was a major difference between a £10,000 sweepstake organised by Duggan, resulting in a substantial private profit, and a Christmas goose club or prize draw organised to raise comparatively minuscule funds for a small sports club or repairs to a parish church. An example of the far-reaching nature of the law is found in an incident from 1926 when the Department of Justice threatened to prosecute the *Limerick Leader* newspaper if it proceeded with a relatively innocuous word puzzle.[30] The legal situation was not to be clarified until legislation permitting sweepstakes to raise funds for public charitable hospitals was enacted in 1930, after which the Department of Justice abandoned its battle to keep ticket sales within the Free State.

THE FINANCIAL CRISIS OF THE VOLUNTARY HOSPITALS

Dublin's voluntary hospitals faced a financial crisis in the 1920s, which threatened their survival. The principal causes were wartime inflation, which greatly reduced the value of their endowments, and Irish independence, after which a number of supporters of the Protestant voluntary hospitals left the country.[31] In addition to international and domestic political upheaval, public demand for new and costlier medical treatments was increasing, a decline in the number of medical students at some hospitals resulted in fewer teaching fees, and the overall cost of running a hospital rose dramatically during the 1920s.[32] A closer analysis of the hospitals that participated in the first Irish hospitals sweepstake in 1930 illustrates clearly the burdens under which the voluntary hospitals laboured during the 1920s. Tables 1.1 to 1.3 show how deficits rose in some of these hospitals as the differential between ordinary income and expenditure increased throughout the decade. The growing demand for hospital services is noticeable in the high number of attendances at the hospitals:

Table 1.1: *Sir Patrick Dun's Hospital: financial position and number of patients treated, 1920–8*

Year	Income (£)	Expenditure (£)	Deficit (£)	Bank debt (£)	No. patients treated	
					Internal	External
1920	9,286	11,545	2,259	6,872	1,400	19,120
1922	7,783	11,651	3,868		1,518	25,677
1924	8,001	10,495	2,494		1,664	31,346
1926	8,221	11,184	2,963		1,813	29,178
1928	8,314	10,118	1,804	9,676	1,633	23,893

Source: Sir Patrick Dun's Hospital Annual Reports, 1914–29.

Table 1.2: *Incorporated Dental Hospital: financial position and number of patients treated, 1920–9*

Year	Overdraft (£)	Total attendances
1920	2,423	15,096
1923	2,664	17,874
1926	3,434	15,772
1929		17,468

Source: Incorporated Dental Hospital *Annual Reports, 1919–30.*

Table 1.3: *St Ultan's Infant Hospital: financial position and number of patients treated, 1919–29*

Year	Income (£)	Expenditure (£)	In-patients	Out-patients
1919–20	1,204	926	53	214
1922–3	3,692	3,084	105	802
1925–6	1,739	2,098	162	2,071
1928–9	1,882	2,555	195	4,763

Source: Teach Ultain Annual Reports, 1919–30.

Although proud of their charitable tradition, a number of hospitals were increasingly forced to ask patients to contribute towards the cost of their treatment.[33] Yet this did not yield very significant amounts. More than a quarter of the patients in Sir Patrick Dun's Hospital, located in and serving one of the poorer districts of Dublin, were treated free, and those who did contribute were able to give only between 2s 6d and 5s per week. Only 24 of the 1,577 admitted to the hospital in 1929 were able to pay the full maintenance fee of three guineas per week.[34] A large amount of the work was done free at the Dublin Dental Hospital, with the dental school bearing the cost of gold used in fillings.[35] Of the two children's hospitals that participated in the first sweepstake, patients' fees accounted for approximately 12.5 per cent of the income of St Ultan's in the 1920s, while 70 per cent of the National Children's Hospital's patients in 1929 were either treated free or contributed less that ten shillings per week, less than one-third of the maintenance cost.[36]

In addition to the limited resources of their patients and the ever decreasing donations from the charitable public, the hospitals' principal sources of income included an annual local authority grant of a couple of hundred pounds, contributions from the ever dwindling Hospital Sunday Fund (a charitable fund collected by Dublin Protestants) and the proceeds from their own redoubled fund-raising efforts – both St Ultan's and Sir Patrick Dun's undertook fund-raising campaigns in the USA in the 1920s.

The financial woes of the hospitals were exacerbated by the physical condition of their buildings, many of which were nearly two hundred years old and in need of much repair; in 1929 the ceiling of the gynaecological landing in the National Maternity Hospital was in danger of collapsing.[37] Their city centre locations, some like the National Maternity Hospital and St Vincent's in unsuitable converted townhouses, made the level of expansion needed to cater for increased numbers of patients very difficult. Internal improvements were equally pressing; by 1922 the x-ray equipment in Sir Patrick Dun's was outdated and the cost of updating it was estimated at £1,000, while the Adelaide spent almost £5,000 remodelling its outpatient and x-ray departments in 1926.[38]

In addition to the individual difficulties of each hospital, the voluntary hospital system in Dublin was extremely inefficient. Too many small, cramped, inadequately equipped hospitals provided unnecessary duplication of treatment. The financially straitened circumstances of the 1920s brought many of the smaller hospitals to the realisation that rationalisation might solve some of their difficulties. In 1924 proposals were made by the governors of Sir Patrick Dun's to amalgamate five city hospitals – the Meath, the Adelaide, Mercer's, Sir Patrick Dun's and the Royal City of Dublin (Baggot Street). Dun's launched a campaign to raise funds for the construction of a new central

Dublin hospital with which it was intended to replace the five smaller ones.[39] The Rockefeller Foundation was also approached and sent a representative to Ireland in May 1924 to examine the issue.[40] At this juncture the foundation was considering assisting medical education and research in Ireland, and the plan to rationalise the Dublin hospitals fitted well with its philosophy of reducing the number of medical schools and reorganising them along modern lines. However, because of the dispute over plans for the creation of a separate medical register for the Irish Free State 'the impression created in the Foundation about Ireland was generally unfavourable'[41], and they decided 'that until the controversy which has arisen over the Medical Register has been satisfactorily adjusted, no further steps will be taken'.[42] In the absence of any other sources of funding, the amalgamation project was abandoned at the start of 1927.[43] The insurmountable issue of finance also prevented a more modest proposal to merge Dun's with the Meath from progressing.[44]

There were some calls for state assistance for the voluntary hospitals. In both 1922 and 1923 a proposed 'golden ballot' scheme was submitted to the government, in an effort to raise funds for the hospitals, but it does not appear to have been sanctioned, and at the AGM of the Coombe Hospital Linen Guild it was proposed that the government provide grants towards the purchase of expensive new medical equipment.[45] While the government was not prepared to undertake the expensive burden of financing the hospitals, many of the hospitals themselves were wary of any such interference and preferred to retain their independent voluntary status.[46]

Such was the extent of the crisis facing the voluntary hospitals in Dublin in the 1920s that many warned they might be forced either to curtail their services or even close down.[47] The hospital in greatest difficulty was the National Maternity Hospital. Much newer than the other voluntary hospitals in Dublin, having been established in 1894, it was housed in a wholly inadequate building and did not have sufficient facilities to cope with the increase in hospital over home births:

> At times during the past year the Master has been faced with the alternative of either refusing admission to maternity patients, or introducing stretchers into wards to accommodate the excess patients, resulting in undesirable congestion which might easily become dangerous.[48]

Table 1.4 illustrates the growing demands on the hospital during the 1920s:

Table 1.4: National Maternity Hospital: admissions, attendances and operations performed, 1923–30

Year	1923–4	1925–6	1927–8	1929–30
Admissions	1,200	1,302	1,343	1,413
Confinements	721	846	866	961
Dispensary attendances	3,142	6,113	6,118	7,843
Gynaecological operations	341	346	378	371

Source: National Maternity Hospital, *Annual Reports, 1928, 1929, 1930.*

Efforts to expand were stymied because of insufficient funds; in 1925 an appeal was launched to raise £10,000 to begin building an extension to the hospital, but by 1928 only £2,208 had been raised.[49] The annual report for 1926 cast a gloomy outlook on the hospital's future: 'the governors must either carry on as best they can for three or four years and then close down the Hospital . . . or else curtail its activities, and . . . limit our charity to a favoured few.'[50] By 1929 it appeared this prophecy would be fulfilled and it was this threat to the survival of the National Maternity Hospital that finally resulted in the legalisation of sweepstakes to raise funds for hospitals.

THE LEGALISATION OF THE HOSPITALS SWEEPSTAKE

The success of ventures such as Duggan's 1922 Mater Hospital sweepstake pointed to a possible remedy for the financial difficulties of voluntary hospitals. However, the decision of the government to enforce the Lottery Act from 1923 onwards appeared to close off this fund-raising route. This resulted in the first effort to legalise sweepstakes in early 1923. The Public Charitable Hospitals (Temporary Provisions) Bill was introduced to the Dáil by Cumann na nGaedheal TDs Dr Vincent White and Seán Milroy. Only the second private bill to be introduced in the Dáil, it is clear that those who drafted it had very little experience writing legislation.[51] Consisting of only five short sections, its aim was stated simply:

> It shall be lawful to hold carry on and conduct sweepstakes and drawings of prizes in Saorstát Eireann [Irish Free State] for the support of public hospitals and convalescent homes in Saorstát Éireann which afford medical or surgical treatment without charge or reward and which . . . are mainly supported by voluntary subscriptions of the charitable public.

The sweepstakes were to be conducted by a committee of hospital representatives who would also decide how to distribute the proceeds. The names of the proposed committee, including Dr Louis Cassidy, master of the Coombe, and surgeons John Stephen McArdle and H. Barniville, indicated the bill had the support of some of the state's leading medical practitioners. The entire amount of prize money would be deposited in a bank in the Free State beforehand. The temporary nature of the bill was stressed in the final section, which stipulated that it would remain in force for just one year after its enactment into law.[52]

From the start the bill encountered strong opposition, both within the Dáil and without. Its principal opponent was the Minister for Home Affairs, Kevin O'Higgins, which boded ill for its success. A deep distrust of sweepstake promoters – 'they were people whom I never suspected of being philanthropists' – led O'Higgins to think it was not possible to eliminate fraud and corruption from the running of sweepstakes and this was his principal reason for opposing the bill.[53] This opinion influenced other TDs to do likewise, including some erstwhile supporters of the bill such as Sir James Craig, an independent TD for Dublin University and a leading Dublin surgeon, who was well aware of the financial woe of the city's hospitals.[54]

The civil servants in O'Higgins's department were also unenthusiastic about the idea of legalising sweepstakes. A memo entitled 'Reasons why any measure introduced for the purpose of legalising sweepstakes should be opposed', drawn up around the same time as the bill, outlined six reasons for rejecting the measure. Sweepstakes were 'subversive of every idea of thrift' because they encouraged people 'to better their conditions other than by their own labour efforts and skill'. If lotteries were illegal in America, Europe and Britain for good reasons, why should they be 'considered laudable in a country with such bad economic conditions, unemployment, and chronic poverty as ours'. The exclusivity of the proposal to legalise only one specific form of gambling was seen as impractical. The vagueness of the proposed regulations governing the running of the sweepstakes and O'Higgins's view that there could be no guarantee against fraud were particularly stressed. Finally, having devoted much time and effort trying to curtail lotteries, the officials in Home Affairs did not relish the prospect of their legalisation: 'The principle of the Bill is wrong inasmuch as it would be the means of opening a door to all kinds of illegalities which enactment after enactment has endeavoured to bar.'[55]

The immorality of legalising gambling and utilising its proceeds for charitable purposes emerged as a powerful argument against the bill. Speaking tongue-in-cheek, William Magennis, professor of metaphysics at University College Dublin and a Cumann na nGaedheal TD for the university, suggested that the bill's supporters simply rob a bank or the wealthy members of the senate, because such a form of theft was no different from running sweep-stakes, which encouraged people to squander money and neglect their work.[56] Denis Gorey of the Farmers' Party feared the country would become like Monte Carlo or Switzerland.[57]

The strongest moral objections came from outside the Dáil chamber, in the guise of the Protestant churches. The charge was led by the Church of Ireland Archbishop of Dublin, Dr John Gregg. Preaching at St Patrick's Cathedral on 25 February 1923, on the theme of 'Take heed and beware of covetousness' from St Luke's gospel, he outlined his objection to making 'charity, however deserving, the ostensible object and justification of a call to the public to put down small sums in the hope of gaining large sums'. His chief condemnation of the proposed legislation was reserved for what he saw as its detrimental effects on society: 'The reiterated appeal to chance over stimulates our minds and excites them unhealthily', leading to an addiction to gambling, unwillingness to do steady work and loss of a sense of the true value of money. Having regard to the object of the intended measure, he felt that if people wanted to support the hospitals they should simply make donations to them.[58] Responding to Gregg's denunciation, one of the bill's promoters, J. S. McArdle, felt that his proposal that the public make donations to the hospital was futile as this would not even raise sufficient money to pay the staff in one hospital, and he questioned Gregg's claim to have knowledge of the social effects of sweepstakes.[59]

The *Irish Times*, a predominantly Protestant and unionist newspaper, supported Gregg's position, believing that the new Irish state needed the virtues of industry, concentration and discipline, rather than a get rich quick attitude.[60] In similar vein the Dublin Methodist Council forwarded a resolution to the government expressing 'its deep regret at the manner in which widespread gambling has in recent months been encouraged by the promotion of sweepstakes' and urging 'upon the Government the necessity for taking strong measures to prevent the further spread of this most injurious practice by all means in its power'.[61]

Roman Catholics had fewer moral qualms about the use of sweepstakes, as evidenced by the number of their clergy who resorted to this form of fund-raising. Catholic theologians were prepared to recognise the legitimacy of lotteries so long as they complied with a number of conditions: the seller must give the buyer the exact chance he purchased, in other words his ticket must be placed in the draw, which in turn should be a fair one; the price paid for the chance must also be fair; and ticket buyers should not spend what they cannot afford.[62] There were, however, some Catholic voices raised in opposition to the sweepstake, most notably in the editorial pages of the *Catholic Bulletin* which complained that 'The extension of that already great national and international evil, the Public Sweepstakes . . . have made Dublin notorious and Ireland a byword over the whole world during the year 1931'.[63] Such views, however, were not widely shared by Catholic clergy or laity.

Those proposing the bill in the legislature argued that, while they did not feel it was an ideal solution – Seán Milroy had hoped the state would come to the aid of the hospitals – it was the only option available in view of the dire needs of the hospitals. While some TDs were unhappy with aspects of the bill – such as its lack of safeguards against fraud and the promotion of gambling – they were prepared to support it for the sake of the hospitals.[64]

The only TD to suggest an alternative form of financing the hospitals was Labour leader Thomas Johnson, one of the most vehement parliamentary opponents of the sweepstake proposal, which he decried as giving permission 'to exhibit the sores of Ireland, and the poverty of Ireland to the world and as a beggar to ask the world to come to the aid of the hospitals of this country'. The plan to sell most of the tickets abroad, particularly in Britain, was a denial of the doctrine of self-reliance and made a mockery of Ireland's newly won independence by making her dependent on England for the support of her hospitals. Johnson's alternative proposed an additional levy of one penny per week for a year on health insurance, half to be paid by the employee and half by the employer, which he estimated would raise £100,000 per year.[65] His proposal had the support of his Labour colleague Cathal O'Shannon, but the majority of TDs were not prepared to consider it.[66]

The bill made it through the first two stages in the Dáil, but when it reached its third stage the vague language in which it had been drafted began to come under closer scrutiny. In particular, the need to ensure that funds were given only to hospitals which predominantly provided free treatment was stressed.[67] The question of what percentage should be set aside to cover expenses was also raised for the first time at this juncture, an issue which would eventually become one of the most controversial aspects of the Irish hospitals sweepstake. Professor William Thrift of Trinity College proposed an amendment that no more than 10 per cent of the prize money would be allotted in expenses. In a cynical move, Kevin O'Higgins supported this amendment in the belief that, if passed, it would kill the bill because no sweepstake promoter would be prepared to settle for so small a proportion for expenses.[68]

The problematic nature of the bill as highlighted at this stage of its passage, led to it being referred to a select committee of the Dáil for closer examination. The committee sought information on both the financial necessities of the hospitals and the expenses involved in running a sweepstake. Among those who gave evidence on the first issue were surgeons J. S. McArdle and Lambert Ormsby, while Richard Duggan, D. J. O'Nolan (brother of Toome sweepstake organiser Fr John O'Nolan), and a representative of P. L. Smyth shared

their collective wisdom on the costs of organising sweepstakes. Not surprisingly, the committee agreed that the 'financial needs of the hospitals could
not be doubted'. However, on the subject of the expense of running a
sweepstake they were naïve enough to believe the evidence of those who had
most to gain from promoting the view that these were expensive ventures for
the organisers. On the basis of dubious evidence from less than impartial
sources the committee recommended that promoters expenses should account
for not more than 40 per cent of total ticket sales. Their other conclusions
included provisions for the auditing of sweepstake accounts and conditions
that the Minister for Home Affairs sanction all sweepstakes, that hospitals
submit audited accounts before receiving any funds and that there be no
statement to the effect that the sweepstakes were in any way directed or
guaranteed by the government.[69] Before the committee's recommendations
could be acted upon the Dáil was dissolved for the 1923 general election and
the bill died along with it.

Six years later in 1929 the idea was revived. On this occasion the prime
mover behind the scheme was the National Maternity Hospital, where inadequate accommodation and lack of sufficient capital to extend had brought the
hospital to the brink of closure. A number of other financially deficient hospitals were invited to promote a private members' bill in the Dáil to legalise
sweepstakes.[70] In November 1929 representatives of seven hospitals – the
National Maternity Hospital, Sir Patrick Dun's, Jervis Street, the Incorporated
Orthopaedic Hospital in Cappagh, St Ultan's, the National Children's
Hospital and Peamount Sanatorium – wrote to W. T. Cosgrave seeking his
support for their scheme. Their main argument was financial; the combined
overdraft of the seven hospitals was £93,000. Arguing that 'the only feasible
way in which funds can be raised for the carrying on of the Hospitals is by a
series of sweepstakes on the principal English races', they proposed to run six
sweepstakes over two years. The additional benefits accruing to the state were
stressed: £10,000 of Irish manufactured goods would be offered as prizes;
between 250 and 400 girls would be employed to handle tickets sales; Irish
Free State printers would benefit to the value of £50,000 and the post office to
£40,000; and the £60,000 it was estimated would be raised for hospital
building projects would also be spent in the Free State.[71]

Official opposition to legalising sweepstakes was still quite strong. Quite
simply, the proposals, irrespective of the offer of goods as prizes, were illegal
under the lottery acts and it was also forbidden 'to maintain an office in the
Saorstat for the purpose of organising a lottery or distributing tickets outside
the Saorstat'. The claims that the scheme would bring considerable revenue to
the state were considered dubious. A provision for selling most of the tickets
outside Ireland was viewed as 'intolerable', presumably because it would entail

promoting lotteries in countries where they were illegal. Finally, the involvement of Justice's *bête noire* where sweepstakes were concerned, Richard Duggan, was clearly unpopular.[72]

While the civil servants in Justice retained strong opposition to legalised sweepstakes, a major change at the head of the department affected the chance of success on this occasion; the assassination of Kevin O'Higgins in 1927 had removed one of the most powerful opponents of the idea. While his successor, James Fitzgerald-Kenney, was not in favour either, he was a much less effective minister. Also, by 1929, sweepstakes seemed to be the only alternative to government funding of the hospitals.[73]

From the viewpoint of the participating hospitals, the scheme was seen as the only option available for raising the large sums required to repair and expand their buildings in order for them to continue in existence. At the annual general meeting of the National Children's Hospital in 1930, the chairman of the board of governors, Lord Powerscourt, lamented how 'We have tried everything we can to get funds to pay our debts, or even get an income to live on, but I am sorry to say that we have failed'.[74] However, one Dublin hospital remained to be convinced that legalising sweepstakes was the only way to finance the hospitals. The Protestant-managed Adelaide:

> could not participate in such sweepstakes as it is a religious institution.
>
> The Board had decided some years ago that it would be wrong to raise money for the Adelaide by such means. The Board see no reason to change their view, that it would be objectionable to the supporters of the Adelaide to take part in any form of gambling.[75]

Financial necessity would not overcome the moral qualms of the Adelaide until 1960.

The bill to legalise sweepstakes was introduced in the Dáil in December 1929. In its initial form it was very similar to the original 1923 one. However, by the time of its enactment in June 1930 it had undergone considerable revision. Once again it was poorly drafted. At one stage the parliamentary draftsman advised that the entire bill be redrafted in the form of amendments to be moved in place of the original sections.[76] The amateur nature of the bill and many of the proposed amendments meant that its passage through the Dáil was not straightforward, entailing two committals to special committee to iron out many of its problems.

The final act, consisting of ten articles, was much more detailed and comprehensive than the original bill which contained only five. A large number of regulations and conditions had been added in the course of its parliamentary journey. Dental hospitals, as well as medical and surgical institutions, would now benefit from the proceeds of sweepstakes. A considerable amount of debate had taken place around the issue of how to define a hospital's eligibility and it was eventually decided they would have to reserve at least 25 per cent of their indoor accommodation for non-paying patients, who were defined as patients who paid, or on whose behalf was paid, no more than ten shillings per week.[77] Fianna Fáil failed to have an extra condition added that would have prevented the participation of hospitals it believed discriminated on religious grounds when allocating beds and appointing staff.[78] This was clearly aimed at Protestant-run hospitals such as the Adelaide and Rotunda; in the course of a Dáil debate Fianna Fáil's P. J. Little complained that Catholics were prohibited from becoming master of the Rotunda.[79]

Opportunity for fraudulent dealings had been a principal concern of Kevin O'Higgins in opposing the 1923 bill. In an effort to close off such loopholes a number of regulations were included governing the deposit of prize money, auditing of sweepstake accounts, information printed on tickets, and distribution of free tickets. Prior to the each sweepstake a sum of money or 'sound marketable stocks, shares or securities' equal to the value of the prizes on offer had to be deposited in a public bank in the state.[80] Within three months of the draw taking place, the accounts of the sweepstake had to be submitted for audit by a qualified auditor or accountant and the published accounts made available to the Oireachtas.[81] In an effort to pre-empt problems with forged tickets, and to give purchasers an awareness of the use to which their money would be put, all tickets would have to have printed on them the names of the participating hospitals and the proportion of proceeds each would receive.[82] Most of these regulations were proposed by Fianna Fáil, which indicated that it would support the bill if such conditions were accepted. It was common practice among sweepstake organisers to allow sellers a free ticket for each book sold, raising the possibility that the promoters could give away as many free tickets as they liked to their friends. An amendment proposed in the Senate by Thomas Farren was accepted which provided that 'no tickets shall be issued free, except by way of reward to a seller of tickets'. The value of such tickets was not to be included when calculating the overall receipts from ticket sales.[83]

As with the 1923 bill, its 1929 descendent proposed that the sweepstakes would be organised by a committee appointed by the hospitals. The composition of this committee and the contents of the scheme for running each sweepstake were laid out in detail in the final act. The governing bodies of the hospitals retained the right to appoint the committee members, none of whom were to receive any payment for their services. The scheme, which would have to be sanctioned by the Minister for Justice, must include detailed particulars of each participating hospital, the value of prizes, ticket prices, the name of the person appointed to audit the accounts and outline how proceeds would be applied to the hospitals.[84]

One very noticeable difference between the original bill and the act as passed was the power conferred upon the Minister for Justice to regulate many aspects of the running of each sweepstake. In the proposed bill his role was simply that of approving the sweepstake scheme. As enacted the Public Charitable Hospitals (Temporary Provisions) Act also gave the minister the power to make hospitals provide evidence of their eligibility to participate and to modify the scheme, which had to be submitted for his sanction before each sweepstake. Contained in his power of sanction over the sweepstake scheme was a measure of control over the method by which the proceeds of each sweepstake were allocated among the hospitals. Clearly it was felt that greater ministerial supervision would also help reduce the opportunities for fraud. It is interesting to note that the only minister responsible for the act was the Minister for Justice, and that as yet there was no role envisioned for the Minister for Local Government and Public Health.

The issue of what constituted legitimate promoters' expenses had proved a major stumbling block in the original proposal to legalise sweepstakes in 1923. While no figures were available, it was assumed that promoters such as Duggan were making considerable personal profits from their ventures and this made many deputies wary of enacting legislation that would be of significant financial benefit to private individuals. When framing the 1930 legislation it was decided to separate the promoters' fee from the expenses covering printing, distribution and salaries. Figures of thirty per cent of the gross proceeds of ticket sales for expenses and seven per cent for promoter's fees were agreed on. The latter figure had been reduced from eight per cent, although an effort to amend the bill in the Senate to reduce it to five per cent failed.[85] In order to ensure that the hospitals received an adequate proportion of the sweepstake proceeds, it was also stipulated in the legislation that they should receive no less than twenty per cent of the gross proceeds of ticket sales.[86] An amendment proposed in the Senate by Thomas Johnson had sought unsuccessfully to increase this figure to forty per cent.[87] The remaining forty-three per cent would constitute prize money.

Because of the need to make sweepstakes attractive to potential ticket buyers, the proposal made in 1929 to include goods of Irish manufacture among the prizes was quietly dropped. However, an amendment was added during the special committee's deliberations which provided for the use of Saorstát Éireann printing, labour and materials 'So far as may be practicable'.[88] Finally, after considerable debate and parliamentary revision, the act was signed into law on 4 June and plans got under way to hold the first legal Irish hospitals sweepstake on the 1930 Manchester November Handicap.

THE FIRST SWEEPSTAKE

Richard Duggan could now practice his trade freely in the Irish Free State. The virtual monopoly he had secured on running hospital sweepstakes in the 1920s made him the obvious choice to run the new legal enterprises. In October 1930 he changed the name of his company from Promotions Limited to Hospitals Trust Limited, making it sound more like a charity, and enlisted as directors a former government minister and an engineer who had served in the British army during the First World War.[89]

Joseph McGrath[90] was born in 1888 in Dublin, where his father was a stonemason. After his education at the Christian Brothers' School in James's Street he went to work for the accountancy firm, Craig Gardner, and later became head of the insurance section of the Irish Transport and General Workers' Union (ITGWU). During the Irish revolution he was a member of the Irish Volunteers and Irish Republican Brotherhood (IRB); took part in the Easter Rising; was elected a Sinn Féin TD for the St James's constituency in Dublin in 1918; served briefly as the first Dáil's substitute Minister for Labour; and was imprisoned on a number of occasions. A close follower of Michael Collins, he supported the Treaty, served as Minister for Industry and Commerce in the provisional government and was seconded to the Criminal Investigation Department as Director of Intelligence during the Civil War, in which role he laid aside his trade union background and 'presided effectively over the harassment, detainment and arrest of Post Office Union officials' during the post office strike of September 1922.[91] On 7 March 1924 he resigned from the government in protest at its treatment of the army mutineers and resigned his Dáil seat in October. Unemployed and with very little money, in September 1925 he was appointed director of labour for Siemens-Schuckert at the Shannon Scheme where he was effective in breaking a strike organised by his erstwhile employers in the ITGWU.[92] In 1927 a libel action against A. & C. Black, publishers of Cyril Bretherton's *The real Ireland*, was settled out of court, in his favour. Bretherton claimed McGrath was complicit in the killing of the republican Noel Lemass after the Civil War. His acquaintance with Duggan probably stemmed from a shared love of the turf. McGrath introduced Duggan to W. T. Cosgrave in 1922 when Duggan was planning the Mater Hospital sweep.[93]

The Hospitals Trust triumvirate was completed by Captain Spencer Freeman. Born in Wales in 1892, but raised in South Africa, he worked as an engineer in the USA and Britain before enlisting in the British army in the First World War during which he was put in charge of the mechanical salvage operation in France. Demobilised with the rank of captain in 1919, he spent some time as a consulting engineer before being introduced to Duggan and

McGrath by his brother, Sidney, a bookmaker who knew them from his association with horse racing.[94]

Operating from temporary cramped quarters in Earlsfort Terrace, Hospitals Trust set to work organising their first sweepstake. The first ticket for this inaugural Irish hospitals sweepstake draw was purchased by the Governor General, James MacNeill.[95] Once more, the majority of tickets were sold outside the Irish Free State.

The British postal authorities sought to intercept sweepstake correspondence entering and leaving their jurisdiction, although Joseph McGrath claimed that Hospitals Trust's operations were largely unaffected: 'As a matter of fact, only this morning we opened about three thousand letters, registered and unregistered, from persons in Great Britain who wished to obtain tickets.'[96] The distribution of prizes overwhelmingly in favour of residents of the UK would appear to confirm this. One part of the United Kingdom where it proved very difficult to prevent circulation of tickets was Northern Ireland. One estimate stated that between 20,000 and 30,000 tickets were sold there to people including politicians, civil servants, and even (it was claimed) the Prime Minister, Viscount Craigavon.[97] Concern at the success of ticket sales in the United Kingdom led to the issue being raised in the House of Commons, where the amount of money leaving Great Britain to fund hospitals in the Irish Free State was becoming a cause of concern.[98] The sweepstake proved equally popular at home. There was a massive rush to buy tickets on the last day before sales closed:

> From an early hour in the morning until closing time at 9 p.m. there was a long queue of people waiting to return their counterfoils or purchase additional tickets. At times the crowd grew to such an extent that the Civic Guards on duty had considerable difficulty in regulating the traffic, while the assistants in the office found their time very much occupied.[99]

Spencer Freeman's exceptional publicity skills turned the draw into a public spectacle. A film company was employed to record the proceedings and a large contingent of English journalists, including the thriller-writer and racing enthusiast Edgar Wallace, attended the draw in the Oak Room of the Mansion House, and the proceedings, which lasted for four hours, were relayed outside by loudspeakers erected at the bandstand in St Stephen's Green. The counterfoils were placed in the drum by nurses from the participating hospitals and the draw itself was made by four blind boys from St Joseph's blind institution in Drumcondra. Garda Commissioner Eoin O'Duffy, who supervised the proceedings, assured the audience that they were totally blind, and for their services each was presented with a large box of chocolates.[100]

The prizewinners were overwhelmingly British: forty English, three Scottish and two Welsh. The Irish Free State did well with eleven winners, and there were also three from Northern Ireland. Six Canadians, four Americans and four South Africans also got lucky, and the remaining winners were from the Isle of Man, South-West Africa, the Philippines, Demerara, Malay and India. The prizes on offer were much greater than anything previously offered in an Irish sweepstake, and put Duggan's £10,000 prizes in his 1920s sweepstakes in the shade. First prize of £204,764 was won by F. R. Prescott, from Belfast, an official in the Northern Ireland Ministry of Agriculture, but he did not get the entire prize money because he had sold two shares to two other Belfast men, Frank Ward and John Torney, and half a share to Ladbrokes. Mr A. P. Dawe of Vancouver scooped £81,905 and £40,953 went to Mrs Selina Hastings of Worksop, for second and third prizes respectively.[101]

For the six participating hospitals it was a windfall which they could not have imagined a few years previously. Jervis Street, Sir Patrick Dun's and the National Maternity each got two-ninths of the hospitals allocation, which amounted to £29,272 each, while the smaller hospitals, the National Children's, St Ultan's and the Dental Hospital, each got one-ninth or £14,636 each.[102] The net proceeds from ticket sales amounted to £658,358. Deductions of £97,340 were accounted for through winning ticket sellers' prizes of £8,351 and commissions paid on the sale of tickets of £88,989. A substantial portion of this latter amount went to Mutual Club Limited, Vaduz, who had a deal with Hospitals Trust to sell tickets outside Ireland and Britain.[103] Hospitals Trust received a fee of £46,085 for conducting the sweepstake. The net expenses of running the sweepstake, including salaries, stationery, postage, accounting and legal fees, travel and rent, amounted to £71,367, or just under eleven per cent of the gross proceeds from ticket sales.[104] The success of the sweepstake in the following years soon made these sums appear modest.

TWO

THE SWEEPSTAKE IN IRELAND
IN THE 1930s

—

May... Sweep Committee takes over O'Connell Street as offices...

July... Government decides to establish a Department of Sweeps and Lotteries and to run a Sweep on the St Leger to abolish Taxation...

August... Mail boat sinks off Dun Laoghaire. Expert gives it as his opinion at Inquiry that counterfoils shifted...

October... Premises formerly known as Guinness's Brewery acquired by Minister for Sweeps and Lotteries as temporary offices pending the erection of adequate office accommodation on the site known as the Phoenix Park...

December... Separate political parties have... been wiped out by the Central Pro-Sweep Party who returned one hundred and twenty one out of one hundred and twenty members at the General Election in October.

('Young Moore's Almanack', *Dublin Opinion* (Dec. 1930), pp. 326–9)

The sweepstake did not quite live up to the expectations of the satirical magazine *Dublin Opinion*, but it became extremely successful in a short period of time and by the mid-1930s was the biggest, most successful and most notorious lottery in the world. Approximately 142 million tickets were sold during the 1930s, amounting to over £71 million. The majority of these were sold illegally in Great Britain and the United States of America. Prizewinners around the world shared £45 million, while £13.5 million was allocated to building and equipping Irish hospitals. The personal profit of the three promoters was estimated at £1.6 million.[1]

The success of the first sweepstake was soon surpassed. Ticket sales for the second sweepstake on the 1931 Grand National grossed £1,761,963, more than two and a half times the figure for the first one. Thereafter, there was a sustained increase in the proceeds, reaching a peak of £4,184,485 for the 1932 Derby. The enactment of the Betting and Lotteries Act in Great Britain in 1934 resulted in a considerable reduction in proceeds for the second half of the 1930s, during which they never rose higher than £2.7 million (see Appendix).

THE DRAW

The sweepstake draw took place a week before the race upon which it was based. A large drum held all of the subscribers' counterfoils while a smaller drum contained the names of the horses entered for the race. Counterfoils were drawn to match horses and the prizes would then be decided on the basis of where the horse corresponding to the counterfoil was placed in the race. From 1931 three draws were held each year, on the Aintree Grand National in March, Epsom Derby in June and one of the principal autumn races – the Manchester November Handicap, the Cambridgeshire or the Cesarewitch.[2]

Higher proceeds resulted in a commensurate enhancement of the prize fund; the first three prizes in the 1931 Grand National sweepstake were £354,544, £177,277 and £118,181. Under a new scheme introduced for the 1931 Derby sweepstake the prize fund was to be divided into units of £100,000, comprising a first prize of £30,000, second of £15,000 and third of £10,000. The remainder was to be shared out among the drawers of non-runners and there would also be a number of consolation cash prizes of £100 each. Thus, the largest prize that could now be won was £30,000, and there would be a number of first prizewinners.[3] While individual prizes were now smaller there were a larger number of winners.

This change in prize distribution appears to have been the result of pressure from the horse racing authorities in Great Britain, who feared that the introduction of the sweepstakes would have a detrimental affect on the races upon which they were run. A very large field had been entered for the 1930 Manchester November Handicap and it was feared that an unwieldy number of horses, including many of an inferior standard, would now be entered for the major races.[4] Fears that the sweepstake would ruin major English horse races were allayed by 1932, when the field for that year's Epsom Derby was considerably down on previous years.[5]

Beginning with the 1931 Derby sweepstake, each draw held in the 1930s had a particular theme. In each case Hospitals Trust's female employees who performed the work of mixing and drawing tickets wore symbolic costumes, dressing as jockeys for the 1932 Derby sweepstake draw, the theme of which was the Derby race itself; in period dress of the 1830s for the 1933 Derby draw which commemorated the Derby one hundred years before; and in hunting costume for the 1933 Grand National draw's focus on the 'Horse in Ireland'. Hospitals Trust's involvement in the London to Melbourne Air Race in 1934 was emphasised in that year's Cambridgeshire draw which highlighted 'Notable events in the history of flight', with the staff clothed as aviators.[6] Aware of the growing importance of the market for tickets in the United States by the mid-1930s, the theme of the 1936 Grand National was 'Americana', with the ticket girls dressed as famous film stars, baseball players, Red Indians, and Uncle Sam. In a reflection of the international situation, 'Peace' was the theme of the March 1939 Grand National draw.[7] The outbreak of the war in Europe necessitated holding a more modest draw for the 1939 Cesarewitch and dropping 'The world's fairest' theme, for which 'it had been planned to build . . . a representation of the trylon and perisphere which are the dominating symbols of the World's Fair in New York'.[8]

The element of luck associated with the sweepstake, large windfalls and the dreams one could realise if successful were reflected in themes such as 'Great treasure stories of the world' (1934 Derby), 'If dreams came true' (1935 Grand National), 'That "drawn the favourite" feeling' (1937 Grand National) and 'Luck' (1934 Grand National).[9] For the latter the walls of the Plaza Hall in Dublin's Abbey Street, where the draw took place, were decorated with traditional symbols of luck including a four-leaf shamrock, a black cat, a new moon, and a swastika – 'a universal luck bringer when points are turned to the right'.[10] The counterfoils were transported to the Plaza by means of Big Tom, a gigantic model of a black cat.[11] Domestic themes were highlighted by focusing on 'Old Gaelic legend' (1932 Cesarewitch), in which the employees were dressed as ladies at Tara's court, galloglasses and elves[12], and the general theme of Ireland (1938 Grand National), which was used to showcase Irish manufactured products.[13] Tickets were distinguished by having the face of a girl on them. In later years this was often a nurse or an employee of Hospitals Trust. During the 1930s the images recalled famous women from early Irish history, including Queen Tailte, Queen Maeve, Grainuaile, Deirdre, and Fionnuala, one of the mythical children of Lir.[14]

The hall in which the draw was held was decorated elaborately by some of the leading artists of the time to reflect the theme. The illustrator and cartoonist Aubrey Hammond designed the setting for the 1932 Grand National draw, which was based on the theme of 'Pegasus', from Greek mythology.[15] Lionel Edwards, best known for his paintings of sporting and hunting themes, designed the backdrop for the 1932 Derby draw, which was a commemoration of the Derby itself. A frieze around the Plaza depicted scenes from the famous Epsom racecourse, including the paddock, parade of horses and Tattenham Corner.[16] Medallions depicting previous Derby winners that decorated the pillars in the Plaza were designed by the sculptor C. Rebel Stanton, who opened a studio in Dublin specifically for the purpose of making them.[17] Much of the artistic work associated with the draws was undertaken by the most famous Irish artists of the day; the setting for the 1932 Cesarewitch draw was designed and painted by Maurice MacGonigal and Harry Kernoff, and those for the 1933 Grand National and the 1935 Cambridgeshire were the work of the Harry Clarke studios.[18]

During 1933 and 1934 most of the artwork was undertaken by Seán Keating. In 1931 Keating had designed the cover of the draw programme used throughout the 1930s, depicting a nurse and a jockey. The settings for four consecutive draws from the Cambridgeshires of 1933 to 1934 were also the work of Keating. His most imaginative work was conducted for the draw on the 1934 Grand National, with the theme of luck. The draw drum was decorated with painted images of playing cards; an effigy of Hoodoo, a symbol of bad luck, was burned on a raft in the river Liffey during the parade transporting the counterfoils to the Plaza; and 3,000 black cats were brought to Dublin for a competition to select the model on which Keating would base his giant black cat, Big Tom.

However, Keating's work for the sweepstake is generally considered to be poor; the figures of the nurse and jockey on the cover of the draw programme were 'more carelessly executed than one would expect in his work at this period'. The ingenuity of the 'luck' draw was an exception, and the work of the Clarke studios was considered 'greatly superior'. The inferiority of this work reflects Keating's financial motivation in accepting the commission, and the time-consuming nature of the work had an adverse effect on his career; the summer of 1934 was the first time in ten years that he did not exhibit at the Royal Academy.[19]

In addition to the thematic costumes of the employees, the drum and other parts of the draw setting were similarly decorated. In 1932 for the Gaelic Ireland theme of that year's Cesarewitch draw the drum was painted to resemble Manannán MacLir's galleon, while for the following year's Derby draw it was transformed into turf in front of the grand stand at Epsom.[20] The theme for a particular draw was sometimes chosen by the public. In 1932 a prize of £200 was offered to men and women of Irish birth or parentage in a competition to design the setting for the Derby draw, while 'The horse in history and legend', chosen for the 1933 Cambridgeshire, was the idea of a Dublin schoolteacher, Andrew Walsh.[21] The pageantry of the draw was designed to attract the maximum public and press attention. The 1935 Cambridgeshire draw, with an 'Arabian Nights' theme, resembled 'a gorgeous procession, with all the pomp and pageantry one expects to see in a Cecil de Mille film "epic"', complete with two camels, numerous donkeys, 'Two ferocious looking black slaves', guarding the drum in its guise as Moorish Place, and 'a pair of Ali Babas'.[22]

To prove that the draw was completely fair, an elaborate process of mixing the counterfoils was introduced. Firstly, the large metal boxes containing the millions of counterfoils to be entered in the drum were paraded from the sweepstake headquarters at Earlsfort Terrace through the main streets of Dublin, accompanied by an armed Garda escort, to the Plaza, where two oval-shaped railway tracks had been laid down, with a mixing machine in the centre of each. The boxes containing the counterfoils were then placed on small trucks which ran along the tracks. One team of female employees, dressed in themed costumes, moved the counterfoil-laden trucks around the tracks, from where a second team removed them via metal scoops and loaded them into the mixing machines. Air was then blasted into the machines, ensuring that all the counterfoils were thoroughly mixed. They were removed and re-loaded regularly and finally transferred to the drum on the day of the draw.[23]

The spectacle of the draw attracted many overseas tourists, and having one's photo taken with the sweepstake drum was part of the itinerary of many celebrities who visited Dublin during the 1930s, including the New Zealand rugby union team, J. C. Graham, the head of Paramount film studios, film stars including Anna May Wong and the cast of *Man of Aran*, and the British singer Gracie Fields, who 'got into the drum to examine it, and, through a workman's mistake, was twirled around inside it until her screams got the drum stopped'.[24] 1932 was a particularly good year for Irish tourism, largely due to the Eucharistic Congress (an international Roman Catholic Eucharistic celebration that brought 10,000 pilgrims to Dublin in June), but also because of 'an unprecedented number of British people who are combining a short holiday with a little sweepstake business'; it was estimated that the sweepstake drew more visitors 'than the Spring Show and Horse Show combined'.[25]

A well-known Irish firm that played a central role in the sweepstake draw was the accountancy house of Craig Gardner & Company (now part of the Price Waterhouse Coopers Group), Joseph McGrath's erstwhile employers. As auditor it was responsible for monitoring the receipt of tickets and money, managing the finances of the draw, arranging payment of prizes to winners and preparing the audited accounts. A representative of the company also helped supervise the draw. The initial reluctance of the company's Protestant partners to become associated with such a major gambling enterprise was soon overcome and the sweepstake contract came to represent a significant portion of the firm's income; collecting an annual fee of £12,000 by the mid-1930s, income from the sweepstake accounted for almost 30 per cent of the fees earned by Craig Gardner's main office in Dublin. Thereafter the fortunes of the sweepstake and those of its auditors were closely aligned and the decline in the income from sweepstakes during the Second World War had a similar detrimental effect on Craig Gardner's profits.[26]

WINNERS

One of the most colourful and controversial winners of the sweepstake was a little-known Italian immigrant ice-cream parlour proprietor from Battersea, London. Born in southern Italy, as a teenager Emilio Scala came to live with relatives in London, where he worked selling ice-cream, and also as an artists' model at the Royal Academy, before opening his own ice-cream parlour.[27] He claimed first prize of £354,544 when Grakle won the 1931 Grand National. Grakle had been one of the favourites for the race and after his ticket was drawn Scala sold three quarters of it to Ladbrokes.[28] However, before he could claim the remaining quarter of his prize, approximately £90,000, an injunction was taken out against him by two London hairdressers, Antonio Apicella and Matteo Constantino, who claimed that Scala's winning ticket was one of a pool of sixty-one tickets held among the three men, and not the sole property of Scala.[29]

The ensuing case was heard in the Irish High Court in October and November 1931. The plaintiffs claimed that they, along with Scala, jointly purchased two books of tickets from a bank in London. They returned to look for more but there were none left, whereupon Scala undertook to write to Dublin for them. When he got these he was to sell some to other acquaintances and put the remainder into the pool held by the three men. They further claimed that all three signed a written agreement, dictated by Scala, containing the numbers of all of the tickets in the partnership, including that of the winning ticket.[30] Refuting these claims, Scala's defence team accused the plaintiffs of perpetrating a forgery by inserting the number of the winning ticket into the agreement after the result of the draw became known.[31]

The case caught the public attention to the extent that it had to be moved to a larger court to accommodate spectators.[32] Interest was heightened by the bizarre nature of some of the evidence. The plaintiffs and their witnesses stated that the ticket holders held a seance in Constantino's house in February 1931 to consult the spirits on their chances of winning, at which Scala was said to have called upon a number of spirits, including Rasputin and Paganini. The deceased Italian composer was asked to '"Raise the table twice if we are to win and once if we are to lose" . . . It jumped twice and they all congratulated themselves'.[33] Apicella's wife noticed that the leg of the table, on the side which was raised, was between Scala's legs and speculated that he, rather than the spirit, had been responsible for its elevation.[34] In his evidence, Scala denied that any such event had ever taken place.[35] Both sides made bitter and damning accusations about each other. Scala's wife denied the sworn evidence of Mrs Apicella that her husband 'horsewhipped [her] and made [her] work like a nigger while he enjoyed himself'.[36]

There was also the mystery of the bogus telegram received by Scala purporting to have come from Hospitals Trust informing him that payment was being deferred because of a stewards' enquiry into the running of the race. Apicella denied he had sent it to frighten Scala, who also denied authorship.[37] A crucial witness in the case was a handwriting expert, Captain Quirke, who, having examined the written agreement containing the ticket numbers, was of the opinion that the number of the winning ticket had been inserted subsequently.[38]

Towards the end of the hearing of evidence a very strange incident of external interference occurred. Arriving home one evening the presiding judge in the case, James Creed Meredith, found a letter awaiting him accusing the plaintiffs of blackmail and forgery in their attack on Scala. The judge was outraged at this 'great contempt of court'.[39] Nor did Meredith have a very high opinion of any of the litigants:

> However he looked at the case there was no escape but that on one side or the other there was the most amazing tissue of lies he ever had experienced ... even if he came to a certain decision he could not close his eyes to the fact that there might be liars on the winning side as well.[40]

He was particularly unimpressed by Scala, who he believed had 'perjured himself to the hilt'.[41] Nonetheless, he dismissed the case brought by the plaintiffs seeking a share in the prize money. A crucial point of law in the decision concerned the validity of English contracts in the Irish Free State, particularly where such contracts concerned activities that were illegal in England, such as sweepstake gambling: 'The Irish Free State Courts could not enforce such contracts except where they had in any case been expressly validated by their own legislature.' Finding in favour of the plaintiffs would set a dangerous precedent: 'if actions of this type could be successfully maintained in this country, Dublin would rapidly become the gamblers' cockpit of Europe.'[42]

When the proceedings had concluded Scala was left with £52,000, a sufficient amount for him and his family to live very comfortably for the remainder of their lives.[43] When his son, Geofredo, was married in St George's Cathedral in Southwark, Swiss Guards from the Vatican were brought in for the occasion. He bought Hamilton Lodge, a mansion in Battersea, which suffered some bomb damage in the Second World War, during which he was interned in the Isle of Man as a native of one of the Axis powers, while three of his sons fought in the British Army.[44] In order to avoid similar legal disputes, Hospitals Trust advised shareholders to ensure they each received a receipt and put all of their names on the counterfoil, or send the full list of shareholders to them if there was not sufficient room on the counterfoil.[45]

Scala was not the only winner to end up in the Irish courts in the 1930s. Judging by the number of disputed ticket cases reported in the newspapers throughout the decade Justice Meredith's fears were realised. Usually such cases centred on contested ownership of a ticket within a family. In March 1933 Meredith once again presided over a case concerning the ownership of a prize, in which Maurice Morrissey of Charlestown, Massachusetts, had bought a ticket in the name of his son, James, for the 1932 Derby sweepstake. When the ticket drew a prize of £1,750 the senior Morrissey sought payment of the prize to himself. Meredith ruled that an arrangement be made to allow him to take a certain portion of the prize and settle the remainder on his children.[46]

In a similar case in July 1933 Cecilia Laura Baines of Luton, England, sued James McLean, a commission agent, and her daughter Cecilia Clara Baines, over a prize of £1,458 won by her husband in the 1932 Cesarewitch sweepstake. Mr Baines had bought the winning ticket in his daughter's name and sold half of it to McLean after it was drawn. The judge ruled that McLean be paid his half of the prize and that the remaining half be invested in the child's name, with the interest to be paid to her mother for the child's maintenance.[47] Mabel McKie of San Francisco was not so fortunate when she sought a share in a prize won by her husband. Divorce proceedings between the couple were underway and a San Francisco court order had allocated community property, defined as that acquired during the marriage, to Mrs McKie. However, the Irish courts held that such an order had no validity in the Irish Free State.[48] The proliferation of legal disputes involving children whose names appeared on winning tickets led Hospitals Trust to warn customers about the consequences of this practice, stating that they were not permitted to pay out prizes to minors.[49]

It is impossible to state categorically what class of people bought sweepstake tickets. Generally, gambling is considered to have its greatest appeal among the working class.[50] The only method of creating a social profile of ticket buyers is to examine the occupations of prizewinners, taking them as a random sample. The winners of first and second prizes in the inaugural sweepstake were a civil servant and a garage owner.[51] Emilio Scala owned an ice-cream parlour, and his fellow prizewinners in the 1931 Grand National draw were a mechanic and a licensed victualler.[52] The Irish prizewinners in the 1931 Manchester November Handicap sweepstake included a shoemaker, a dressmaker, a merchant, haulage contractors, a postman, the wife of a railway signal painter, road workers with Dublin County Council, five Gardaí, and a surveyor.[53]

Analysis of American and Canadian winners in the latter half of the 1930s reveals a similar profile, with a concentration among the working and lower middle classes, particularly manual workers, factory hands, and clerical workers.

There were very few winners at the extreme ends of the social scale; of a sample of 176 winners, there was only one unemployed person, and five employees of the Works Progress Administration, a federal relief agency set up to provide temporary employment in public works during the great depression. Very few professionals appear to have gambled on the sweepstake, with one doctor, lawyer, teacher, engineer, and broker appearing in this sample of north-American prizewinners.[54]

This is by definition a very small sample of those who bought tickets. Nonetheless, it does not suggest that they were bought predominantly by the poorer classes. The reasonably high price of tickets, ten shillings each (US$2.50), may have served to exclude some of the poorer members of society, although as the 1930s progressed it became much more common for gamblers to form syndicates to buy tickets, thus allowing people to buy shares in a ticket. There is little evidence that the introduction of the sweepstake led to any great increase in poverty or deprivation. In September 1931 a Roman Catholic priest denied that the worst fears of its opponents were being realised:

> It is not my experience, nor that of many social workers, however, that the Hospital Sweepstakes have done much to create dissatisfaction with the usual slow, prosaic ways of making a living, or to detach any considerable number of people from their ordinary business, or to concentrate their attention, to the prejudice of it, on methods of getting rich quick and without any trouble.[55]

HOSPITALS TRUST LIMITED

The principal work of running Hospitals Trust was the responsibility of its managing director, Joseph McGrath, who employed a number of his fellow Irish revolutionaries, including circulating manager, Charles Dalton, a senior Dublin Brigade figure during the War of Independence; former Sinn Féin organiser Jack O'Sheehan, who became director of publicity; P. J. Fleming, the manager of the Foreign Department, who had been active in the IRA in Laois and Kilkenny; and 1916 veteran Eamon Martin, who was controller of sales. Although McGrath had been a senior pro-Treaty politician, many of his closest associates in the sweepstake had taken the republican side, including Martin and Fleming. The most important of these ex-revolutionary comrades was Frank Saurin, who served as McGrath's personal assistant until his death in 1957, carrying out much of the day-to-day administration of the sweepstake on McGrath's behalf.[56] McGrath's personal control of the company was solidified after the death of Richard Duggan in 1935.

The sweepstake quickly resulted in McGrath building up very extensive personal wealth, something that became one of its most controversial aspects. By 1933 he had accumulated a sufficient profit to purchase Cabinteely House, a mansion in south county Dublin, for £15,000. He extended this property with the purchase of the neighbouring Brennanstown estate for £3,350 in 1940. By the time of his death in 1966 he possessed one of the largest private estates in the country, encompassing a large part of south Dublin between Carrickmines and Foxrock. Much of his fortune was invested in his growing bloodstock empire, that included stud farms in Kildare (Brownstown) and Meath (Trimblestown) and Glencairn Gallops in Dublin, formerly owned by the notorious Tammany Hall 'Boss', Richard Croker. The sweepstake profits were also reinvested in a number of indigenous Irish industries, such as the Irish Glass Bottle Company and Donegal Carpets.[57]

When Fianna Fáil assumed office in 1932 questions were asked about the excessive fees paid to Hospitals Trust (see Appendix), possibly reflecting some suspicion of McGrath's close links to the opposition Cumann na nGaedheal Party. The new Minister for Justice, James Geoghegan, had reservations about sanctioning the scheme to run the 1933 Grand National sweepstake, feeling that the provision to pay a fee equivalent to six per cent of proceeds from ticket sales to the promoters was excessive, and the Department of Justice felt 'that the point has been reached when there should be a very substantial reduction in the remuneration of the promoters'.[58]

This view was rebutted vigorously by McGrath, who cited in his company's defence the capital outlay needed to organise each sweepstake, the legislative provision requiring that a sum of money equal to the value of prizes be deposited in a bank prior to the draw taking place, the financial risk posed to Hospitals Trust if a sweepstake failed, Hospitals Trust's corporation profits tax liability, and expenditure on premises (the purchase of the former Pim's building on Exchequer Street and lease of the Plaza for holding draws). He also reminded the self-sufficiency conscious Fianna Fáil government that Hospitals Trust invested some of its profits in native Irish industry, highlighting an initial investment of £16,000 in restarting the Irish Glass Bottle Company in Ringsend.[59]

Anxious to avoid any interference with the sweepstake that might be detrimental to the hospitals, Lord Powerscourt defended the financial *status quo* of the enterprise, highlighting the need to facilitate the illegal sale of tickets outside Ireland: 'having regard to the fact that the sale of tickets & return of counterfoils is illegal in all countries outside the Free State, they [Hospitals Trust] have to maintain an elaborate secret network of communications *at their own expense*' [original emphasis].[60] The strength of Powerscourt's defence of Hospitals Trust appears to have stalled any immediate plans that the government might have had to tackle the issue of reducing its remuneration.[61]

Powerscourt's claim that Hospitals Trust used the funds allocated as expenses and promoters' fees to ease the passage of tickets into jurisdictions where their sale was illegal, including payment of commission to selling agents and bribes to police officers and customs officials, was incorrect. Due to a most unusual clause (section 2) contained in the legislation establishing the sweepstake these payments could be made without any reference to them appearing in the audited accounts:

> When calculating for the purposes of this Act the amount of the moneys received from the sale of tickets, the value of tickets issued free of charge by way of reward to a seller of tickets shall be excluded from the calculation, *and there shall be deducted from the nominal selling price of all other tickets all commissions, prizes, and other remuneration given in relation to the selling of such tickets.*[62] [my emphasis]

This provision allowed the government to distance itself from the underhand activities that were necessary to secure a sizeable foreign market for tickets. Because such payments were deducted separately and not subject to audit, it is impossible to state exactly how much money was spent.[63] The only politician to highlight this anomaly was the sweepstake's most strident political opponent, Thomas Johnson:

> It seems to me . . . that what the auditor is required to audit is the amount of money that is placed to the credit of the Hospitals Commission by the people who organise the sweep, and not . . . the amount of money that comes into the possession of the organisers of the sweep.[64]

The success of the sweepstake turned Hospitals Trust into one of the country's largest and most profitable indigenous businesses. Starting life in the modest premises of Number 13 Earlsfort Terrace in Dublin, by the end of 1932 it had nine offices located throughout the Free State. The Foreign Department was housed in 40 Upper O'Connell Street, and the principal secretarial work involving indexing and filing of counterfoils and dealing with correspondence was undertaken in numbers 11 to 17 Exchequer Street. Ticket offices for direct cash sales to the public were located in 33 and 38 Dame Street and the Plaza Hall in Abbey Street, which was also the scene for draws until it was destroyed by fire in 1935. Outside Dublin there were offices in Cork, Limerick and Waterford.[65] The destruction by fire of the Plaza in April 1935 caused an accommodation crisis, as it was just over a month until the Derby sweepstake draw.[66] The draw returned to the Mansion House.

By the mid-1930s the volume of business being undertaken in a variety of different buildings scattered across Dublin city highlighted the need for a larger, more permanent premises within which all activities could be conducted. In 1937 a suitable site in Ballsbridge was identified.[67] As the Associated Hospitals Sweepstake Committee felt that Hospitals Trust could not be expected to undertake the construction of such a large project, special legislation was passed by the Oireachtas sanctioning the use of the Hospitals Trust Fund to construct the new sweepstake premises, which would then be rented by Hospitals Trust.[68]

Constructed between 1937 and 1939, and covering approximately four of the eleven and a half acres of the site, the building was designed in the new international style that was popularised in the 1930s and emphasised functionality over decorative ornamentation and maximised light and open interior spaces.[69] The work of John J. Robinson, a partner in the firm Robinson & Keefe, who specialised in church architecture and had been architect to the Eucharistic Congress in 1932[70], it was 'Basically a warehouse with an office addition'.[71] Aware of the danger posed by fire in the wake of the Plaza experience, most of the building was single storey to reduce this risk. Covering 96,000 square feet and built to accommodate up to 4,000 workers, it had 'probably the greatest staff capacity of any [building] in Ireland', and was equipped with air-conditioning, a compressed air system to allow for vacuum cleaning, and a canteen with a capacity of 1,000.[72] The steel and concrete underground strong room was guaranteed by the manufacturers as being both explosive and blow lamp proof.[73] Unfortunately it was not flood proof and was 'totally submerged' by floodwater during Hurricane Charlie in 1986.[74] Outside three acres of gardens were reserved for recreational purposes. Plans to add an elaborate extension to hold draws 'in a vast art deco hall surmounted by a tower, that would have looked more at home on Sunset Boulevard than the Merrion Road', had to be abandoned because of the Second World War.[75]

EMPLOYMENT IN HOSPITALS TRUST

The need for a building that could accommodate up to 4,000 workers was an indication of the huge workforce necessary to conduct the business of Hospitals Trust. Staff numbers fluctuated, and a large number of temporary staff was hired for a couple of months at a time in advance of draws. The vast majority of the work was clerical: filing counterfoils, issuing receipts, and dealing with correspondence. During the draw a considerable number of costumed female employees transported counterfoils and mixed them thoroughly prior to depositing them in the draw drum.

Earlier in his life Joseph McGrath had worked for the country's leading trade union, the Irish Transport and General Workers' Union. However, his role in crushing strikes by post office workers during the Civil War and labourers on the Shannon Scheme in the 1920s, indicated that his days as an advocate of workers' rights were behind him, and his attitude to labour relations in the sweepstake did little to endear him to his erstwhile trade union compatriots. Even before the first sweepstake draw had taken place complaints were being made about 'sweated labour' in Hospitals Trust, where the female employees worked from 9 a.m. to 6 p.m., in contrast to civil servants who worked from 9.30 a.m. to 5.30 p.m. for better pay.[76] Dissatisfaction with employment conditions persisted throughout the 1930s.

In 1937 the company threatened to sue the *Irish Catholic* newspaper for libel after it published an article entitled 'Where workers are sweated', alleging that competitions were organised to encourage employees to work faster, for which prizes of cash and silver cups were awarded and photographs of the winners publicly displayed, activities compared to those adopted in the Soviet Union.[77] The Irish Women Workers' Union (IWWU) also complained about the adoption of such methods.[78] The fact that employees were often compelled to work on Sunday in the lead up to draws was another bone of contention for both the *Irish Catholic* and the IWWU.[79]

The precarious nature of some of the seasonal employment was also a cause of concern to unions.[80] The IWWU complained that 'Permanent hands were put out on slackness this year, all of them in sore need of the work', and 'well off people are kept in constant employment while people who must work to live are thrown out'.[81] The union's general secretary, Louie Bennett, also complained that permanent staff were relegated to temporary status to be replaced by previously temporary workers.[82] Such was the trade union movement's dissatisfaction with working conditions in Hospitals Trust that it considered a boycott of the sweepstake by unions.[83]

The relatively low wages paid to the mostly female workforce concerned the unions. In January 1931 an official of the Dublin Trades Union Council complained that 'some of the girls were receiving a wage which was very much below the standard paid to recognised Trade Union clerical assistants'.[84] Admitting to having 'no official knowledge of the "standard" rates of pay', Joseph McGrath was satisfied that he was 'paying a very reasonable rate'; the starting weekly wage for female workers was thirty shillings per week, while some of the more experienced staff received forty shillings or more.[85] Therefore, most female employees earned between £78 and £104 per year. In comparison, the majority of women employed in the civil service in 1934, were paid at a rate of between £104 and £157 per year.[86] Thus, Hospitals Trust's highest wages were at the lower end of the civil service scale. In January 1932, the IWWU secured an increase of five shillings per week for its Hospitals Trust members.[87] Nonetheless, complaints about low wages persisted.[88] In 1939, as the volume of subscriptions to the sweepstake declined dramatically because of the worsening international situation, the IWWU was incensed at the decision of Hospitals Trust to cut wages by 40 per cent.[89] Labour's James Everett, who complained frequently in the Dáil about pay and conditions in the sweepstake, alleged in 1940 that letters of complaint by employees about their wages were censored: 'The Press were threatened by the Hospitals Commission that if these letters were published all advertisements would be withdrawn from the daily papers.'[90]

Concerns were also raised about alleged discrepancies in rates of pay. According to the IWWU, 'girls doing exactly the same work received different wages'.[91] The controversial issue of the substantial salaries paid to certain employees was pointed to by way of contrast when highlighting how poorly some clerical staff were paid: 'while huge salaries are paid in certain directions, the temporary staff are often employed for 16 or 17 hours a day at 30s or £2 a week.'[92]

In spite of such reservations about working conditions, the fact remained that Hospitals Trust was one of the largest employers in Dublin, and in the straitened financial circumstances of the 1930s many were anxious to find work there. The vast majority of the workforce was female, at a time when Irish society was not receptive to the idea of paid employment for women, partly on social grounds but also because of 'the acute competition which existed for jobs in a society where many young adults were forced to emigrate'.[93] Joseph McGrath justified the preference for female labour on the grounds that the nature of the work was more suited to them, and denied trade union claims that it was for 'economic reasons', meaning that women could be paid lower wages than men.[94] He also claimed that there was insufficient accommodation available for male workers.[95]

Given the difficulty which many men in Dublin had in finding suitable employment during the economically depressed 1930s, the trade union movement agitated for an improvement of the gender balance among employees of Hospitals Trust. The Dublin Trades Union Council passed a motion seeking 'to have a proper percentage of male clerks employed at Trade Union rates', drawing attention to the employment of married women 'when there were numbers of clerks who were unemployed married men with families'.[96] Unions also sought to spread the workload by having overtime abolished, which McGrath assured them he was trying to eliminate, while pointing out that those working overtime were given 'the rate of double time and a half, in addition to a good meal'.[97]

Recruitment practices were also controversial. A connection to McGrath was always considered a good chance of landing a sweepstake job. His acquaintances were inundated with requests to use their influence to secure work in Hospitals Trust.[98] In a meeting with representatives of the Dublin Trades Union Council in February 1931, he admitted that some jobs were filled through patronage.[99] Some fairer recruitment practices appear gradually to have been introduced during the 1930s. In 1932, 700 candidates sat an exam for clerical positions, and in 1933 representations from the government resulted in Hospitals Trust seeking employees through the labour exchanges.[100]

Unions advocating preferential treatment for unemployed male clerks, along with the IWWU which sought to protect female labour in the sweepstake, were united in their dislike of pin-money employees. In 1939 Labour TD James Everett 'alleged that there are people receiving £10 a week merely as pin-money – officers' wives and so on'.[101] Some years previously McGrath had admitted to having some such employees on his staff but denied that the practice was as widespread as the unions believed.[102] Nevertheless, there was a public perception that such practices existed; a priest in Drogheda lamented that 'There are some women with jobs in the Sweep who are taking the money from the deserving poor women, married or otherwise whose husbands have salaries. These women want money for cocktails etc., and are turning away from religion'.[103]

Securing official representation for the staff in Hospitals Trust was a priority for the trade union movement, not least because of the large proportion of the Dublin labour market which its 4,000 employees accounted for. McGrath denied union requests that only those who belonged to trade unions be employed.[104] Apart from the IWWU, whose numbers in Hospitals Trust were not extensive, the Irish Union of Distributive Workers and Clerks also had some members employed there.[105] While the hostility of Hospitals Trust management was largely responsible for the failure to unionise staff, the attitude of some of the staff also appears to have been a factor, with the IWWU complaining of 'employees who are too proud to be members of a Trade Union'.[106]

PUBLICISING THE SWEEPSTAKE

The advent of the sweepstake coincided with the development of indigenous radio broadcasting in Ireland, and it did not take the promoters long to realise the importance of radio as a method of publicising their product. With the state unwilling to subsidise its own station, 2RN, to any great extent, it became dependent for its survival on commercial support in the form of sponsored programmes, one of the most famous and long running of which was that of Hospitals Trust. The first of these was a 'Jolly, Bright, Musical and Surprise Entertainment', broadcast on Sunday 19 October 1930.[107]

2RN initially received a fee of £5 per hour from the sponsors who were responsible for providing the content, which usually consisted of light musical entertainment. Opinion among listeners and radio administrators was divided on the contribution of sponsored programmes. Neither of the directors of Irish radio in the 1930s liked them. Seamus Clandillon felt that 'From a programme point of view they are a nuisance and are regarded by listeners as an impertinence', and his successor, T. J. Kiernan, was believed to be 'anxious to eliminate entirely the Irish Hospitals Trust nightly sponsored hour'.[108] Others were concerned about the influence exerted by the sponsors; *Irish Radio News* 'feared that . . . the control of the Irish service will pass into the hands of British commercial firms', in reference to the sponsoring of programmes by non-Irish enterprises, such as the British food manufacturers Crosse & Blackwell.[109]

Opinion on the quality of Hospitals Trust's sponsored programme varied. Maurice Gorham, who served as director of Radio Éireann in the 1950s, claimed that 'Only the Hospitals Trust . . . continued to put on programmes of a higher standard'.[110] The *Irish Radio News* critic, 'A Z', was initially impressed by the offering of Hospitals Trust, complimenting one of its programmes which was 'well conceived, showed good continuity, and did not bore at all'.[111] However, it was not long before contrary opinions from listeners appeared in the weekly *Irish Radio News*; one complained that 'The programme sponsored by the Hospitals Trust seemed most inappropriate for a Sunday evening'.[112] After a year of the sponsored programme experiment, 'A Z' was becoming similarly disillusioned: 'In the beginning I had great hopes for them, but really they can at times be quite dull.'[113]

In some circles sponsored programmes were seen as unpatriotic. The Gaelic League objected to the predominance of what it described as 'jazz'. The Labour TD for Clare, Patrick Hogan, complained that 'the sponsored programmes do a good deal of advertising of foreign culture . . . and . . . are not at all desirable for broadcasting from an Irish station'.[114] Hospitals Trust drew the ire of the nationalistic Hogan in 1937, when it hired an English compère for its show: 'I found myself listening to what I thought was an English programme. Even the voices were decidedly and distinctly English . . . Has it been necessary to go across to England to find people to run the sponsored programme?'[115] There was also some opposition to the principle of using radio programmes to promote the sale of goods such as sweepstake tickets.[116]

The initial experiment with sponsored programmes ended in April 1932, but following the erection of a high-power transmitter at Athlone in 1933 they recommenced with Hospitals Trust now broadcasting two half-hour programmes on Wednesday night and Sunday afternoon. The new programmes largely took the form of radio concerts and included a range of contemporary artists.[117] However, this new style did not endear itself to all listeners; N. O'Doherty of Castleconnell, County Limerick, complained of repetition of tunes, and similarly 'Boyne Water' from Drogheda, was fed up of hearing 'Stormy weather' and 'How deep is the ocean'.[118] *Irish Radio News's* 'A Z' criticised the preponderance of 'crooning', and others wanted to hear more Irish music and dancing.[119] The neighbouring BBC considered Hospitals Trust's programme to be 'a rather nondescript collection of gramophone records, somewhat lamely billed as variety'.[120] Not all opinions were negative, however; 'Slievenamon' from Tipperary felt that the sponsored programmes provided variety and only regretted that they did not last until midnight, and according to the Fine Gael TD, Dan Morrissey, 'were it not for the sponsored programmes it would not be worth tuning into Athlone at all.'[121]

The government was not happy with the quality of Hospitals Trust's sponsored programme. T. J. Kiernan had 'considerable, and . . . continuous trouble with the Trust in his efforts to raise their programmes to a proper standard'; it was felt that Hospitals Trust 'seems to have no conception of radio entertainment of a higher order than jazz, crooning, [and] songs reflective of, or associated with, London night life'. This is not very surprising, as Hospitals Trust saw the sponsored programme more as a form of advertising than entertainment. Its explanation for the Anglocentric content was that the programme was aimed at listeners, and by definition customers, in Great Britain. Following a threat from the Department of Posts and Telegraphs to 'take over the framing of the programmes' the quality of content improved.[122]

Opposition to the sponsorship of programmes by non-Irish companies resulted in the promulgation of new regulations in 1934; henceforth only programmes advertising Irish Free State goods and enterprises would be broadcast.[123] Aware of the importance of sponsored programmes for advertising sweepstake tickets abroad, the Department of Posts and Telegraphs was willing to facilitate Hospitals Trust as much as possible:

> In view of the fact that the programmes sponsored by the Irish Hospitals' Trust constitute the only means of publicity advertising [for] the Hospitals Sweepstakes outside the Saorstat, and having regard to the importance of the Sweepstakes, special arrangements should be made with the Hospitals Trust, if the promoters should so desire, for continuance of their advertising programmes on suitable terms.[124]

Hospitals Trust entered into a contract directly with Radio Éireann (as 2RN had been renamed in 1932) giving it an hour every weekday, for which it paid £60 and copyright fees of £2 and ten shillings, becoming the principal broadcaster of sponsored programmes and generating considerable revenue for the station. Income from advertising, in effect sponsored programmes, rose from a mere £1,350 in 1932 to £35,000 in 1938, by which time it accounted for almost one-third of all Radio Éireann's revenue, second only to licence fees.[125]

Apart from the sponsored programme, some of Hospitals Trust's radio broadcasts in the 1930s were quite innovative. In November 1930, after the inaugural draw on the Manchester November Handicap had taken place, speeches from a celebratory dinner in the Gresham Hotel were broadcast, and for the benefit of those who had not heard or read the draw results, 2RN's regular announcer, Máiréad Ní Ghráda, spent ninety minutes reading them out on radio 'being revived by a bottle of Veuve Clicquot sent over from the dinner at the Gresham'.[126] In March 1935 the entire draw for the Grand National sweepstake was broadcast, in an effort to circumvent new British restrictions which prohibited newspapers from publishing the results.[127]

Horse racing was closely linked to the sweepstake and Hospitals Trust was anxious that its customers know the racing as well as the sweepstake results. In its early years 2RN refused to announce racing results and betting prices; the Minister for Posts and Telegraphs during the early 1920s, J. J. Walsh, considered racing 'to be the deadliest element in the life of this country'.[128] However, Hospitals Trust was not prevented from announcing these prices during the course of its programme and went a step further in the promotion of horse racing on radio when it hired commentators to re-enact the horse races, beginning with the Lincolnshire and the Grand National in March 1938.[129]

The publicity generated for the sweepstake through the sponsored radio programme was as important to Hospitals Trust as the sponsorship fee was to Radio Éireann. Radio ownership expanded at a considerable rate in 1930s Ireland; the number of radio licences rose from 26,015 in 1930 to 180,563 in 1940, and as there was widespread licence evasion the actual ownership figures would have been much higher.[130] In any event most people in Ireland, whether they possessed a radio or not, knew of the sweepstake, and the small population meant that the domestic market was minuscule. Hospitals Trust's principal interest in radio was the access it provided to Britain. This became especially pressing after 1934, when the Betting and Lotteries Act banned newspaper publicity of the sweepstake in Britain, resulting in a noticeable reduction in ticket sales. The value of lost publicity was estimated at between £200,000 and £300,000 per sweepstake.[131]

To compensate for this loss Hospitals Trust turned to radio as 'The only alternative to press publicity'. Initially, Spencer Freeman sought permission to licence a radio ship to 'cruise in different parts of the world and be a sort of floating radio station'.[132] This 'fantastic' idea was dismissed disdainfully by the Department of Posts and Telegraphs as 'nothing less than a "wireless" pirate on the High Seas sailing under a Saorstát flag', and contrary to the principle of establishing radio stations for the benefit of the citizens of the country in which they operated. It would also have been in breach of both domestic legislation and international regulations governing broadcasting.[133]

In 1934 Hospitals Trust became associated with George Shanks, an English entrepreneur, who sought permission to establish a commercial radio station in Ireland. He proposed establishing a European-style double chain broadcasting system in the Free State, whereby his new commercial station would handle all commercial broadcasting and advertising, thus allowing Radio Éireann to become 'a purely National Station, free from all publicity', similar to the BBC, which did not allow advertising. Initially, it was planned to use the existing Cork transmitter on a temporary basis, then, using a wavelength which had been allocated to Yugoslavia but was not being used by them, to erect a new high-power transmitter. The benefits to the state included freeing Radio Éireann from the need to carry commercial broadcasts, the access which Irish firms would enjoy to the wider market which could be reached by means of the strong transmitter, and the revenue accruing to the exchequer in the form of income tax on the earnings of the private company that would run the station.[134]

Philip O'Reilly, Hospitals Trust's solicitor, was said to be involved with the Shanks scheme, and Shanks was also thought to be acting as an adviser to the directors of Hospitals Trust.[135] Given the BBC's eschewal of advertising, this station was clearly aimed at broadcasting advertisements into Britain. With legislation then going through Westminster that was to eliminate Hospitals Trust's newspaper publicity in Britain, this venture was obviously attractive. The Catholic Truth Society of Ireland was also approached about renting an hour for religious broadcasting on the proposed commercial station.[136] Shanks had some very influential backers, including Frank O'Reilly of the Catholic Truth Society, and the principal of Blackrock College, Fr John Charles McQuaid, who described him as 'very honourable: a good Catholic with singularly right views on our nation'.[137]

The proposal was supported by the Minister for Industry and Commerce, Seán Lemass, but opposed strongly by the arm of the state responsible for broadcasting, the Department of Posts and Telegraphs, whose minister, Gerald Boland, objected to the principle 'of the establishment of a high-power station under non-Governmental control, to be used for broadcasting outside the Saorstat by almost exclusively non-Saorstat advertisers'. Civil servants in the department were opposed to it on technical grounds. It was widely believed that the proposal contravened the International Radio Telegraph Convention of Madrid, of which the state was a signatory, and which stated that 'In principle the power of broadcasting stations must not exceed the value which permits in an economic manner of the maintenance of an effective national service of good quality within the limits of the country concerned'. The objective of the new station was also anathema to Posts and Telegraphs' opinion of the purpose of radio broadcasting:

> The broadcasting of propaganda, whether political or commercial from one country with the deliberate view of reception in other countries, against the wishes of those countries is contrary to the view held by the majority of responsible Governments.

Shanks's plan to establish a high-power station was considered implausible, as there already was one in the state at Athlone. New legislation would be required as the existing law governing ownership of radio stations, the Wireless Telegraphy Act (1926), allowed only the Minister for Posts and Telegraphs to establish and maintain ownership of broadcasting stations in the state. The fact that many advertisements for English manufactured goods would be broadcast into the Free State was also distasteful to Posts and Telegraphs.[138] In the end, its disapproval outweighed the support of Lemass and the cabinet dismissed the Shanks proposal.[139] It was resubmitted and rejected again in 1950.[140]

Following this failure Hospitals Trust bypassed the use of intermediaries and proposed building and operating a radio station by itself.[141] This station would be aimed primarily at a British audience, but there was also a suggestion of erecting a short-wave transmitter that could broadcast to the increasingly important market in north America. Hospitals Trust proposed to build the station at its own expense, hand control of it over to the government on completion, and then lease it for an annual fee. The government would own the station for the duration of the sweepstake and afterwards should it cease. The proposed content appeared to be an extended version of the sponsored programme, featuring 'instrumental and vocal items of a light and popular character', as well as light opera, the more popular pieces from grand opera, the lighter works of the great composers, waltzes, tangos, 'and the more tuneful and unobjectionable dance music apart from the type known as "hot jazz" or the crooners'. It was also hoped 'to form at least one full orchestra of such high class as to build up Irish prestige throughout Europe'. Hospitals Trust sought to make the proposal more appealing to the government by emphasising the benefits which would accrue to the country in general, such as increased employment for both radio staff and musicians, the boost it would give to tourism, and the increased prestige the Irish Free State would enjoy from having a more powerful radio station.[142]

The reactions to this scheme were identical to those in the Shanks case, with Lemass in favour and Posts and Telegraphs implacably opposed on both technical and policy grounds. The proposal was incompatible with the international regulations governing wireless broadcasting. A conference held in Lucerne in 1933 had allocated wavelengths to all stations in Europe; there was no suitable wavelength available for the proposed new station, and it was felt that a claim for a new wavelength would not be considered and could not be justified. While there were no such regulations restricting the creation of a short-wave station, there were considerable technical difficulties involved in such an enterprise.[143] Any alteration to the legislation vesting sole control for radio stations in the Minister for Posts and Telegraphs was considered antithetical to government policy which favoured the retention of the state's monopoly. Posts and Telegraphs also anticipated international objections to the establishment of a short-wave radio station purely for the purpose of advertising the sweepstake in countries where the sale of tickets was illegal.[144]

The strength of these objections again resulted in the rejection of Hospitals Trust's request and the company now began to explore other avenues to increase its radio publicity. The biggest problem with the existing Irish station was that, at 60 kilowatts, it was not powerful enough to reach parts of the east and south-east coast of Britain, where many sweepstake customers resided. A brazen suggestion that the station, based at Athlone in the Irish midlands, be moved to the east coast to improve access to the further reaches of Britain, was dismissed on the grounds that the Athlone site had been chosen in order to give a satisfactory service to all parts of Ireland. Service to the more remote parts of the west of Ireland would be adversely affected by moving the station eastwards. Posts and Telegraphs made it abundantly clear that the principal purpose of Irish radio was to serve the needs of the country's citizens and not the sweepstake.[145]

The decisions that there would be only one government-controlled domestic radio station and that it would remain in Athlone, left Hospitals Trust with one option, which was to seek an increase in the power of that station. Joseph McGrath offered to undertake the cost of re-equipping the Athlone station in return for its power being raised to 120 kilowatts and its mast moved in a more south-easterly direction.[146] It was considered desirable that any finance put up by Hospitals Trust for the upgrading of the station be channelled through increased fees for its sponsored programme, in order that 'no private parties should directly finance a state work as such a procedure would imply a kind of private ownership of state property'.[147] The proposal was in line with existing government plans to improve the strength of the station, especially as a new 100 kilowatt BBC Northern Ireland station was due to begin broadcasting in the near future: 'from the point of view of State prestige, it would be undesirable to have a "Regional" Station in Northern Ireland of greater power, and giving a better public service, than the national station in the Saorstat.'[148]

Finally, in 1936 it was agreed that the power of the Athlone station would be increased to 100 kilowatts. A new three year contract was entered into with Hospitals Trust, whereby the fee for its sponsored programme was raised from £60 to £85 per hour, and allowing it to broadcast from 9.30 p.m. to 10.30 p.m. each night.[149] Capturing this peak-time listening hour was a considerable boon for Hospitals Trust, but produced criticism from those who saw it as detrimental to the development of Irish radio. Commenting on the broadcasting of music in the Free State, Eamonn Ó Gallchobhair, music correspondent of the short-lived review *Ireland Today*, lamented the restrictions which leasing this hour to Hospitals Trust imposed on remaining broadcasts: 'symphony concerts . . . must commence at half past seven – an hour that is unsuitably early from all points of view . . . relays of dramatic performances from theatres like the Abbey must needs be confined to, at most, a couple of acts of a play.'[150]

Hospitals Trust's strenuous efforts to increase its radio coverage after 1934 was an indication of the serious adverse effects of the restrictions on its publicity introduced in Britain under the 1934 Betting and Lotteries Act (chapter 4, pp. 100–2). There was also a noticeable increase in other initiatives by Hospitals Trust at the time, in an effort to compensate for the loss of valuable newspaper publicity. In 1934 and 1935 it sponsored a rugby league challenge cup, a trophy based closely on the design of Gaelic football's Sam Maguire, which was competed for in Dublin between Wigan and Warrington in 1934 and Wigan and Leeds in 1935, with Wigan victorious on both occasions.[151]

Holidaymakers visiting Clacton-on-Sea and other British seaside towns in the summer of 1934 got a glimpse of Big Tom, the giant black cat who had formed the centrepiece of the 1934 Grand National draw, when he went on a tour of Britain, collecting in aid of local hospitals.[152] At Hastings he was employed as a backdrop for judging the Miss Europe beauty pageant, before departing for Hollywood where he was used as publicity for the MGM film about the sweepstake, *The Winning Ticket*. Travel arrangements had proved difficult: 'he arrived in a rather bedraggled condition after his long sea journey. However, the Hollywood magicians got to work and re-dressed Tom so that he was bigger and more beautiful than ever.' He was also a lot noisier: 'by means of sound apparatus installed in his internal organs (or the place where they would be if he had any) he played splendid selections of Irish airs.'[153]

The marriage of Joseph Buckley and M. B. Townend in Huddersfield on Easter Sunday 1935 was celebrated with the bride and groom wearing wedding costumes which had been used for the 1935 Grand National draw. They had won the costumes in a radio competition, the idea of Joseph McGrath's wife. Ironically, the wedding was conducted in a Methodist church, the denomination most opposed to gambling.[154]

Hospitals Trust's most ambitious publicity venture was the sponsorship of an aeroplane in the London to Melbourne air race to be held in October 1934 to mark the centenary of the Australian state of Victoria.[155] Most of the leading aviators of the day had entered.[156] The pilot chosen to undertake the mission was the famous Irish aviator, Colonel James Fitzmaurice, who in 1928 as co-pilot of the *Bremen* had completed the first east to west crossing of the Atlantic Ocean. The selection of machine was left to Fitzmaurice. Unable to find a British machine conforming to his desired specifications, he chose one manufactured by the American firm Bellanca.[157] The engine chosen was a Double Row Pratt & Whitney Wasp Junior, which had previously been on the US army's secret list, but which Fitzmaurice convinced them to de-list in order for him to use.[158] The plane had other innovative features, such as 'a new direction-finder developed by the US Navy which excited much interest'.[159] Fitzmaurice's preference for an American manufactured plane was not a popular decision in Britain.[160]

Officially christened *Irish Swoop*, the plane was just completed in time for the race but without sufficient time for a final airworthiness test to be conducted.[161] Initially it was not felt that this would pose any major problem. However, on the eve of the race *Irish Swoop* was sensationally disqualified from the race in a dispute over its airworthiness and permissible fuel load. A furious Fitzmaurice appealed the ruling but this was dismissed a matter of hours before the start of the race and *Irish Swoop* never got off the ground.[162] Prior to his withdrawal, Fitzmaurice had been installed as favourite, with odds of 8/1.[163] The sponsors of the Irish entry were angry at the lateness of the Royal Aero Club's decision and felt they had been misled into believing there would not be a problem with their machine.[164] However, there was little sympathy among the other competitors, many of whom also had been forced to reduce their fuel loads. It was felt that if concessions were made to Fitzmaurice, others would have sought similar dispensations, resulting in chaos, as the race was about to start.[165] Nearly thirty years later he was still bitter about the event: 'it was barefaced robbery of the meanest description on a flimsy technicality.'[166]

A week after the race officials from the US Embassy and Air Commerce Bureau tested *Irish Swoop* at Lympne aerodrome in England, and it was given a full certificate of airworthiness, but an attempt by Fitzmaurice to undertake the London to Melbourne route on his own was aborted when the plane encountered brake trouble and had to be sent back to the US for further tests and improvements.[167] Sold to Jim Mollison, and renamed *Miss Dorothy*, it knocked almost five hours off the record for the west to east crossing of the Atlantic when it flew from Newfoundland to Wales in just over thirteen hours in October 1936.[168] The *Irish Swoop* debacle had been costly. Instead of a publicity coup it turned into a humiliating embarrassment. There were also legal and financial implications. In 1935 Bellanca sued Hospitals Trust for £2,260, claiming that the plane had never been fully paid for, and when it was sold to Mollison further legal complications arose over its ownership.[169]

POSTAL ARRANGEMENTS FOR HOSPITALS TRUST

The example of sponsored programmes shows how government departments were prepared to make special arrangements to facilitate the sweepstake. Posts and Telegraphs also made special provision for the transmission of Hospitals Trust's post. Leading up to the inaugural sweepstake the department granted a request for the use of private box facilities. The same concession was granted to nineteen 'reputable traders' acting as ticket agents. In return Hospitals Trust provided armed guards to accompany the postal collectors.[170] A request for a special delivery of post arriving on Sunday's mail boat, for which Joseph McGrath offered to pay the overtime expenses, was also granted.[171] The establishment of the sweepstake put a considerable additional strain on Dublin's postal service; in November 1930 it was estimated that 'Almost since the Trust was formed an average of from 8,000 to 10,000 letters have been posted daily from Monday to Friday and about half that number on Saturday'. Three daily collections, averaging 2,000 items each, were made from Hospitals Trust's offices. The additional volume of postage also translated into considerable extra revenue for the postal service; between June and November 1930 Hospitals Trust was estimated to have spent £6,233 on postage stamps.[172]

The illegality of the sweepstake in many of the countries to which tickets and literature were posted gave rise to concern within Posts and Telegraphs. Article 45 of the International Postal Convention made it an offence 'to send by post . . . any articles whatever of which the importation or circulation is forbidden in the country of origin or destination'; such packets were to 'be treated as prescribed by the inland regulations of the Administration which discovers them'. The Post Office solved its dilemma by deciding to take no action unless specifically ordered to do so. It would wait on other arms of the government to take action first: 'The Post Office position in the matter will then be quite clear. If it recognises the traffic it will stop it, but even for this a warrant from the Department of Justice will apparently be required; otherwise it can take no action.' Preventing illegal sweepstake mail from reaching Ireland in the first place was seen as the responsibility of the country of origin. If it escaped notice there and arrived unmolested in the Irish Free State, the Post Office declared itself willing to deliver it to its destination.[173]

Foreign postal authorities soon became suspicious of mail addressed directly to Hospitals Trust and a system of designated receivers was instituted, whereby communications were sent to certain names and addresses around Dublin. The Post Office had a list of these and knew that post addressed to them was to be diverted to Hospitals Trust instead. This system was not without its problems, especially when mail was undelivered resulting in failure to issue receipts for counterfoils; irate sweepstake customers then threatened legal action against Posts and Telegraphs for interfering with their mail.[174] Nonetheless the minister approved of the system, adhering to the department's policy of assisting Hospitals Trust, expressing 'the wish that the Department should do everything possible within the regulations to facilitate the Hospitals' Trust'.[175]

Hospitals Trust soon began to abuse its concessions. Officials in the department complained that many of the receivers' names and addresses were fictitious. Examples of such non-existent addresses were numbers 1 to 9 Heytesbury Street, Dublin, grounds occupied by the Meath Hospital. Alternative versions of the General Post Office, including Henry Street Post Office and Nelson's Pillar Post Office, were also used. Post Office authorities were concerned that the use of such fictitious addresses would cause problems for them with foreign administrations who often sought proof of delivery.[176] The department's patience was stretched to the limit in 1936 when Rita O'Donoghue of Blackrock, County Dublin, a receiver for sweepstake contributions from the USA, whose post was delivered to a fictitious 'Irene Donnelly', PO Box 3, Dún Laoghaire, asked for a separate post office box for each sweepstake.[177] An exasperated civil servant complained at length to the secretary of Posts and Telegraphs about the effrontery of Hospitals Trust's agents in seeking the department's collusion:

> It is one thing for the Department to close its eyes to the use of an assumed name in connection with a Private Box, when it is known that no illegal purpose is intended and that the spirit of the rules is not infringed; it is quite another matter to become an active party to the adoption of the fictitious name, thereby putting the Department quite out of court with outside Postal Administrations and rendering it impossible for us to tell them in the future, as we have actually told them in the past, that we would ensure as far as practicable that no officers of the Department would be a party to the violation of foreign postal laws.

O'Donoghue's request was rejected, signifying that the Department of Posts and Telegraphs had clearly reached the limit of its readiness to accede to Hospitals Trust's increasingly demanding requests.[178]

Another way in which Posts and Telegraphs, along with other government department, assisted in the safe arrival of post destined for Hospitals Trust was through forwarding foreign correspondence that was addressed to the government. In 1935 the Department of the President of the Executive Council (later the Department of An Taoiseach) began to question the probity of continuing to send on such communications. Michael McDunphy, assistant secretary to the cabinet, believed it was 'wrong that this Department should permit itself to be used as an intermediary or cover for the transmission of correspondence which, if sent through the ordinary post from these countries would be subject to confiscation or other penal action'. He was also concerned about the department's liability for undelivered mail.[179] Even worse was the 'dangerous situation [that] would arise if a disputed claim to ownership of a winning ticket were made by a person who claimed to have sent the money and counterfoils through this Department'. He was also concerned for the reputation of the head of government's department abroad, wishing to avoid 'anything which might appear to countenance an evasion of the law of other countries by their citizens'.[180]

In November 1935 a letter was drafted by the President's department to accompany any sweepstake-related mail that would henceforth be returned to its sender, stating that 'the Department of the President cannot in any way act as agent or intermediary' for Hospitals Trust. Joseph McGrath suggested an addition: 'Your communication is on this occasion being sent to Hospitals' Trust Limited in order that you may not be inconvenienced. You must understand that in future communications of this nature cannot and will not be dealt with through this Department.' Opinion within the civil service on this suggestion was divided, with the President's department opposing its inclusion but the Department of Industry and Commerce favouring it in order to avoid injuring Hospitals Trust's foreign business.[181] No decision was taken on the issue by the cabinet and a compromise was adopted whereby post containing cheques, postal orders and money orders made payable to parties other than the President, along with bank notes, were sent to Hospitals Trust's Foreign Department. Blank, rather than headed notepaper accompanied this money in order to distance the government from it officially. Any cheques or orders made payable to the President were returned to the sender. A separate file was opened for each sweepstake and maintained, until all remittances were acknowledged by Hospitals Trust. This eased some of McDunphy's fears about the department's liability for lost items.[182]

Throughout 1936 and 1937 the President's department continued to receive sweepstake subscriptions, mostly from the USA; between 1 January 1936 and 11 September 1937, 48 letters containing a cumulative total of over £506 were received. One correspondent, Mr Devlin of Tacoma, Washington, who 'appears to be using this office as an agency for the transmission of money and counterfoils', sent fourteen of these letters along with £152.[183] The continued flow of such post led to the Taoiseach revisiting the issue in 1938: 'The view is strongly held that steps should be taken immediately to terminate this state of affairs.'[184] The timing of this coincided with direct pressure from the US government for the Irish government to take action against Hospitals Trust's violation of American anti-lottery laws, and was probably a factor in the Taoiseach's desire to curb the practice.[185] In order to minimise any loss of business to Hospitals Trust, cabinet secretary Maurice Moynihan, wondered 'If it should be practicable to furnish to the Sweepstake authorities a list of the names and addresses of people who have transmitted remittances and counterfoils through Government Departments' so that Hospitals Trust could advise them to send them by other means in future, but this was considered likely to lead to renewed pressure from Hospitals Trust for the government not to change its policy, as well as necessitating extra work for civil servants.[186] Finally, in May 1938, it was agreed that all future sweepstake-related correspondence received by government departments would be returned to the sender accompanied by a printed slip stating that: 'Government regulations do not permit of Departments of State being used as a transmitting agency for counterfoils or cash remittances in connection with the Hospitals Trust Sweepstakes. Your letter and enclosure are accordingly herewith returned.'[187]

Moynihan warned that the government's decision would result in renewed pressure from Hospitals Trust not to implement this new policy. The ruling was said to have come 'as a bombshell' to Joseph McGrath, who complained about the government's failure to consult him. His displeasure was compounded by the publication of an article highly critical of the sweepstake in the popular American magazine *Collier's*, in June 1938, not long after the new government policy was adopted.[188] To assuage Hospitals Trust's annoyance, and reassure foreign customers as to the probity of the sweepstake, the printed slip accompanying returned communications was amended:

> Sweepstakes promoted by Hospitals' Trust Ltd., are legal and in accordance with the provisions of the Public Hospitals Act they are supervised by a committee appointed by the governing bodies of the benefiting hospitals. They are not, however, conducted by the State or by any Department thereof, and, since Government regulations do not permit of Departments of State being used as transmitting agencies for counterfoils or cash remittances in connection with the Sweepstakes, your letter and enclosure are returned herewith.[189]

FRAUD AND FORGERY

The success and reputation of Hospitals Trust was put at risk in the mid-1930s by the discovery of fraudulent dealings involving some of its agents. In June 1932, Henry Glynn, a Kent-based foreign exchange broker, and Robert Pierce, his Dublin-based associate, were both tried on a charge of 'converting to their own use £222 entrusted to them as payments to the Irish Hospitals' Sweepstake'. Pierce pleaded guilty and received a six-month prison sentence, while Glynn was acquitted on a technicality because he had been charged under the wrong legislation.[190] A second forgery case heard in the Irish courts in 1932 involved Joseph Nolan, who was charged with forging 7,000 receipts and cheques totalling £617 arising from the 1932 Cesarewitch sweepstake.[191] Another such case surrounding the 1932 Cesarewitch sweepstake was discovered in Manchester, where police recovered a small printing press believed to have been used for printing fake receipts.[192]

In 1935 a potentially serious libel suit was brought against Hospitals Trust by one of its South African-based agents, James Robb Stanhope, who sought £60,000 in compensation for an alleged breach of contract and negligence in failing to acknowledge receipt of a bank draft for £22 10s and 52 counterfoils that he had returned for the 1932 Grand National sweepstake draw. Stanhope claimed that the failure to include the counterfoils in the draw had destroyed his reputation as a professional seller of lottery tickets in South Africa. The defence argued that only two counterfoils had been received and included in the draw, and that Stanhope's bank draft had never been received. Stanhope's original suit was rejected in the High Court by Justice Hanna, who awarded judgement and costs to Hospitals Trust on the grounds that sweepstakes were illegal in South Africa.[193] In a subsequent appeal, the Supreme Court reversed part of Hanna's judgement, allowing that Stanhope 'was entitled to bring an action in respect of the alleged breach of a contract capable of being performed lawfully in the Irish Free State, and, accordingly, that there should be a new trial', but he does not appear to have sought one.[194]

Joseph Andrews, then an employee of Hospitals Trust's Foreign Department, subsequently claimed that both the counterfoils and the drafts had been received, but were entered in different sections of the accounts and no connection made between them. In his opinion 'Stanhope had the strongest of cases for some compensation'. He also claimed to have discovered the discrepancy, which he brought to the attention of both P. J. Fleming and Dr de Burgh Daly, who was handling the internal investigation into it, and who he accused of 'influencing the evidence' of witnesses to ensure their knowledge of the discrepancy was not revealed in court.[195]

The Irish hospitals sweepstake was an instant success. This owed much to the ingenuity of its publicity and the co-operation of the Irish state. Although a private company, Hospitals Trust was facilitated to an exceptional degree by the arms of the state responsible for broadcasting and postal arrangements, as well as the Department of Justice which protected its monopoly on running large-scale lotteries. Both of these factors contributed to its phenomenal success selling tickets abroad, which will be examined later.

THREE

THE DEVELOPMENT OF IRISH
HOSPITALS IN THE 1930s

—

THE SUCCESS OF THE SWEEPSTAKE

The introduction of the sweepstake transformed the Irish hospital system during the 1930s. As the sweepstake achieved instant success and subscriptions to it rose dramatically during its first few years, so too did the dividend accruing to the hospitals. The six hospitals that participated in the inaugural draw shared a total fund of £131,671. This figure rose to £438,490 by the time of the next sweepstake on the 1931 Grand National and continued to rise until it reached a peak of £1,032,121 after the Derby draw in 1932 (see Appendix).

Such a windfall had the effect of enticing more voluntary hospitals to take part. Even before the inaugural sweepstake had taken place, the Coombe Maternity Hospital had decided to participate in subsequent ones.[1] The Royal City of Dublin Hospital in Baggot Street, annoyed at not being consulted about the establishment of the sweepstake, initially 'washed their hands of the new scheme', declaring it not to be a 'desirable method of raising money for charitable purposes'; it was not long before the success of the sweepstake brought a reversal of this policy.[2] Similar moral objections to the use of the proceeds of gambling to fund Protestant voluntary hospitals were soon set aside in the face of the lucrative prize on offer; an anti-sweep combine formed by the Adelaide, Mercer's and Dr Steevens' did not survive very long.[3] The Church of Ireland Bishop of Limerick, Dr Vere White, warned 'we must not do evil that good should come',[4] and in his role as a governor of Barrington's Hospital objected to the decision of its board of governors to join the sweepstake.[5]

The prominent Jewish gynaecologist, Dr Bethel Solomons, had tried to convince Mercer's Hospital to raise funds through a sweepstake during the 1920s but encountered strong opposition; in August 1931 the board of Mercer's applied for inclusion in forthcoming sweepstakes.[6] By that time Solomons had become master of the Rotunda Maternity Hospital, bringing it into the sweepstake in 1933 in the face of stiff opposition from many of its governors, including the Church of Ireland Archbishop of Dublin, Dr J. A. F. Gregg; those governors were either unaware or unwilling to recall that the Rotunda was initially built on the proceeds of a lottery.[7] Similar decisions, often reluctantly taken, were made by Dublin's Royal Victoria Eye and Ear and Meath hospitals and Barrington's Hospital in Limerick city.[8] Yet, in a small minority of hospitals moral quibbles still overcame the desire to share in the new-found wealth generated by the sweepstakes. The Adelaide remained firmly opposed to involvement for another thirty years.[9] Donnybrook's Royal Hospital, which catered for incurable diseases, remained outside until 1960.[10] The Victoria Hospital and St Patrick's Incurable Hospital in Cork also refused to become involved for some time.[11] One Protestant who did not share the opinion of her co-religionists was Dr Kathleen Lynn of St Ultan's Infant Hospital, one of the hospitals that participated in the sweepstake from the start; she complained in her diary of 'Silly articles in [the] paper ab[ou]t hospitals & sweeps, surely they shoul[d] have sense to see there is no sin in chance as such!'[12]

Hospitals other than those covered by the definitions laid down in the Public Charitable Hospitals Act also lobbied for the right to benefit from the sweepstake, necessitating the passage of special amending legislation. During 1931 and 1932, three such acts were passed to allow eye and ear, cancer and orthopaedic hospitals, and sanatoria to become eligible to receive funds.[13]

Rate-supported local authority hospitals also began to agitate for inclusion.[14] The original legislation was inadequate to deal with the demands of a wider array of hospitals to be included in the sweepstake. To deal with this situation, Minister for Justice, James Fitzgerald-Kenney, introduced new legislation, under which a committee of experts would be established to 'inquire into the eligibility of every individual hospital which wishes to participate'. The bill also took into account the demands of the local authority hospitals; one-third of the hospitals' share of the sweepstake surplus would be allocated to the Minister for Local Government and Public Health to be used for improving these institutions. The minister appears to have agreed reluctantly to this latter provision, stating his fear that such an allocation might be used for the relief of rates.[15]

The Public Charitable Hospitals (Amendment) Act of 1931 established a Committee of Reference which would advise the minister on how best to allocate the funds among the voluntary hospitals. The absence of such a body had become problematic for the organisers of the early sweepstakes; the Associated Hospitals Sweepstake Committee, composed of representatives of the participating hospitals, was finding it increasingly difficult to decide upon an equitable distribution of the sweepstake surplus as the number of participating hospitals increased.[16] The committee had the power to visit the applicant hospitals and to inspect their buildings and equipment, but it had no jurisdiction over the proportion allocated to the local authority hospitals, the distribution of which was at the discretion of the Minister for Local Government and Public Health.[17] The overall effect of this act was to bring an element of organisation to the distribution of sweepstake funds among the participating hospitals in an effort to curb some of the wanton spending of the voluntary hospitals.

Immediately after the inaugural sweepstake the six participating hospitals announced their plans for development. The hospital in direst financial straits, the National Maternity Hospital, intended to pay off its substantial overdraft of £13,000 and set aside the remainder of its £29,272 towards the cost of constructing a new hospital. The National Children's Hospital, St Ultan's and the Dublin Dental Hospital also planned to clear overdrafts.[18] Having paid off their debts, the National Children's Hospital was considering the idea of a home in the countryside to help the recuperation of its patients, and St Ultan's, operating from a very limited and unsuitable building in Charlemont Street, that was described more appropriately as an antique than a hospital, wanted to construct a new purpose-built hospital.[19]

The rather small Sir Patrick Dun's, which had previously considered amalgamation with some of the other Dublin hospitals, now produced elaborate plans to transform itself, including the construction of an entirely new outpatient department, a new modern hospital with 200 beds, a new pathology department and isolation block, and the conversion of the existing outpatient department to a dedicated venereal disease unit. The hospital's annual report for 1931 reported proudly that each ward was now fitted with hot and cold running water, each landing had sterilising apparatus, the floors in the fever wing were being re-laid, a complete house telephone system had been installed, gas stoves had replaced fires in the kitchens, and among the new equipment purchased was an oil fuel burner, a portable x-ray, and a destructor for surgical dressings. The exterior of the hospital was not neglected either: it had been re-painted and the gate lodges had been reconstructed. Such work was facilitated by the total of £108,578 Dun's had received from the proceeds of the first three sweepstakes.[20] Other hospitals' plans included the purchase of x-rays and other equipment, completion of building projects, and expansion of accommodation for both staff and patients.[21] The wish-list drawn up by the master of the Rotunda included improvements to accommodation for outpatients and paying patients, extending pathological, consultant and paediatric services, and improvements to administration and communications within the hospital.[22]

As the money coming in from the sweepstake expanded the hospitals' spending plans became more elaborate and haphazard. There was a complete absence of co-ordination among the hospitals with regard to their plans for expansion. Dublin contained a sizeable number of small voluntary hospitals located in close proximity to each other and many of them frequently applied for grants for the same purpose, leading to unnecessary duplication of service in the city. Hospital governors also appear to have been unaware of exactly how much money there was in the sweepstake pot and how many hospitals were competing for it; the historian of the National Maternity Hospital has pointed out that 'Towards the end of 1932 the total sums claimed for various schemes amounted to at least seven times the enormous amount of money actually available'.[23]

The hospitals were dissatisfied with the discrepancy between their demands and the grants allocated. In January 1931 the chairman of the Baggot Street's Royal City of Dublin Hospital's sweepstake subcommittee complained about its projected allocation for the forthcoming Derby sweepstake and of the method upon which the allocation was decided; as this would be its first sweep, and some of the other participants had already benefited from previous ones, Baggot Street considered itself worthy of receiving at least ten per cent of the available surplus. The hospital's representatives were reminded by Lord Powerscourt that they had agreed in advance to this system, and were left with no alternative but to accept their allocation.[24]

The benefits of the sweepstake to the Dublin voluntary hospitals were soon obvious. The Coombe made its decision to participate in September 1930; it subsequently received grants of £26,391 and £41,901 from the 1931 Grand National and Derby sweepstakes respectively.[25] On entering the scheme the Meath brought with it a 'shopping list' for repairs and equipment totalling £188,319, of which £150,406 was awarded.[26]

The case of the National Maternity Hospital, the threat to whose survival led to the legalisation of the sweepstake, best highlights the benefits of the sweepstake funding. By 1931 the governors had the resources to purchase adjoining buildings at numbers 32, 33 and 34 Holles Street, as well as renew the lease on its existing premises. This would allow for a doubling of the hospital's bed accommodation to 120 and the creation of an endowment fund of £100,000. By 1938, the hospital had tripled in size to become the largest maternity hospital in the state.[27]

However, the sweepstake windfall had a detrimental effect on other sources of funding. In December 1930 participating hospitals were expelled from the Hospital Sunday Fund.[28] The House of Industry (comprising the Richmond, Whitworth and Hardwicke hospitals) had an annual government grant of £5,000 withdrawn.[29] Those who had previously made charitable donations to the voluntary hospitals now adjudged such subscriptions to be superfluous in view of the hospitals' new-found source of wealth. St Ultan's noted that 'with the advent of the Sweeps our subscriptions diminished'.[30] In 1931 it received £284 in general subscriptions, augmented by grants of £225 from Dublin Corporation and £50 from Rathmines Urban District Council; by 1935 these first two figures had declined to £69 and £125 respectively and the grant from the Rathmines Council had ceased after 1931.[31] Similarly, subscriptions and donations made to Sir Patrick Dun's decreased by half from £2,000 to £1,000 in the first year of the sweepstake.[32] The parsimonious Provincial Bank in Limerick stopped its annual subscription of £1 to Barrington's on the grounds that 'they could not see their way to subscribe to a Hospital which benefited under the Sweepstake Fund'. It was restored only after the hospital threatened to take its business elsewhere.[33] By 1934 when the sweepstakes had become well established and were at the peak of their success, the chairman of the Hospitals Commission estimated that voluntary donations to seven hospitals in Dublin had declined by over two-thirds.[34]

Patients who had previously made a contribution towards the cost of their treatment no longer considered the hospitals to be in need of such financial assistance. While this was attributed partly to the depressed economic conditions of the early 1930s and consequent high unemployment, most hospitals shared the belief of the National Children's Hospital that patients 'expected to pay less, or nothing at all, owing to our good fortune in getting the Sweepstakes money'.[35] This view was echoed by St Ultan's, where the total portion of patients treated free of charge rose from 67 per cent in 1933 to 77 per cent in 1938.[36]

While the decline in alternative sources of income was principally the result of the impression that hospitals no longer needed the money, the Irish voluntary hospitals were not alone in experiencing a fall off in charitable donations in the 1930s. In Great Britain, philanthropic contributions to voluntary hospitals declined noticeably from the mid-1930s, due to a combination of increased taxation and the introduction of contributory schemes to offset the cost of hospital treatment.[37] Therefore, the Irish voluntary hospitals might also have been the victims of a changing trend generally in charitable contributions to voluntary hospitals in the 1930s.

In addition to the clamour for inclusion from a variety of hospitals, nursing organisations also sought to share in the benefits which the sweepstake was bringing to the Irish hospital service. Yet another bill amending the provisions of the Public Charitable Hospitals Act was passed in 1931 permitting the Minister for Local Government and Public Health to apply one twenty-fifth of his allocation for local authority hospitals to nursing organisations, defined as institutions or organisations whose sole purpose was 'the nursing of and providing of nurses for poor persons suffering from physical diseases or injuries of women in childbirth'.[38]

THE COMMITTEE OF REFERENCE

The Committee of Reference established in 1931 had three members, whose remuneration and expenses were deemed part of the overall expenses of running each sweepstake.[39] The appointments were largely political. The first committee, appointed by Cumann na nGaedheal, was chaired by Peter Hughes, a former Minister for Defence. He was joined by Vincent Kelly, an architect, and Henry Mangan. The secretary of the committee was a retired Irish army officer, Felix Cronin.[40] When a new committee was appointed in 1933 by Fianna Fáil it was composed of supporters of that party: Denis Allen, a former Fianna Fáil TD for Waterford who had lost his seat in the 1933 general election; Liam O'Doherty, an accountant who had served as Fianna Fáil's director of elections in north Dublin during the 1933 election; and Michael Doran, an engineer employed with Ford in Cork.[41]

The first Committee of Reference was appointed in October 1931 and its first duty was to decide on the allocation of funds from the 1931 Manchester November Handicap Sweepstake. It undertook an impressive amount of work, visiting forty-four participating hospitals in a sixty-day period, to inspect their premises, equipment and management structure. Hospital governors were also invited to submit estimates of the financial grants required to pursue their projects. Such details were discussed in meetings between the committee members and the various governors of each hospital, and the architectural plans for hospital construction were studied.[42]

Having completed its review the committee decided that the most equitable means of distributing the sweepstake surplus was to base it on the total financial needs of each hospital, derived from a number of criteria including repayment of loans and overdrafts, building work, furniture, equipment and investment for endowment purposes. Hospitals that had already received awards from the previous three sweepstakes had the value of those grants deducted from their new awards. The gross amount claimed by the hospitals was £8,206,245, reduced to a net of £6,936,222 when the sum allocated in previous sweepstakes was deducted. The committee awarded a total of £3,986,942, 57 per cent of the net amount claimed by the hospitals, the vast majority of which (£2,764,509) was allocated for building works. Wisely, the next largest sum (£1,992,386) was set aside for investment to generate income for the hospitals.[43]

In compiling its first report on the 1931 Manchester November Handicap sweepstake, the committee undertook a survey of the Irish hospital system, which highlighted a number of deficiencies. In one area only, 'the care of the individual patient', were Irish hospitals seen as having made progress, and even this had its negative side as it was achieved at the expense of neglecting the needs of the community as a whole. In contrast to their compatriots in Great Britain and the USA, they were slow to adopt modern methods of statistical analysis and scientific research. Provision in certain specialist areas, most notably paediatrics, obstetrics, orthopaedics and fevers, was inadequate. The committee's criticisms were based largely on its first-hand experience of processing the funding claims submitted to it by the hospitals. These proposals outlined starkly the lack of co-ordination of services both within the voluntary hospital sector itself and between the different types of hospitals, all of which resulted in 'Duplication of institutions and facilities in some areas, absence of both in others, leading to extravagance, waste and confusion'. There was also a notable absence of a 'follow-up' system or of hospital social service departments; once patients had received their treatment the hospitals deemed their obligations to have been met.[44]

In order to rectify such deficiencies, the committee recommended that a complete survey of the hospitals be undertaken that would include the compilation of a detailed statistical record of the entire population of the country, including the number of factory and agricultural workers; the health, social and economic conditions of the population; the number of physicians and surgeons available; and the level and causes of mortality. Every hospital in the state would be examined in detail to produce statistics of their bed capacity and occupancy, volume of work undertaken and a full statement of annual accounts. Such a survey was needed 'before the claims of the individual hospitals can be fully examined and their needs accurately estimated'.[45]

Having considered the most pressing needs of the hospitals, the committee deemed the provision of adequate bed accommodation to meet the demands of patients for treatment to be 'the chief problem confronting the voluntary hospitals'. In contrast to the priorities of the hospitals themselves, the committee did not deem construction of new buildings to be as important, and discouraged extensive building plans, largely because such projects were 'apt to be hastily conceived and carried out without close and expert study of the problems involved'. Hospitals that had already committed themselves to extensive building projects ran the risk of being unable to complete such work in the event of the discontinuation of the sweepstake.[46]

The second report of the committee, on the 1932 Grand National, reiterated many of these points, especially the need for better co-ordination of services and treatment to avoid unnecessary duplication or neglect. The self-interest of individual voluntary hospitals, at the expense of the good of the overall system, was alluded to: 'loyalties may become misguided and pernicious if the main objectives are obscured by an anxiety to preserve existing interests.' Once again the inadequacy of plans for building projects submitted by the voluntary hospitals to the committee was criticised: 'they lack a familiarity with the needs of the various groups who live and work in the institution, including patients, doctors, nurses, as well as lay and professional workers. They indicate also a want of understanding of the technical procedures of a hospital.' Yet again the financial claims of the hospitals were extravagant and unrealistic, exceeding the grants made by almost £3 million.[47] A similar discrepancy between claims and awards also existed in the case of funds distributed after the next sweepstake on the 1932 Derby.[48]

The imposition of this form of central control over the distribution of the sweepstake surplus did not meet with total agreement from the voluntary hospitals, who saw it as unwarranted government intrusion in the voluntary sphere. The major cause of dissent from the hospitals was the delay in distributing grants which ensued because of the time required for the committee to undertake its review of hospital needs and decide their subsequent allocations. By August 1932 the surplus from the 1931 Manchester November Handicap sweepstake was still outstanding, forcing the Minister for Justice to release one third of it to placate the hospitals which were clamouring for their money.[49] Complaints from the Chairman of the Associated Hospitals Sweepstake Committee, Lord Powerscourt, were met by the new Fianna Fáil Minister for Justice, James Geoghegan, with the acerbic response that if his hospitals were not prepared to wait for their money, there were plenty of other institutions that would be glad of it.[50]

A complaint from St Mary's Orthopaedic Hospital in Cappagh, north Dublin, was a large part of the reason for the delay. Cappagh's claim for an endowment out of the proceeds of the 1931 Manchester November Handicap sweepstake was rejected because it was deemed to be profitable. As it was run by a religious order, many of whose nuns worked in the hospital as both nurses and domestic staff, it made considerable savings on salaries in a way not open to all other hospitals. There was a national school attached to the hospital but the funding received from the Department of Education for the school was not declared as an external source of income.[51] In an effort to reverse the committee's decision, the hospital sought to play the religious card, hoping it might have some effect on the new Fianna Fáil government:

> If the protestant hospitals such as Harcourt Street and the Orthopaedic Hospital are endowed, they can take in free patients. The Boards of Health will send the Catholic children to these hospitals as they will not have to pay for them. The result will be that those Catholic children will be deprived of religious instruction for an important part of their lives. This may be turned to advantage for proselytising. We have had a few cases of children whose faith was endangered in this way.[52]

The Committee of Reference showed no obvious interest in the spiritual well being of Cappagh's would-be patients and refused a second claim for an endowment; it was the only one of the 48 participating hospitals to have its claim denied.[53]

The delay in allocating the sweepstake surplus was exacerbated by the change in power which saw the installation of a new Fianna Fáil government in February 1932 that was determined to review the entire method of allocation. Rumours even suggested that they were planning to nationalise the voluntary hospitals.[54] This delay, and the discontent it generated within the voluntary hospital sector, was ammunition for the sweepstake's enemies, especially among the English popular press. Plans drawn up in the latter half of 1932 to introduce new legislation governing the allocation of sweepstake funds also resulted in a delay in distributing the proceeds of the 1932 Grand National and Derby sweepstakes.[55]

The Committee of Reference produced three reports. The fact that the criticisms and observations contained in their final report mirrored those made in its first indicated how little success the committee had with its plans to exert greater control over the administration of the voluntary hospitals. This failure to make any significant progress highlighted the need for more radical change, to which Fianna Fáil had pointed during its time in opposition. After the 1932 general election that party had its chance to introduce the changes it desired.

THE PUBLIC HOSPITALS ACT (1933)

Soon after taking office the Fianna Fáil government began to formulate plans for new legislation to govern the entire sweepstake enterprise, resulting in the enactment of the Public Hospitals Act in July 1933. A memorandum drawn up by the Department of Local Government and Public Health in September 1932 declared that there was 'a pressing need for a complete survey of the entire hospital system of the country'. The existing method of distributing funds was seen as inadequate and if continued likely to lead to the loss of a unique opportunity to overhaul hospital organisation in the state. Citing many of the criticisms voiced by the Committee of Reference, it was felt that these would never be rectified by the action of the hospitals themselves; such co-operation and co-ordination would have to be imposed on them by an external body. To avoid any suggestions that this implied unwarranted intervention by the state in the administration of the voluntary system it was made clear that it would not be either 'desirable or feasible for the State to assume even remotely any additional liability in connection with hospitals or to take any action that would appear subversive of the voluntary principle'.[56] The secretary of the Department of Local Government and Public Health was at pains to reiterate that it was not the government's intention to interfere overtly in the running of the voluntary hospitals: 'it is not intended that the minister will be empowered to enforce amalgamations or reorganisation', though he did intend for the minister, through the medium of a proposed Hospitals Commission, to 'influence the Voluntary Hospitals by advice and recommendations'.[57]

The government's twin desires were to seize the unique opportunity offered by the sweepstake to construct a first-class hospital service, and to prevent the wasteful use of resources. To achieve these ends a new system was suggested for the purpose of controlling the distribution of sweepstake surpluses in the future. The Committee of Reference was to be replaced by a Hospitals Commission nominated by the Minister for Local Government and Public Health, with functions similar to those of its predecessor. It would also have powers to inspect participating institutions and have full access to their financial records.[58]

The Hospitals Commission was established in part for the purpose of conducting a full audit of the Irish hospital system. Therefore, its functions were more wide ranging than those of the Committee of Reference. It was charged with enquiring into and recording 'information in relation to [hospital and nursing] facilities, the needs of the people for such facilities, and the adjustment of such facilities to such needs'. It was also invested with the power to investigate and report on 'every matter relating to hospital or nursing facilities referred to them by the Minister' and to make recommendations 'for the improvement and coordination' of hospital facilities in the state.[59] The power of the Hospitals Commission to plan the future hospital system of the state was limited to dealing only with hospitals that participated in the sweepstake.[60]

The commission's final duty was to advise the minister on the administration of a new Hospitals Trust Fund into which all sweepstake funds would be pooled.[61] This new fund centralised the collection and distribution of sweepstake funds, removing the existing binary system whereby the Committee of Reference recommended allocations to the voluntary hospitals, while the Minister for Local Government and Public Health controlled the share for local authority hospitals and nursing organisations. While the principle of public hospitals benefiting from the sweepstake had been established in 1931, their portion was still very small compared to that of the voluntary hospitals. By merging the allocations for both voluntary and local authority hospitals the government effectively removed the superior benefits enjoyed by the voluntary hospitals, and allowed the local authority hospitals to compete equally for sweepstake funds. Given that the sweepstakes had initially been established as a result of agitation from within the voluntary hospital sector, and had been intended solely for its benefit, the usurpation of the fund for general use was not greeted warmly.[62] Responsibility for the management of the Hospitals Trust Fund would rest with another new five-member body, the National Hospital Trustees (subsequently known as the Hospitals Trust Board), to be appointed, as with the Hospitals Commission, by the Minister for Local Government and Public Health.[63]

The creation of this new hierarchy resulted in a more structured process for the application and distribution of sweepstake funds. Participating hospitals would now apply to the Minister for Local Government and Public Health for a grant from the Hospitals Trust Fund. This application would be adjudicated upon by the Hospitals Commission which would make a recommendation to the minister. However, the minister was not bound by this recommendation; the act stated that the minister would merely 'have regard to the report of the Hospitals Commission on such application'.[64] The new act also gave the minister considerable discretion to allocate funds without any reference to the Hospitals Commission.[65] Ruth Barrington has highlighted the controversial nature of this provision, especially as such expenditure was not subject to sanction or supervision from either the Department of Finance or the Comptroller and Auditor General.[66] One noticeable feature of the new act was the greater power given to the Minister for Local Government and Public Health. In 1930 most of the responsibility for the sweepstake lay with the Minister for Justice. Henceforth, that minister's role was limited to sanctioning the sweepstake scheme, a realisation that the sweepstake now came more within the purview of Health than Justice.

The new legislation envisaged some significant changes from the existing system. The scope of spending future funds was also widened considerably to cover 'the whole field of health work in both its preventive and curative aspects'.[67] This allowed funds to be used for supporting medical research and for institutions such as county infirmaries and county homes, psychiatric hospitals, and homes for unmarried mothers. The vagueness of the original 1930 act had led to much confusion about what types of institutions could participate, necessitating the various amending acts passed in 1931 and 1932. Therefore, it was hoped that the new act would remove such doubts.[68] Introducing the bill in the Dáil, the Parliamentary Secretary (Junior Minister) for Public Health, Dr Con Ward, stated that this was also intended to prevent 'the neglect of other less popular areas of curative medicine'.[69] The only institutions exempted were those that were privately owned and profit making. Provision was also made for the application of sweepstake funds to set up hospital libraries.[70]

Initiating the second reading of the bill in April 1933, Ward cited the reason for introducing the bill as the need to address 'the problems of administration and organisation arising out of the rapid and unprecedented financial success' of the sweepstake. He also admitted the intention of using sweepstake funding to undertake a complete reorganisation of the hospital system, stating that the government had a duty to ensure that the sweepstake funds were put to the best and most efficient use for the benefit of hospital patients. The duplication of services and resulting neglect of other forms of treatment were noted in particular. Lest the voluntary hospitals fear that the government intended to dictate how they would be run, the commitment to retaining the voluntary principle was now stated in public: 'As regards legal control, the Minister does not propose to invade the domain of voluntary effort.' Yet, the voluntary hospitals were warned that there was a need for the amalgamation of some institutions. Since the establishment of the sweepstake there had been numerous calls for the funding to be put to use to cure many other ills within Irish society, in particular that of slum housing in the major cities. Ward used the occasion of the bill's introduction to state categorically that there would be no diversion of funds for any such purposes.[71]

One important change which was made at the committee stage of the bill was the deletion of the prohibition on the use of sweepstake funds to pay the maintenance expenses of hospitals. Presumably this prohibition had initially been inserted to ensure that sweepstake funds were not wasted on paying the day-to-day costs of running the hospitals. Following its removal, civil servants still appeared satisfied that the act reserved sufficient power to the Minister for Local Government and Public Health to ensure that this did not happen.[72] However, as hospital deficits continued to mount during the 1930s this would prove not to be the case.

Fine Gael was unconvinced by Ward's commitment to retaining the independence of the voluntary sector. Denouncing the measure as 'practically unworkable', James Fitzgerald-Kenney declared that it would sound 'the death knell of all voluntary hospitals in this country'. He also attacked what he saw as the retrospective nature of the bill; sweepstake funds which had been collected for an original purpose, i.e. voluntary hospitals, would now be used to fund a variety of other activities.[73] Opposition was also voiced from within the ranks of Fianna Fáil. Thomas Kelly complained that the sweepstakes were being made permanent, while M. J. Kennedy took a swipe at employment practices in Hospitals Trust, claiming 'it is a well-known fact . . . that in some cases three or four people out of the same wealthy family are in positions in the Sweepstakes' offices'.[74] In the Senate the opposition focused on the lack of transparency surrounding the running of the sweepstake. Again, the chief opponent was Thomas Johnson, who failed to have an amendment adopted that would have made the provisions of the scheme for running the sweepstake public.[75] He was the only parliamentarian to highlight the anomalous section 2 (p. 33).

THE HOSPITALS COMMISSION

A level of continuity was retained between the new Hospitals Commission and the Committee of Reference with the appointment the three members of the outgoing body, Michael Doran, Denis Allen (who remained until 1937) and Liam O'Doherty to the new commission. They were joined by Edward Kelly, a county councillor from Monaghan, and two medical doctors, John Madden and Joseph O'Carroll (who resigned in March 1935). In 1937 Dr Seumas Ó Ceallaigh and a Fianna Fáil county councillor from Mayo, Michael Kilroy, were added. The first secretary of the new body was Dr Andy Cooney, also well known in republican circles.[76] Opposition was voiced to the failure to include any women members: 'All advanced thought on matters connected with hospitals maintains that, for all-round efficiency, the nurse's point of view must be ascertained as well as that of the doctor.'[77] The chairman, Michael Doran, received an annual stipend of £1,000, the medical members got £800 each, and the ordinary members £600. There was also a clerical staff of seven.[78]

The commission's first task was to prepare a report on the hospitals for the year 1933 to 1934. Immediately on commencing work in September 1933 it undertook to visit and inspect 98 hospitals, including some that had not applied for sweepstake grants, where discussions were held with governors as to 'the part the hospitals of the future might be expected to play in the life of the community'. The commission was not impressed by the level of ignorance displayed by hospital authorities regarding the new system for allocating sweepstake funds which had been put in place under the Public Hospitals Act:

> the Commission has experienced and still continues to experience much difficulty in getting many hospital authorities to recognise these changes . . . A considerable proportion of the Committee's time has been absorbed in explaining these changes in the allocating of Sweepstake funds . . . which a superficial study of the Act in question should have rendered unnecessary.

The commission's frustration at such ignorance and gratuitous time wasting was palpable and would be noticeable in other instances also.[79]

The financial situation inherited by the commission from the Committee of Reference was as follows. The total claims made by hospitals amounted to over £11 million, of which £2,762,501 had been awarded, leaving unsatisfied claims of over £8.5 million. At the time of the formation of the Hospitals Commission in September 1933, £1,214,000 remained to meet these outstanding claims. In its first published report the commission was scathing about the extravagance, selfishness and disregard for organised hospital provision displayed by the voluntary hospitals during the first three years of the operation of the sweepstake: 'Each hospital appreciated that there was enough money available for its particular scheme and did not see why it should not get it, remaining indifferent to the fact that some 60 other hospitals held the same view, regarding their own individual claims.'[80]

The bulk of the commission's first report comprised a blueprint for the future organisation of the country's hospitals, based on the extensive inspection undertaken. The most radical and controversial plans related to the rationalising of the number of hospitals in Dublin city, which in 1933 had 25 public hospitals, of which 12 were general and 13 specialist, including children's, maternity, cancer and fever hospitals. In addition, there were seven convalescent homes. The existence of such a large number of general hospitals, which had already been commented upon unfavourably by a commission in 1854, was 'indefensible', uneconomic and inefficient in the view of the Hospitals Commission.[81]

To rectify this situation the commission considered two alternative methods of organising the capital city's hospitals. The first envisioned the formation of a federation, whereby 'each hospital would retain its identity on its existing site, whilst becoming a member of a group of federated hospitals for common purposes, such as combined purchasing, exchange of patients, etc.'. Alternatively, some of the smaller hospitals could be amalgamated, an idea that had been considered by some of the voluntary hospitals themselves during the 1920s. Amalgamation was the option favoured by the Hospitals Commission. Federation was unsuitable because some of the older voluntary hospitals already required rebuilding, it would not result in any noticeable saving on administrative costs, and the limited bed accommodation would hinder specialisation. In general, the commission felt many of the existing voluntary hospitals were too small to function efficiently: 'Experience in other countries has shown that the most economic unit is a hospital possessing five to six hundred beds.'[82]

Under the amalgamation scheme proposed by the commission, Dublin city would have four large general hospitals, two each on either side of the River Liffey. One of those on the south side would consist of a new unit formed from the amalgamation of Sir Patrick Dun's, the Royal City of Dublin, Mercer's and the Meath, in spite of objections from the latter which the commission chose to disregard. This recommendation drew upon the previous efforts of these hospitals to amalgamate during the 1920s.[83] The issue was revisited during the early 1930s; in September 1931 the governors of Sir Patrick Dun's resolved unanimously to consult their compatriots in the Royal City of Dublin on the subject of a merger of both institutions.[84] The arguments made by the governors of Dun's in 1932 foreshadowed the thinking of the Hospitals

Commission. As they then existed many voluntary hospitals were unable to afford or justify the services of full-time specialists such as pathologists, bio-chemists and radiographers. Larger units would also lead to fewer overheads and increased efficiency generally, and modern transport obviated the need for hospitals to be in multiple locations.[85] Not all of Dublin's leading medics were in agreement with the Dun's board. Richard Atkinson Stoney of Trinity College Dublin expressed the view that the finance required to build and equip a modern hospital, combined with the attendant scrapping of the existing hospitals, 'would be a very wasteful procedure', and the benefits that these hospitals brought to medical education would also be lost.[86]

Following discussions between representatives from both hospitals Dun's governors agreed to the idea in January 1932, although they warned of the potential difficulties which the venture might encounter, in particular the need to repeal the School of Physics Act which would require the consent of both Trinity College and the Royal College of Physicians of Ireland. Although the medical staff of the hospital appeared to be getting cold feet, moves towards a possible amalgamation with one or more hospitals continued. Professor Thomas Gillman Moorhead, the chairman of Dun's governors, had discussions on the subject with board members from other hospitals in 1933, and in 1935 agreement had been reached on the division of Sir Patrick Dun's estate in the event of amalgamation taking place.[87]

The second general hospital for south Dublin was to be an expanded St Vincent's to be built on an entirely new site. St Vincent's escaped with its identity completely intact because it was owned and administered by the Sisters of Charity and as such there would be too many legal difficulties involved in combining it with a number of other hospitals controlled by voluntary boards. North of the Liffey the existing Mater and Richmond Hospitals were to be extended and redeveloped on their existing sites. In addition to these two general hospitals, Jervis Street was to be retained as the principal accident hospital for the city, due to its central location and the extent of redevelopment which had been undertaken and was nearing completion. Another factor contributing to the retention of these existing hospitals was their status as teaching hospitals.[88]

The scheme outlined by the commission for the reorganisation of the Dublin hospitals was based on the principle of retaining the voluntary hospitals. An alternative would have been to develop the municipal St Kevin's Hospital (formerly the workhouse hospital of the South Dublin Union, now St James's Hospital) as one of the south city's flagship general hospitals. While the commission gave consideration to this option, it came down heavily in favour of retaining the pre-eminence of the voluntary hospitals. It recognised that they 'have always been the spearhead of hospital service in this country' and that a very close relationship existed between them and the city's medical schools. In recommending 'the development of the principal Dublin Voluntary Hospitals as against the creation of a Dublin Municipal Hospital', the commission stipulated that this would be dependent on the cooperation of the voluntary hospitals with the plan in order 'to ensure that the public interest would be safeguarded'. In a thinly-veiled threat, the voluntary hospitals were warned that the Public Hospitals Act gave the minister power 'to attach conditions to grants from the Hospitals Trust Fund'.[89]

Dublin city also had an abundance of specialist hospitals, many serving the same purpose, with three maternity (the National Maternity, the Rotunda and the Coombe) and four children's hospitals (National Children's, St Ultan's – which catered for infants, Temple Street and the Incorporated Orthopaedic). The commission felt that 'there would appear to be no reason why the treatment of children in a city the size of Dublin could not be carried out in one central Children's Hospital'. However, it recognised that any plans to so rationalise hospital treatment of the city's children would fall foul of 'Conflicting interests'. These interests were not specified but presumably referred to the religious differences between the management of some of the hospitals: Temple Street was under the control of the Sisters of Charity whereas St Ultan's was founded and run by a prominent Protestant doctor, Kathleen Lynn.

In addition, most of them had already undertaken development projects with the proceeds of previous sweepstakes; the National Children's Hospital had effectively been rebuilt at the cost of £38,000 and Temple Street had similarly expended £33,000. Such money would be wasted if the hospitals were closed in favour of the creation of an entirely new hospital. In light of these obstacles, the commission conceded that the 'desirable result' of constructing one new children's hospital for Dublin was 'impracticable'. However, the fact that the National Children's Hospital and St Ultan's were situated close to each other and there was close co-operation between the medical staffs in both institutions raised the possibly of amalgamating them. While the commission did not make a concrete recommendation in this regard, it was 'engaged on an exploration of the possibilities of such an amalgamation'. In keeping with the overall view of the commission that there were too many children's hospitals in Dublin city a proposal from 'a group of doctors practising in Dublin' for the construction of yet another one, to be based in Lower Mount Street and to serve the neighbourhoods of Westland Row, Ringsend, Irishtown, City Quay and Mount Street, was unsurprisingly rejected.[90]

In contrast to the situation regarding children's hospitals, the commission did not seek any rationalisation or amalgamation of the city's three maternity hospitals, partly because the National Maternity Hospital was well on the way to being rebuilt. The principal argument against such a change was that the nature of the service provided required that maternity hospitals be situated in different areas for ease of access.[91] The commission's chief recommendation concerning Dublin's maternity services was that there should be an increase of 158 in the number of maternity beds available to cope with the increased demand for hospital accommodation for expectant mothers. It was hoped that by 1944 half of all child births in Dublin city would take place in a maternity hospital.[92]

Shifting its focus away from the capital, the commission suggested the establishment of a system of regional hospitals to serve the 'acute medical and surgical' needs of the rest of the country. New regional hospitals would assume precedence over the existing 26 county hospitals. While recognising the contribution of county hospitals in the past, the commission did not regard the county as the best entity on which to base hospital development, largely due to the arbitrary nature of many county boundaries, whereas

> The grouping of three or four counties together for hospital purposes, in suitable centres, would enable not only better and more up-to-date central and special services to be provided, but would enable a more complete hospital medical staff to be employed, at less cost to the ratepayers of such grouped counties than the restricted services and personnel that one county can at present afford.

Four main regions were identified for the provision of such centralised services: Dublin city, serving the city itself and surrounding counties of Wicklow, Kildare and Meath along with certain cases from the Leinster and border counties; Cork city, serving Cork, Kerry and Waterford; Galway, serving Galway, Mayo and Roscommon; and Limerick, serving Limerick, Tipperary and Clare. Further consideration would be given to the designation of Sligo as a fifth regional centre, to provide for Sligo, Donegal and Leitrim. The regional hospitals would still be backed up by the existing network of county and district hospitals, which could deal with maternity and certain medical and acute surgical cases.[93]

To equip Cork city as the regional centre for the southern counties, it was recommended that a completely new hospital be built, to be under the public control of the South Cork Board of Public Assistance. The existing semi-voluntary North and South Charitable Infirmaries, and the voluntary Mercy Hospital, would all benefit from upgrading, but in light of the plan for a new hospital there would be no serious reconstruction of them undertaken. The urgent need for a new maternity hospital was also identified.[94]

Galway city provided the only example of a centralised hospital service in the Free State in the shape of the rate-supported Galway Central Hospital.

Plans were submitted to the commission for the construction of a new hospital but no decision had yet been made. To serve the county of Galway ministerial sanction had been given to the completion of a district hospital at Clifden and the construction of another in Ballinasloe.[95]

Limerick city was a microcosm of Dublin; the existence of four general hospitals (Barrington's, St John's, the County Infirmary, and the City Home and Hospital) to serve the population could not be justified. Rather than granting awards for the development of these existing institutions, the commission favoured the development of 'one Central Hospital situated convenient to Limerick City'. These plans would lead to considerable resentment and opposition, especially in the case of Barrington's: 'The Medical Staffs in particular were strongly of the opinion that a large central hospital combining the activities of existing hospitals would not be a forward step.' Their opinions were not looked upon favourably by the commission: 'Whatever justification there may exist for this view among lay men and women on the Boards of these hospitals, its existence amongst the Medical Staffs is regrettable in the extreme and completely at variance with progressive hospital and medical opinion in other countries.' Limerick city's small voluntary maternity hospital in Bedford Row was in an 'extremely unsuitable' location and its 26 beds were 'inadequate'. Therefore, the provision of a new maternity hospital for the Limerick region was recommended.[96]

Having dealt with the geographic provision of general hospitals, the Hospitals Commission turned its attention to the issue of making adequate national provision for certain specific illnesses. Three voluntary sanatoria in Dublin and Wicklow catered exclusively for TB patients, while general and local authority hospitals also dealt with many cases. Pulmonary TB was the most common version of the disease in Ireland, but provision for non-pulmonary cases, in both adults and children, was also adjudged to be inadequate. In order to cater for the high incidence of TB the commission recommended the provision of an additional 346 dedicated beds. It also proposed 'a coordinated scheme for anti-tuberculosis work', which would not be achieved until the late 1940s and early 1950s.

The 1930s saw notable developments in the use of radium and x-rays to treat cancer, the third highest cause of mortality in the state. Yet, treatment of this disease left much to be desired: 'the fight against cancer in Ireland has hitherto been carried out in a more or less desultory fashion.' While there were two specialist cancer hospitals in Dublin, St Anne's and Hume Street, 'the greatest amount of total cancer treatment [was] carried out in the General Hospitals.' There was also an insufficient supply of radium in the state. 'Financial stringency' was the principal factor responsible for this inadequate provision. Henceforth, cancer would have to be approached from

a national rather than local or regional standpoint. Rather than simply purchasing additional supplies of radium and doling it out to the general
hospitals, the commission favoured 'some form of Central Institute, where
only specialists in radium treatment would have access to an adequate supply'.
A new cancer strategy was clearly needed, but because of the short window
available to the commission to prepare its first report, it was unable to make
any definite recommendations at this stage.[97]

VOLUNTARY HOSPITAL DEFICITS

Increasing deficits in the budgets of voluntary hospitals were to emerge as the
biggest obstacle to the Hospitals Commission's plan to use the sweepstake
money to establish an effective health service in the Irish Free State during
the 1930s. While the 1933 Public Hospitals Act allowed for the use of the
available surplus to clear such deficits, the framers had no indication of how
much of the surplus would eventually have to be set aside to cater for the
ordinary expenditure of these hospitals. The combined deficits of the voluntary
hospitals almost doubled in the four years from 1933 to 1937, rising from
£54,868 to £103,966 during that period (Table 3.1). The figure rose to £115,257
in 1938 and £156,975 in 1939.[98] The Dublin general hospitals were responsible
for the largest increases, with their combined deficit rising by 147 per cent in
the five years from 1933 to 1938. In the same period the deficit of the capital
city's specialist hospitals rose by 71 per cent, while in the provinces those of
general hospitals rose by 81 per cent, and specialist hospitals by 75 per cent.
Such deficits would have been even higher if the hospitals did not 'derive an
appreciable amount of their income from invested Sweepstake funds in their
possession'; without this source of income it was estimated that the 1938
deficit figure would have been £166,362, over £50,000 more than the actual
deficit of £115,257.[99]

In its first general report the Hospitals Commission stated that it would
be unable to 'bear any large capital expenditure on individual building
schemes' for 'some considerable time' because of the need to set aside funds
for endowment and maintenance.[100] In 1935 it warned that 'the abnormal rate
of increase' of deficits was a major concern as the need to spend increasingly
larger sums on maintaining the hospitals inevitably meant there was less of
the sweepstake surplus available for the large capital programmes envisaged.[101]

In an effort to make the hospitals economise in future the commission
announced that payment of the 1935 annual deficit would be based on bed-
occupancy rates for 1934, leading to complaints from the hospitals about the

refusal to pay the full deficit.[102] The commission's warning was not heeded and hospital expenditure during 1936 showed 'a marked increase' over that for 1935.[103] Further punitive measures were taken by the commission: hospitals that failed to return acceptable accounts were not entitled to full benefit, as the Mater Hospital discovered when it failed to differentiate what proportions of its deficit had been incurred by its public hospital and private home respectively.[104] Jervis Street was refused a claim for salaries of newly appointed medical staff because it refused to consult beforehand with the commission.[105] However, such actions had no obvious effect and hospital deficits continued their upward spiral. The warning against this trend became a standard feature of all of the Hospitals Commission's reports. The third general report, dealing with the year 1937, lamented the growing dependence of the voluntary hospitals on the sweepstake fund to cover their deficits: 'Unless measures are taken to limit the deficits . . . it is not easy to see how, with their present tendencies, the voluntary hospitals can avoid becoming more dependent on the Hospitals Trust Fund.'[106]

Table 3.1: Total annual deficits of voluntary hospitals, 1933–9 (£)

Year	Total deficits	Increase over previous year	Increase since 1933
1933	54,868	—	—
1934	58,469	3,601	3,601
1935	78,841	20,372	23,973
1936	88,012	9,171	33,144
1937	103,966	15,954	49,098
1938	115,257	11,291	60,389
1939	156,975	41,718	102,107

Source: Hospitals Commission, *Sixth general report, 1942, 1943 and 1944* (Dublin, 1946), p. 5.

The commissioners laid the blame for the rapidly increasing expenditure firmly at the door of the hospitals themselves: 'in many of the hospitals there is a marked tendency to relax that ever-watchful supervision of spending which is so essential for the economic administration of such institutions.'[107] The implication was clear: safe in the knowledge they would be bailed out by the sweepstake funds the voluntary hospitals allowed their spending to spiral out of control with impunity. The commission's secretary, Dr Andy Cooney, complained that 'it is only since the practice of paying deficits has been introduced that these deficits have each year continued to increase in alarming proportions'.[108]

The inadequate administrative procedures governing hospital budgets were considered to be a large part of the problem. In a thinly veiled threat the hospitals were warned that if their refusal to modernise their administrative structures and rein in expenditure continued their voluntary status might be jeopardised:

> For the sake of the voluntary status of the hospitals and their tradition of voluntary service, it is desirable and not untimely that the governing authorities of each institution should have brought home to them the necessity of exercising a business-like and conscientious control of expenditure, as otherwise an alternative method of dealing with the deficit question will have to be considered.[109]

The commission called regularly for the introduction of 'effective internal control within each individual institution' to help curtail excessive spending. Its frustration at the apparent failure of the hospitals to act upon this recommendation was expressed on numerous occasions: 'it does not appear . . . that there has been any marked improvement in hospital administrative methods in the matter of supervision of expenditure'; 'hospital working expenses generally could be considerably reduced if a greater effort was made by hospital managements to adopt business methods of control under the various heads of expenditure.'[110] Hospital administrators who acceded to every request for equipment from their medical staff were identified as some of the biggest culprits: 'Requisitions for expensive medical supplies and equipment by members of hospital medical staffs are generally accepted without questioning whether less costly substitutes would serve the purpose equally well.'[111] The reluctance of medical staff to consider paring back such requests was also blamed: 'Medical staffs in hospitals are inclined to be resentful of any steps which are taken to supervise expenditure on drugs and appliances, taking the attitude that their work is so all-important for the welfare of the patients that no interference in the way of checking expenditure could be tolerated.'[112]

Alarmed at the prospect of growing voluntary hospital deficits swallowing up an increasingly larger portion of the sweepstake funds, in 1936 the Hospitals Trust Fund was divided into two parts. A Special Purposes Fund containing £2 million in both cash and investments was formed specifically to provide income to satisfy annual deficits. The remainder of the fund became the General Purpose Fund and all grants, other than those for maintenance purposes, were paid out of it. However, the failure to curtail deficits meant that by 1938 the Special Purposes Fund had to be augmented to £3 million.[113]

Hospital administrators defended themselves against the commission's claims of wasteful extravagance and administrative incompetence by pointing

to the increase in the size of their institutions as sweepstake-funded construction came on stream and by highlighting the effects of inflation. In 1935
the commission acknowledged that the 'slight increase in average daily bed
occupancy' during the year justified 'a proportionate increase in expenditure',
noting, however, that this should have been offset by 'a decrease in the average
number of free patients'.[114] In the case of the Rotunda Maternity Hospital,
the increased expenditure between 1934 and 1936 was attributed to improved
diet for both patients and nurses; the greater consumption and increased price
of medicines and disinfectants; more widespread use of x-rays; increased fuel
prices; the installation of additional electrical appliances; an increased bill for
salaries and wages consequent on the employment of new staff; and the
overhaul of the hospital chapel's organ.[115] Such explanations were echoed by
Sister Brigid of the Mater Hospital, who highlighted a 4 per cent increase in
bed occupancy, a 6.5 per cent increase in the cost of living index, the employment of 42 new staff, and an additional 1,566 outpatient attendances between
1936 and 1937.[116] To highlight the increased expenditure on foodstuffs alone,
the registrar of Sir Patrick Dun's compared the relative prices of basic foods
between 1934 and 1938, reporting that the cost of a gallon of milk had
increased by one penny, a 4lb loaf of bread by two and a half pence, a pound of
butter by one and a half pence, and a hundredweight of potatoes by one
shilling.[117] Physicians highlighted how improvements in medicine also contributed to working deficits; according to Professor Henry Moore of UCD and
the Mater Hospital: 'New and more efficient remedies and improved methods
of diagnosis and treatment are nowadays being rapidly introduced into medical
practice, they are frequently more expensive than older ones.'[118]

The rising deficits reduced the proportion of the sweepstake surplus
available for hospital development, much to the frustration of the medical
profession. In 1938 Moore complained about the difficulty encountered by
the hospitals in acquiring sweepstake funds, for which he blamed the
Department of Local Government and Public Health: 'The Department
holds, I understand, over six million pounds for hospital development; it is
difficult, and often impossible, to extract a penny from it, in our case even for
hospital debt.' The specific case to which he was referring was that of the
Mater Hospital, where he was a physician, and which he claimed had received
'no money . . . out of the Hospital Trust Fund' since 1932 'with the exception
of £20,391 for annual deficits in working expenses'. He believed the Mater was
being penalised for the savings it made from 38 nuns acting as unpaid nurses
and the surplus profit made by its private hospital.[119] The Minister for Local
Government and Public Health, Seán T. O'Kelly, responded promptly that
the difficulties Moore and the Mater were experiencing were largely due to
the voluntary hospitals' failure to curb their deficits.[120] Moore accepted that

deficits should not be paid automatically without some investigation of their causes, but persisted with his assertion that the Department of Local Government and Public Health remained to be 'convinced of the urgency of hospital enlargement in Dublin'.[121] The dissatisfaction of the Dublin medical profession clearly stemmed from their lingering resentment at the usurpation of sweepstake funds for the general development of the Irish hospitals, a view expressed indignantly by Dr Kathleen Lynn in her private diary: 'Sean T. answered Dr Moore & Rowlette, v. unconvincing, assumes L[ocal] G[overnment] D[epartment] has a right to Sweep funds wh[ich] they have confiscated & says they must [not?] allow "waste", the Govt officials being judges of Hosp. requirements!!!'[122]

Prior to sanctioning payment to cover the voluntary hospitals' deficits for 1938, the commission undertook a close examination of the books of some of them. The main expense appears to have been increased bed occupancy and Sir Patrick Dun's was criticised for 'being run at an excessively high cost in this regard'.[123] In 1938 Dun's returned a debit balance of £13,215, rising to £15,008 in 1939.[124] Higher commodity prices generally, wage increases, improved diets, the need to replace surgical instruments, increasing demand for patent drugs, new procedures such as x-rays, and general structural repairs accounted for most of the additional expenditure.[125]

The experience of voluntary hospitals in the United Kingdom during the 1930s appears to lend some credence to the arguments put forward by the governors of the Irish voluntary hospitals to explain their increasing deficits. In their study of 72 London voluntary hospitals in the interwar years Martin Gorsky and John Mohan found that 'there was a persistent risk of income shortfall throughout the period, with at least half of all hospitals in deficit in 1921, 1930, 1938 and 1939'. As a result the hospitals were forced increasingly to rely on external borrowing to make up for this shortfall in income. While their findings agreed with the more recent interpretations that there was not 'a universal financial crisis in London's voluntary hospitals', it was clear that many of them 'faced very serious difficulties. There were recurrent shortfalls of income in some institutions coupled with rising debt levels.' These financial difficulties became more acute towards the end of the 1930s.[126]

Echoing one of the arguments made by the Irish voluntary hospital administrators, they found that 'the greatest pressure on current spending was exerted by the rising cost of staffing'.[127] In wider-ranging research on voluntary hospitals throughout Britain such additional expenditure has been attributed to larger hospital capacity which created the need for more staff, the introduction of an eight-hour day for ancillary staff, an increase in the number of salaried resident medical officers, and higher wages for nurses as they became more professionalised, were expected to have a wider range of skills, and sought to have their remuneration kept in line with other 'white blouse occupations'.[128] In addition to the extra demands for salaries and wages, hospital deficits in Britain were explained by the need to purchase new and expensive scientific apparatus, the adoption of more scientific management procedures to deal with administration, diagnosis and treatment, and the increased use of x-rays, pathological and bacteriological laboratories and radiology. The costs incurred in this way were even greater for Britain's teaching hospitals.[129]

The spiralling voluntary hospital debt, and the repeated failure of the hospitals to stem it, had reached such a point by 1939 that the Hospitals Commission was forced to recommend major changes in the method of allocating sweepstake funds to pay deficits. The worsening international crisis and the potential threat which it posed to the continued success, if not actual survival of the sweepstake, made the necessity of addressing deficits all the more pressing. The introduction of a proper annual budgeting system in each hospital was recommended, along with increased inspection of institutions by the commission, and also the possibility of hospitals appointing internal auditors. However, the commission, in line with its view that excess expenditure was largely the fault of the hospitals themselves, favoured more of a stick than a carrot approach. Its principal recommendation was to put a cap on the amount available to satisfy deficits: 'The amount of the total grants to be paid annually in respect of the maintenance deficits of the Voluntary hospitals from 1940 onwards shall be kept within a defined maximum figure.' That figure would be calculated on the basis of the deficit figures for 1940. Hospitals were to be forced to submit their budgets for a particular year by the middle of October in the previous year, and would only receive their grants once their audited accounts had 'been examined by the commission and the deficits approved by the Minister'.[130]

The repeated warnings of the commissioners were to no avail, with the deficit figure of £156,975 for 1939 being 'out of all proportion to previous years even allowing for an all round increase in commodities'. The commission reiterated its 'dissatisfaction with the systems of management in many of the hospitals'. Adequate procedures to supervise 'expenditure and consumption of commodities in a businesslike way' could have prevented 'a large proportion of the increased expenditure'. The Minister for Local Government and Public Health was advised to urge upon the hospitals – especially with a European war in the offing – the need to economise and avoid wasteful use of fuel, food and domestic items, be judicious in the use of medicines that might become necessary in the event of a national emergency, avoid increasing staff and personnel, limit expenditure on construction to essential work, and ensure that 'the greatest care is taken of existing equipment'.[131]

A previous recommendation of the commission to cap the Special Purposes Fund appears not to have been adopted; a further £564,407 was added to it during 1939, and the auditors were recommending another augmentation by £450,000. To meet future deficits it was estimated that a figure of up to £5.25 million would be required, and even that might not be sufficient. Realising that its repeated admonitions to hospitals to economise were not being heeded, and that such economising by itself would not be sufficient to stem the increasing voluntary hospital deficits, the Hospitals Commission recommended fundamental changes to the structure of hospital funding. It suggested the introduction of both hospital contributory schemes, which had become widespread in the United Kingdom during the interwar years, and of hospital insurance schemes, popular in continental Europe, that allowed patients to contribute to the cost of hospital treatment by paying into health insurance schemes.[132] France provided a particularly successful example of such medical insurance schemes; legislation passed there in 1928 made workers and the lower middle class eligible for insurance, so that by 1940 more than half of the population was covered.[133]

The adverse affect of the war on sweepstake income was another factor behind the decision of the commission to recommend investigating alternative sources of funding for hospitals. However, the commissioners were aware of the potential obstacles to the introduction of either of the schemes suggested. The principal difficulty would be the population itself which would be reluctant 'to make extra contributions for hospitals when the Sweepstakes have already provided so much'. The latter option of introducing health insurance was seen as somewhat premature, but the extension of existing national health insurance schemes to cover hospital benefit was considered much more possible. This would be easier since the variety of different schemes that had proliferated since the 1920s had finally been unified under one National Health Insurance Society.[134]

As long as there was a steady income from the sweepstake the problem of rising deficits did not appear to be critical. However, the drastic decline in sweepstake income after the start of the war eventually forced the Minister for Local Government and Public Health to act upon the recommendations of the Hospitals Commission to curtail the proportion of sweepstake funds that could be used for maintenance deficits. In September 1939 it was announced that 'for the year 1940 and each subsequent year the total amount to be paid out of the Hospitals Trust Fund to meet the deficits shall be kept within a defined maximum figure'. The recommendations of the commission that hospitals submit prior budgets upon which the deficit payments would be calculated was adopted as the method of allocating grants.[135]

To protect themselves against a possible shortfall under this new system the hospitals appear to have submitted extravagant budget estimates for 1940;

the secretary of the Hospitals Commission complained 'that owing to the uncertainty of the prevailing conditions . . . hospitals have budgeted on an abnormal basis'.[136] Also to soften the blow, the hospitals requested the payment of an early instalment of their grants. Though reluctant to concede this principle, the commission was forced to acknowledge that in the straitened circumstances created by the Emergency they had little choice other than to accede to this request.[137] The outbreak of war and subsequent restriction of the sweepstake forced the postponement of any drastic efforts to curtail the funding of hospital deficits. The problem would continue throughout the war years and beyond.

PROGRESS OF THE HOSPITALS COMMISSION'S PLANS

Spiralling voluntary hospital deficits proved to be a major obstacle to the achievement of the ambitious hospital construction plans of the Hospitals Commission. Its *Second General Report*, published in 1937, stated that a considerable part of the development recommended in the inaugural report was 'on the way to realisation', while an 'equally considerable portion' was at 'the stage where development may be expected within a reasonable period'. However, the commission's ambitious plans for the radical redevelopment of voluntary hospitals in Dublin city had encountered difficulties owing to 'the many conflicting interests which are the inevitable consequences of the Voluntary Hospital system'.[138] Some important improvements were made to the Dublin hospitals: the new outpatient department of the Mater was completed and the construction of a new gynaecological operating theatre was under construction; the operating suite at the Richmond Hospital had been rebuilt with the addition of an extra theatre; and the Rotunda got a new outpatient department.[139]

Legislation had been put in train to achieve some of the commission's more complicated plans. Heads of bills had been prepared by the governors of Sir Patrick Dun's, Mercer's and the Royal City of Dublin hospitals to arrange their proposed amalgamation, along with the Meath Hospital, even though the latter institution was maintaining its opposition to the venture.[140] Plans to amalgamate the National Children's Hospital and St Ultan's Infant Hospital had fallen foul of the Roman Catholic Archbishop of Dublin and influential Catholic doctors who wanted an entirely new children's hospital under Catholic management.[141]

Improvements to the local authority hospital sector were slower. A sum of just under £5 million was required to complete development of the schemes outlined by the commission; however, there was only £1.5 million available in the Hospitals Trust Fund. Therefore, the commission warned that the amount required would 'not be forthcoming for a considerable time' and urged caution in 'allowing a large number of these schemes to proceed'. Priority would have to be given to the more important types of local authority hospitals, in particular those catering for acute diseases.[142]

The slow pace of progress in hospital development could be compensated for if a greater level of co-ordination was undertaken among the hospitals, both voluntary and local authority. In its first report the commission highlighted how such cooperation could assist in ending much of the unnecessary duplication of service that existed, especially in Dublin. Judging by the commission's next report very little had been achieved in this regard; in the meantime, co-ordination of work between the voluntary hospitals alone was deemed 'negligible' and blamed largely on the 'individualistic outlook of most Voluntary Hospitals'.[143]

Progress in hospital construction was also hampered by the poor quality of the proposals submitted by the hospitals: 'In few cases did the preliminary plans harmonise the ideal with the practice and give evidence of close co-operation between Architect, Hospital Management and Medical Staff in the search for an efficient and economical layout.' As a result expensive alteration of schemes was necessary and this only caused further delay. To avoid similar problems in future the commission felt there should be architectural competition, especially for the construction of large hospitals.[144]

By the time the commission published its *Third general report* in 1938 the investment of sweepstake funds in the development of local authority hospitals was starting to have results. The first new county hospital to be built with sweepstake funds was opened at Mullingar, in County Westmeath, in April 1936.[145] New county hospitals had either been completed or were near to completion in Monaghan, Nenagh, Ennis, Mallow, Castlebar, Cashel and Tralee. Together they accounted for 692 new beds. Smaller district hospitals, with a cumulative total of 320 beds, were provided in Ennistymon, Millstreet, Clifden, Kenmare, Mohill, Ballina, Belmullet, Swinford, Youghal, Midleton, Dingle and New Ross. One hundred and four new beds were provided in fever hospitals located in Ballina, Belmullet, Swinford and Abbeyleix, while 192 beds were now available to treat TB in specialist hospitals and sanatoria in Tralee, Limerick and Rathdrum. Extensions and improvements had also been undertaken to psychiatric hospitals in Ballinasloe, Castlebar, Kilkenny, Killarney, Letterkenny, Mullingar, Portlaoise and Sligo.[146] This was impressive progress for the four years since the establishment of the commission. When representatives of the Rockefeller Foundation visited Ireland in 1942 they rated the new county hospitals as 'amongst the most modern structures to be found anywhere'.[147]

In addition to the above mentioned projects, construction was underway on new county hospitals in Kilkenny, Portlaoise, Tullamore, Roscommon and Sligo; on district hospitals for Killarney, Listowel, Gorey and New Ross; a psychiatric hospital for Castlerea; and fever hospitals for Naas and New Ross. The redevelopment of Dublin city's voluntary hospitals proceeded much more slowly; construction of extensions to the Rotunda and National Maternity Hospital had been delayed by an industrial dispute within the building trade and an extensive search was underway to find a new site for a fever hospital in Dublin.[148]

The discrepancy between the pace of local authority hospital development and that of voluntary hospitals was alluded to in the fourth report of the commission, dealing with the year 1938. As with the deficit problem, the blame for this was also laid at the door of the voluntary hospitals themselves who were accused of submitting unrealistic schemes and failing to consent to the involvement of the state in the plans for their development:

> One of the greatest causes of delay in the development of the voluntary hospitals has been the difficulty of reconciling the demands which the state, as a trustee of the people's hospital rights, finds it necessary to make on the voluntary hospitals, with the tenacity with which those hospitals cling to their time-honoured claim for complete individual independence.

In spite of such recalcitrance the commission was able to report some progress: the Roman Catholic Archbishop of Dublin had acquired a sixteen-acre site from Dublin Corporation that was part of a new public-housing development in Crumlin on the south side of the city, upon which a completely new children's hospital was to be built; legislation was being prepared to merge four of the smaller Dublin voluntary hospitals on the southside; and a site for the new hospital that would replace them had been found south-west of the city.[149]

THE DUBLIN HOSPITALS BUREAU (BED BUREAU)

As part of its attempt to encourage closer cooperation among the state's hospitals, and in particular among Dublin's voluntary hospitals, the Hospitals Commission recommended the establishment of a 'Hospital Information and Bed Bureau' to ensure that poorer patients would be guaranteed admission to hospital.[150] The Department of Local Government and Public Health began planning the establishment of such a bureau in 1936, aware that they were likely to encounter substantial opposition from the voluntary hospital sector:

> If the bureau is established on the lines suggested by the Hospitals Commission it will give rise to a storm of protest from the Voluntary Hospitals. After all they are Voluntary Hospitals whilst the bureau on the lines suggested would undoubtedly be a State Department . . . and I am convinced the Voluntary Hospitals would not stand for it.[151]

Dr Andy Cooney, a strident critic of the voluntary hospitals, retorted that any such opposition would be 'unreasonable and untenable', pointing out that such an innovation should be welcomed by the voluntary hospitals as it would help preserve their status from the alternative of a municipal hospital. In order to placate the voluntary hospitals he suggested that the bureau would be composed of representatives of both the hospitals and the Minister for Local Government and Public Health, thus ensuring a significant level of influence for the former.[152]

A committee composed of representatives of the four proposed Dublin general hospitals submitted a draft scheme for the bed bureau to the minister in November 1936, recommending that it be managed by a voluntary committee comprising two representatives of the four hospitals and a representative of the Medical Officer of Health for Dublin City. Along with powers to employ staff, acquire premises and appoint subcommittees, the bureau would maintain a list of available beds in the participating hospitals, advise hospitals on admissions, collate statistics and arrange for the transfer of unsuitable patients to alternative accommodation. In terms of actual operation the bureau which would be open 24 hours a day, would have a telephone connection to all of the participating hospitals and be limited to Dublin city only. Patients would apply for admission through their doctor and, as far as possible, would be treated in the hospital and by the doctor of their choice. Only free, part-paying and urgent cases would go through the bureau and the decision on whether to continue the treatment of non-paying patients would be taken by the governing authority of the hospital to which they had been admitted.[153]

The commission did not find this proposed scheme satisfactory. In the first place it failed to address the three main problems which had given rise to the need for the bureau: difficulties experienced by both doctors and local authorities finding accommodation for their patients in Dublin hospitals; difficulties encountered by poorer patients seeking hospital admission; and inadequate internal recording and statistic keeping by the hospitals. The proposed constitution of the bureau was also objectionable: it was weighted overwhelmingly in favour of the voluntary hospitals, did not provide for co-ordination between voluntary and local authority hospitals and referred only to general hospitals, ignoring specialist hospitals. Nor was the commission satisfied with the proposed functions of the bureau, in particular the limitation of its activities to Dublin and the selectivity of dealing only with free and part-paying patients. Instead, the commission favoured a bureau whose activities would be national.[154] Civil servants in the Department of Local Government and Public Health spent much of 1937 revising the scheme to bring it more into conformity with the wishes of the commission. The voluntary hospitals still proved recalcitrant, forcing the secretary of the Department, James Hurson to threaten to proceed with the alternative of developing a municipal hospital for Dublin, in place of the voluntaries.[155]

Hurson's threat tapped into a palpable fear among Dublin's leading medics that a flagship municipal hospital for the city was going to be developed. In the June 1936 edition of the *Irish Journal of Medical Science* Professor Henry Moore endorsed the Hospitals Commission's choice of developing the existing voluntary hospitals over the municipal hospital option. However, he was convinced that a significant threat still remained to the future of the capital city's voluntary hospitals:

> The position of the voluntary teaching hospitals in Dublin is being threatened and dangerously threatened. There is, I understand, an organised movement at present exerting pressure in various high places in order to force the awarding authority [i.e., the Hospitals Commission] to establish a new municipal hospital of 600 beds under the control of the Dublin Board of Assistance.

Arguing against any such plans he highlighted the importance of the educational functions of voluntary hospitals (St Kevin's, the municipal hospital in Dublin, was not a teaching hospital). Because of their centrality to medical education, better research was produced by the voluntary hospitals, and their teaching functions also attracted the best medical staff. The financial problems that would ensue from the development of municipal hospitals were also cited. Specialists were not paid for their voluntary hospital work, relying instead on the income generated by their private practices, raising the question of who would pay specialists in a state hospital. Free treatment of patients in municipal hospitals would lead to an increased burden on taxpayers. The only argument in favour of the development of a municipal hospital that Moore was prepared to concede was that it allowed for 'the more prompt placing of poor patients in hospital', a deficiency that could be rectified in the voluntary hospitals by the provision of additional bed accommodation.[156]

Moore's views were endorsed by his colleagues. William Doolin, who believed that the development of a municipal hospital 'would mean the arrested development of medical teaching in Dublin for years to come', complained about 'a particularly obnoxious campaign' that was alleging poor patients were being refused entry to voluntary hospitals, and he was only prepared to accept a bed bureau if it was administered by the voluntary hospitals and not the civil service.[157] Professor T. G. Moorhead also lamented the existence of a mistaken perception that 'voluntary hospitals are unwilling to admit free patients' and warned that 'it would be a direct breach of faith with those who have brought the sweepstakes into existence if the voluntary hospitals are not extended'.[158] That such trenchant opinions were expressed was a clear indication that there was genuine fear within the medical profession in Dublin that the future of the voluntary hospitals in the city was in jeopardy, in spite of the Hospitals Commission's clear preference for the voluntary over municipal option. The scaremongering of 1932, when fears were expressed that Fianna Fáil would nationalise the hospitals, appeared still to have some resonance.

In 1937, at the height of the wrangling over how the bed bureau would operate, Moore repeated his concerns for the future of Dublin's voluntary hospitals: 'If we are to have a state controlled medical system, there will inevitably be a departmental mentality which will retard progress at the expense of the suffering section of the community.'[159] His defence of the voluntary hospitals was supported by the editor of *The Irish Times* who also believed 'that a determined effort is being made behind the scenes to secure the establishment of a municipal hospital in the City of Dublin'. The strident opposition of the leading Dublin medics was reiterated at the charter dinner of the Royal College of Surgeons in Ireland in February 1938.[160]

The existence of this belief that a conspiracy was afoot to replace voluntary hospitals in Dublin with a municipal institution was turned to the advantage of the Department of Local Government and Public Health in its negotiations with the voluntaries over the constitution and jurisdiction of the bed bureau. The threat of the Hospitals Commission's recommendation being overturned in favour of the municipal option finally forced them to concede to the wishes of the department that it would have a greater measure of control over the bureau's activities. Not long after Seán T. O'Kelly announced finally that he would accept the recommendation of the Hospitals Commission to develop voluntary hospitals for Dublin city, final agreement on the format of the bureau was reached.[161] The remit of the Public Hospitals Act did not cover its establishment and operation, necessitating the introduction of specific new legislation.[162] The Public Hospitals (Amendment) Act, passed in May 1940, extended the powers of the Hospitals Commission, allowing it to:

> establish and maintain in relation to any two or more hospitals a bureau whereby the admission to some one of such hospitals of persons requiring hospital treatment will be facilitated and whereat information as to the accommodation available from time to time in such hospitals can be given to medical practitioners and other interested persons.[163]

The act also provided a complaints procedure for patients who felt they had been unfairly denied access to a hospital.[164]

MEDICAL RESEARCH

One aspect of the Hospitals Commission's inaugural report that came in for criticism was its lukewarm support for funding medical research.[165] The commissioners felt that the 'pressing needs of the hospitals must come first'. Prioritising hospital development led to the abandonment of a plan to establish a central institution dedicated to medical research, which was considered to be too costly. The funds accumulated in the Hospitals Trust Fund up to that point were simply inadequate to finance both hospital development and medical research and the former was clearly the priority of both the Hospitals Commission and the government.[166] The commission was only prepared to go as far as providing a £10,000 grant towards research, for one year initially.[167]

In 1925 Henry Moore had sought funds from the Rockefeller Foundation to build a medical research wing at UCD and establish a medical research council.[168] In 1932, two years after the establishment of the sweepstake, the Royal Academy of Medicine in Ireland (RAMI) first suggested the application of sweepstake funds towards medical research. Under the academy's proposed scheme, five per cent of the hospitals fund would be set aside to endow medical research until that sum reached £150,000. This sum would then be invested by the Minister for Local Government and Public Health and the interest used for research purposes, based on the advice of a medical research council, to be composed of nominees of the minister, the four principal universities, the Royal Colleges of Surgeons and Physicians and the Royal Academy of Medicine.[169] At a time when local authority hospitals and nurses were also arguing their case for a slice of the sweepstake funding, the Department of Justice was unwilling to entertain another competitor; the RAMI was informed curtly that, as there were no plans to so amend the legislation governing the sweepstake, there would be no point in the minister receiving a delegation from the academy to discuss their proposal.[170] When this refusal was queried by Eamon de Valera, Justice washed their hands of it further, arguing that it was a subject more suitable for the Department of Local Government and Public Health. It was also suggested that the RAMI could consider sponsoring a private bill of its own in the Dáil.[171] While nothing further appears to have been done, de Valera agreed to meet Henry Moore to discuss the subject.[172]

Following the Hospitals Commission's decision to make £10,000 available for medical research, the Medical Research Council of Ireland (MRCI) was established in January 1937, after negotiations with the minister, the commission, the Associated Hospital Sweepstake Committee, the RAMI, and the state's medical schools. The £10,000 was divided among fifteen full- and part-time researchers for the coming year. In 1938 the council was awarded an annual grant of £5,000 a year for the next five years.[173] This paltry sum was not adequate to allow it to fund significant new research. In 1939 it had hoped to be able to make three new grants but was unable to do so; instead, the limited funds available were reserved to ensure the continuation of existing projects.[174]

The limitation placed on the council by the small size of its grant, and the lack of any guarantee of continued funding, was extremely frustrating:

> £5,000 a year is not adequate for the efficient discharge of its functions. The stringency consequent on this limitation in funds, and the absence of any assurance that the endowment will be continued for a long period makes it impossible to plan for more than one year in advance.[175]

The Hospitals Commission explained that the restriction on the MRCI's grant was a result of the limited resources of the Hospitals Trust Fund and when greater progress was achieved in hospital development it would be possible to consider an endowment.[176] Throughout the war years the MRCI's annual grant remained at £5,000, augmented at times by small private grants, such as £300 given by Joseph McGrath on behalf of Hospitals Trust Ltd in 1944 'for expenses in connection with the distribution of penicillin, preparation of ointment, solution, etc.' and the provision of penicillin supplies by the American government.[177] The severe curtailment of income from the sweepstake during the war would ensure that the MRCI's hand-to-mouth existence would continue for some years. In spite of the paltry and precarious nature of its funding the MRCI undertook a number of important projects during the its early years. In 1940, for example, a project it funded discovered a new serum for treating diphtheria.[178] It also funded investigations into diseases of the blood, TB, liver and adrenal function, vitamin deficiency and diabetes as well as training in research methods.[179] By the mid-1950s a leading medical academic, Patrick Meenan, still considered the resources of the MRCI to be 'grossly inadequate'.[180]

HOSPITAL LIBRARIES

Another ancillary service that was made possible by the availability of sweepstake funds, but which suffered from the same lack of guarantees about its future as the Medical Research Council, was the hospital library service. The movement to provide libraries for hospital patients had been pioneered in the USA. During the nineteenth century 'collections of library materials for patients ... existed in US hospitals', but the campaign to have them widely available gained much ground between 1906 and 1914 under the leadership of Edith Jones, who considered bibliotherapy to be of particular benefit to psychiatric patients. The provision of a library service for hospitalised American servicemen during the First World War was particularly successful and proved to be 'a major catalyst for the development of patients' libraries in general hospitals, because it demonstrated that books and reading can contribute to recovery from physical as well as mental illness'. Similarly, in Great Britain the Red Cross established a library during the great war. After the war this became an ex-servicemen's hospital library and later was made available to civilians and known simply as the Hospital Library; by the end of the 1920s this service was supplying nearly 250,000 publications, including books, magazines and newspapers to more than 2,000 hospitals.[181]

The person largely responsible for the introduction of hospital libraries in Ireland was the Jesuit priest, Fr Stephen Brown. In September 1930, as a member of the newly established Library Association of Ireland, he attended the annual conference of the British Library Association in Cambridge, where he was influenced by one particular discussion on hospital libraries.[182] At the LAI's annual conference in June 1933 he 'urged the necessity of extending library service so as to provide not only for the man in health but also in the event of illness necessitating his confinement in hospital', and referring to the development of patients' libraries abroad, stated that 'Properly administered libraries ... have come to be regarded as an indispensable part of the equipment of a modern hospital'. The meeting passed resolutions urging hospital authorities to recognise the importance of such libraries and the need for them to be administered by professional librarians, and called upon public libraries to assist such libraries in their communities. A committee of the association was established to put forward the case for the introduction of a proper hospital library system in the state.[183]

At the same time as this conference was being held, the Public Hospitals Bill was completing its legislative journey through the Senate. Lobbying by Fr Brown resulted in Oliver St John Gogarty moving a successful amendment providing for a grant to be made from the Hospitals Trust Fund 'to establish a lending library for supplying books for the use of patients or inmates in hospitals'. The Minister for Local Government and Public Health reserved the power to 'specify the purposes for which such library grant is to be expended' and to withdraw the grant if its use was not in accordance with conditions laid down by him. There was no reference in the act to the amount of the hospital library grant or to the proportion of the Hospitals Trust Fund that would be set aside for it.[184]

Soon after the enactment of the Public Hospitals Act, the Library Association of Ireland set to work drawing up a scheme for the operation of hospital libraries. Their proposal submitted to the Minister for Local Government and Public Health in January 1934 estimated that a capital sum of £5,000 would be required to establish the service and run it for the first year. The subsequent administration would necessitate the investment of a sum that would produce an annual income of £2,000. Premises to function as a central depot would also have to be acquired. This depot would house a 'Permanent stock of serious books to be lent under certain guarantees', and a floating stock from which individual hospital libraries would build up their own collections gradually. In addition to the central depot, each hospital would have its own library, which in the case of larger hospitals would require the services of a professional librarian. It was made clear that the depot would not interfere with the arrangements operating within the hospitals themselves.[185] Initially the Library Association of Ireland had been concerned that their proposal might be interpreted by hospitals as unwarranted external interference.[186]

The scope of the scheme alarmed the Hospitals Commission which believed that it 'involved a larger sum of money than the commissioners felt disposed to recommend'. Instead the commission suggested that £10,000 be set aside to finance the scheme for a three-year trial period, after which it could be re-examined.[187] Although the Library Association was prepared to accept this modified scheme the Hospitals Commission was still anxious about the service's continued dependence on the Hospitals Trust Fund, expressing a preference that its existence not be contingent on future grants from the fund.[188] In spite of their reservations, the commissioners recommended the modified plan to the minister and a committee was established to garner public interest and support for the venture, encourage the participation of the hospitals, acquire premises, appoint staff for the central depot, and acquire books.[189]

As a result of the limited finance not all hospitals were able to participate; initially the service was restricted to hospitals classified as voluntary or semi-voluntary. The Hospital Library Council, under the chairmanship of Fr Brown, came into operation in 1937; the first book issued under the new service was *Péig*, the eponymous reminiscences of Blasket Island resident, Péig Sayers.[190]

In February 1940 a deputation from the Hospital Library Council met officials from the Department of Local Government and Public Health to discuss the financial prospects of the library service. £2,400 of the original grant of £10,000 remained, with another £2,000 still to be drawn down from the Hospitals Trust Fund. This was deemed sufficient to continue the service until the end of 1940 and to begin to extend it to rate-aided hospitals. In order successfully to continue to provide a sustained service the council asked for a guaranteed annual income of £2,500 up to the end of 1946, which would allow it to supply books to all hospitals.[191] This was refused by the minister who pointed out that 'in present conditions and having regard to the extent of the commitments of the Hospitals Trust Fund it is not possible to approve of any extension of the activities of the Council to hospitals and institutions that cannot be registered under the existing scheme'.[192] The grand plans of the Hospital Library Council to have a library in every hospital in the state – voluntary and rate-aided – by the end of 1946 had to be put on hold until after the war at least.

A modified request for a grant of £4,300 to cover the years 1941 and 1942 was also turned down; in its stead £2,150 was offered to cover 1941 alone.[193] Henceforth the Hospital Library Council would have to make an annual application for its grant. The government's refusal to guarantee the future of the service for more than a year at a time provoked fears for its future. A meeting of hospital representatives in June 1941 passed a unanimous resolution urging 'upon the Minister for Local Government and Public Health the need for an assurance that the Library Service for patients in hospitals will be continued and further developed in its present form during the minimum period of five years, 1942–1946'.[194]

The precarious funding basis of the service militated against the Hospital Library Council's plans to extend its remit beyond the voluntary sector. In 1938 the council regretted having to turn down requests from public and psychiatric hospitals to participate.[195] Similar requests were also rejected in 1942.[196] Eventually in 1945 the council succeeded in convincing the department to allow TB patients in non-voluntary hospitals to benefit from the scheme.[197] Fears that the service might be ended abruptly at any point during the war proved unfounded and a grant of just over £2,000 was given to it each year until the end of the Emergency. Nevertheless, the council was unhappy with its lack of a guaranteed future, the effort expended each year in re-applying for its grant, and the lack of funds to extend the service beyond the voluntary hospital sector.

In spite of the financial constraints under which it laboured for most of its first decade, the Hospital Library Council succeeded in establishing a satisfactory library service, albeit limited largely to voluntary hospitals. Its success can be judged by the number of hospitals that registered to join and by the number of volumes supplied. Thirty-eight hospitals participated in 1937, rising to seventy-eight by 1942, while the stock rose from 7,060 to 38,270 books in the same period. This latter figure had increased to 47,171 by 1945.[198] The decision of the Adelaide to join the service in 1943 is particularly noteworthy, in light of its opposition to the sweepstake. The response from hospitals was very favourable. The council found 'All hospitals are enthusiastic in their appreciation of the Service'.[199] In spite of space restrictions most hospitals tried to provide good accommodation for their libraries.[200] Hospitals with long-stay patients, such as TB hospitals where patients were often able-bodied and quite bored, and children's hospitals which also had to provide educational services, were especially praise-worthy of the new service. A patient who had spent six years at the children's orthopaedic hospital in Cappagh arrived 'barely able to read' but by the time she left was familiar with the works of 'Pearse, Benson, Kickham, Sheehan, Chesterton, Belloc and Francis Thompson'.[201]

Plans by the new Department of Health to reorganise the Hospital Library Council during the late 1940s never came to fruition and the service continued until 1977, by which time it was deemed to be 'totally inadequate and sub-standard'. The Public Hospitals (Amendment) Act 1976 provided grants from the Hospitals Trust Fund to 'any person controlling or about to establish a lending library for supplying books for the use of patients or inmates in hospitals'. By then the Hospital Library Council transferred its remaining stock to the voluntary hospitals, which assumed the responsibility for supplying their own books.[202]

FOUR

THE SWEEPSTAKE IN GREAT BRITAIN IN THE 1930s

—

GAMBLING, LOTTERIES AND SWEEPSTAKES IN BRITAIN IN THE 1920s

In 1918 the House of Lords sought to end the almost century-long prohibition on lotteries in Great Britain when it passed the Lotteries (War Charities) Bill to allow registered war charities to raise funds by means of public lotteries. However, the measure was rejected in the House of Commons by 81 votes to 77, and lotteries remained illegal.[1] Private lotteries, such as the Stock Exchange's annual Derby sweepstake, were exempted from the ban because they were 'confined to members of societies and clubs and not advertised as open to the public'.[2]

Hospitals in Britain suffered financially in the 1920s and the Home Secretary received a number of entreaties to consider amending the law to allow hospitals to raise funds through lotteries. However, the Conservative Home Secretary, Sir William Joynson-Hicks, refused to budge on the issue, stating in 1924 'I do not see my way to initiate any legislation on the subject, and I doubt if any legislation is required in the public interest'. This remained government policy until the end of the decade and resulted in police action to prevent hospitals holding tombolas and the suppression of a sweepstake organised by Barking Hospital.[3]

The growing pressure on the Home Secretary to consider changing the lottery laws resulted from the realisation that they were no longer suitable for regulating gambling in the changed nature of post-war British society. The 1920s witnessed a huge increase in the popularity of gambling in Britain, due in part to the increase in wages, overtime and leisure hours, and evidenced by the popularity of the football pools, introduced in 1922, and greyhound racing with electric hares, which was started in 1926[4]; the number of greyhound-racing tracks which provided facilities for betting had increased from one in 1926 to 226 in 1932, and the totaliser had been introduced there 'without security against fraud or dishonesty'.[5] The introduction of greyhound racing, a phenomenon of the mid-1920s, was claimed by some to 'have been introduced primarily to exploit the gambling-spirit'.[6] The opening of tote clubs which provided for cash betting in many large towns and the continued problem of illegal street betting compounded the difficulties generated by the increased popularity of gambling.[7]

The realisation that supposedly private sweepstakes, such as those organised by the Stock Exchange and the Calcutta Turf Club on the Epsom Derby, had effectively become public lotteries was a further factor in the argument that it was time for a revision of the lottery law. In 1929 the Attorney General advised the Home Secretary that the time had come to take action against such sweepstakes: 'I should regard the Stock Exchange and Calcutta Sweeps, and similar sweeps, as being public lotteries, and I should consider that we ought not to allow them to continue.'[8] This threat resulted in the Stock Exchange taking pre-emptive action to save its sweepstake; the regulations for its 1930 Derby sweepstake were altered by limiting the prize fund to £100, increasing the price of tickets to £25, and marking tickets as 'not transferable'. The Home Secretary was satisfied that if these new regulations were adhered to the sweepstake could continue.[9] The blurring of the distinction between public and private lotteries, and the lack of uniformity in administering the law throughout Great Britain, led the Home Office to conclude that government policy on lotteries was no longer workable.[10]

The increased popularity of gambling in Britain in the 1920s also resulted in an increased fear of its detrimental effects on society, which may have been the principal reason for the government's continued reluctance to contemplate a change in the lottery law, in spite of the growing evidence of such a need.[11] In July 1930, Labour's Home Secretary, J. R. Clynes, was still adhering to the policy of his predecessor, believing that there was no need to appoint a committee to examine the lottery laws.[12] 1930 was also the year in which the Irish hospitals sweepstake was introduced, and this eventually forced the hand of the British government to amend the century-old lottery laws.

THE SWEEPSTAKE IN BRITAIN

The problem of Irish sweepstake tickets circulating illegally in Great Britain became a very serious one for the British authorities in 1930, when the legalisation of the Irish sweepstake introduced such gambling on a grand scale. In the run-up to the inaugural sweepstake, the *Daily Express* reported that 'A flood of tickets for the sweep have reached England and Scotland, and can be bought almost anywhere', and quoted Joseph McGrath as saying that 95 per cent of applications for tickets were from England.[13] Almost 57 per cent of prizewinners in this sweepstake were British (Table 4.1). An analysis of the country of residence of sweepstake winners during the 1930s shows that almost two thirds, and more that three quarters in the case of the 1932 Derby sweep, of prizes in each draw were won by British residents. Given the random nature of the draw, these figures probably correspond quite closely to the proportion of tickets sold there. Therefore, the success of the sweepstake in its early years clearly depended on its market in Great Britain.

Undoubtedly, the popularity of the sweepstake in Britain owed much to the large number of people of Irish descent living there. In 1931 the Irish-born population of England and Wales was 381,081, accounting for 1.4 per cent of the total population, while in Scotland 124,296 Irish-born citizens made up 2.6 per cent of that country's population. These figures grew during the 1930s as the numbers of Irish emigrating to Britain increased, partly due to a corresponding decline in emigration to the USA, where the depression curtailed employment opportunities. 13,200 Irish people emigrated to Great Britain in 1932, a considerable increase on the previous year's figure of 9,800. This jumped further to 16,400 in 1934, 22,100 in 1935, and 32,300 in 1936.[14]

It was not difficult to buy an Irish sweepstake ticket in Britain in the early 1930s. According to the Metropolitan Police they could be obtained easily in Mooney's Irish Bar on The Strand, the Oxford Street branch of Lloyds Bank, which acted as an agent for Irish banks, Ladbrokes and other well-known bookmakers, the Forum Picture House on New Street, and a number of other businesses located throughout London. The Catering Branch of the Transport and General Workers' Union acted as an agency for distributing tickets in the 1930 Manchester November Handicap sweepstake.[15] The Newspaper Club, which had been established by the editors of the *Daily Express* and *Morning Post*, was reportedly an agent also.[16]

Ease of travel and organisational links between both countries made the transfer of tickets relatively easy and detection by the British postal authorities correspondingly difficult.[17] It was very easy for travellers between Ireland and Britain to conceal sweepstake tickets in their luggage.[18] When customs officials at Holyhead began to search the luggage of travellers between Ireland and Britain for surreptitious tickets it produced an outcry in the House of Commons; the Conservative MP, Colonel Charles Howard-Bury, who had a residence in Ireland, complained indignantly that 'the luggage of passengers arriving from the Irish Free State, including their private papers, is being ransacked in search of sweepstake tickets, their cheque books are opened and examined ',[19] while Sir William Davison demanded the prompt return of 'the old green flag of the 2nd Battalion Connaught Rangers [seized] on its way from Ireland to the Old Comrades' Association regimental dinner in London, on the grounds that Irish sweepstake tickets were enclosed with the regimental colours'.[20] The 1933 Cambridgeshire sweepstake proved so popular that the London, Midland and Scottish Railway Company scheduled an extra boat for Dublin, on the eve of the draw, carrying 1,800 people, many of them returning counterfoils and subscriptions to the sweepstake organisers in Dublin.[21]

Many potential subscribers considered the Irish High Commission in London an obvious source of information about how to obtain tickets. In addition to verbal and written queries from people wishing to buy tickets, which were re-directed to the Hospitals Trust offices in Dublin, the High Commission also received substantial amounts of money in subscriptions from Manchester and Liverpool.[22] Even the High Commissioner himself, J. W. Dulanty, forwarded a sweepstake remittance for a friend through the Department of External Affairs.[23] The staff of the High Commission was unsure of its role as a sweepstake intermediary; the sale of tickets in Britain was illegal, but the sweepstake had been established by an act of the Oireachtas (Irish Parliament), and they were unsure of the extent to which they should assist its activities.[24] Their dilemma was not helped by a suggestion made in the *Sunday Express* by Lord Castlerosse that the office of the High Commission be used to transmit private correspondence to the Irish Free State, resulting in a number of people requesting that counterfoils be returned to Ireland through the commission's office. T. J. Kiernan, secretary of the commission, suggested writing to the British press to inform them that the office could not be used for such transmission.[25]

The British government sought in vain to use the powers of the Post Office to curb the flow of sweepstake correspondence between Britain and Ireland. The principal tool in the post office's anti-lottery armoury was a warrant issued by the Home Secretary in 1920 authorising the Postmaster General 'To detain and open any postal packets observed in course of transmission by post believed to contain advertisements or circulars relating to lotteries promoted in the United Kingdom or abroad'.[26] In November 1930, the Assistant Postmaster General, S. P. Viant, told the House of Commons that 9,031 letters had been opened by the Post Office and £6,960 returned to would-be subscribers to the 1930 Manchester November Handicap sweepstake.[27] In order to evade detection by the postal authorities, Hospitals Trust advised its customers in Britain not to correspond directly with it but to send their subscriptions through a bank, business house, participating hospital or acquaintance resident in the Irish Free State.[28]

The number of British subscribers and prizewinners in the Irish sweepstake during the early 1930s was evidence of the inability of the Post Office to prevent citizens of Great Britain contributing to it. The following table shows the proportion of sweepstake prizes won by residents in Great Britain between 1930 and 1934:

Table 4.1: Percentage of Irish hospitals sweepstake prizes won by British residents, 1930–4

Sweepstake	Percentage of prizes won by British residents
1930 Manchester November Handicap	56.96
1931 Grand National	65.69
1931 Manchester November Handicap	65.89
1932 Grand National	65.20
1932 Derby	76.09
1932 Cesarewitch	69.05
1933 Grand National	61.99
1933 Derby	68.88
1933 Cambridgeshire	56.00
1934 Grand National	61.25
1934 Derby	57.51
1934 Cambridgeshire	44.90

Source: calculated from lists of names and addresses of the prizewinners printed in the Irish daily newspapers after each sweepstake draw.

Thus an average of almost two-thirds of sweepstake prizes was won by British residents in the first half of the 1930s.

The Irish sweepstake appears to have taken over the British market for illegal lotteries in the 1930s, to the detriment of established rivals. By 1932 the Calcutta Turf Club's Derby sweepstake was reported to have 'sunk to very small proportions' because of the competition from the Irish sweepstake, which had also killed off smaller lotteries from continental European countries.[29] The Deputy Commissioner of the London Metropolitan Police concurred that the popularity of the sweepstake reduced 'the activities of the fraudulent sweepstake promoter'.[30]

The national government's Liberal Home Secretary, Sir Herbert Samuel, told the Commons that an estimated £3,785,000 had been contributed by British people to the 1932 Derby sweepstake; and the following year approximately £2.5 million was subscribed to the 1933 Derby sweepstake. The total subscribed to the nine sweepstakes held until then was estimated at £21.2 million.[31] The attitude of the sweepstake promoters was that most of this money eventually made its way back into Britain in the form of prize money and also to purchase equipment for the building and refurbishment of the Irish hospitals, and through more indirect channels:

money originating from salaries and sweep expenses, which is spent on British merchandise, British-provided entertainment, and British holidays.

In addition, a large percentage of foreign and Empire-won prizes is spent by the winners on British merchandise and left in British banks.[32]

The British government was unconvinced by such logic, claiming that the amount won in prize money was only about two-thirds of that subscribed.[33] A comparison between the estimated value of British contributions to the sweepstake with the known value of exports from the Irish Free State to Great Britain indicates the value of sweepstake contributions as an invisible export to the Free State's economy:

Table 4.2: The value of exports to Great Britain from the Irish Free State (Éire), and the estimated value of British sweepstake contributions, 1931–9

Year	Exports to GB (incl. re-exports) (£)	Est. value of sweepstake Contributions (£)
July–Dec 1931	17,373,782	1,963,423
1932	22,846,918	7,941,470
1933	15,844,552	5,546,703
1934	15,000,540	4,920,169
1935	16,242,961	2,700,494
1936	16,443,731	2,586,606
1937	18,587,461	2,423,328
1938	19,911,623	1,847,336
Jan–June 1939	9,350,220	1,007,321

Source for value of exports: Deirdre McMahon, *Republicans and imperialists: Anglo-Irish relations in the 1930s* (London and New Haven, 1984), Appendix ii (b).

The amount of money leaving Britain at a time of economic depression was becoming a source of concern and annoyance to the British government. This was exacerbated by the refusal of the Fianna Fáil government to repay land annuities after 1932, and the imposition of 25 per cent stamp duty on the hospitals' share of sweepstake proceeds in 1933. William Peters, the UK Trade Commissioner in Dublin, and the only official representative there in the absence of diplomatic presence, felt that:

There is something almost comical in the situation. The Irish Free State Government is withholding a sum of £5,000,000 per annum from the United

Kingdom, the United Kingdom government has had to pay the £5,000,000 and is trying to get it back in one way or another from the Irish Free State; the citizens of the United Kingdom are, in the meantime, sending fresh millions to the Irish Free State, a percentage of which goes to the Irish Free State Government.[34]

The prospect of a Fianna Fáil victory in the 1932 general election had occasioned alarm throughout Whitehall and when the government implemented its election pledge to withhold the annuities the 'feelings of collective outrage which swept through the Treasury ranks were matched only by a grim determination to resist de Valera to the bitter end'. Relations between the new Irish government and the national government in Britain were especially poor, particularly in regard to Prime Minister Ramsay MacDonald and the minister with responsibility for Anglo-Irish relations, Home Secretary J. H. Thomas. The British reaction to the success of the Irish sweepstake is more easily understood when seen in this context of strained Anglo-Irish relations in the early 1930s.[35]

The extent to which British money was funding Irish hospitals did not go unnoticed by cash-strapped hospitals in Britain. Sir Gordon Campbell, the chairman of St Bartholomew's Hospital in London, wanted to organise his own sweepstake, which he saw as the best means of stopping money leaving Britain.[36] In view of the large proportion of sweepstake contributions emanating from Britain, it was suggested that the promoters should give a proportion of the proceeds to British hospitals.[37] Some needy hospitals appealed directly to the Irish government for assistance.[38] London's Royal Eye Hospital based its request for £30,000 to rebuild the hospital on the service it provided to the Irish population of London: 'This Hospital serves that part of London in which the majority of Irish people reside and nearly 25% of our patients attending here are Irish or of Irish descent.'[39] All such requests were met with the simple rebuff that the legislation establishing the sweepstake permitted the funds raised to be used only for hospitals in the Irish Free State.[40]

Not all British hospitals shared this envy of the sweepstake and many were anxious lest the Irish example be adopted in Britain. Philip Inman, House Governor of the Charing Cross Hospital, was concerned that the introduction of a hospitals sweepstake in Britain would lead to a loss of idealism.[41] Lord Londonderry, who was to emerge as one of the strongest parliamentary opponents of the sweepstake, feared that the introduction of such a system would 'dry up' the 'charitable fountain'.[42]

Protestant religious leaders joined both the government and the British hospitals in their opposition to the activities of the Irish sweepstake in Britain. The large windfalls accruing from the sweepstake were anathema to Protestant ideals of earning money as a reward for work. The use of the ill-gotten proceeds of gambling for such charitable purposes as building and equipping hospitals was also strongly opposed. Rev. J. Hutchinson-Cockburn of Dunblane Cathedral in Scotland saw the sweepstakes as 'a symptom of our times; they have given enlarged opportunity for the vice of gambling, which flourishes all the more because times are hard and money scarce and men and women are hopeful even to folly', and complained that sweepstake promoters were 'destroying the voluntary generosity of the nation, and degrading the world with an orgy of gambling'.[43]

The British press began to reflect this growing concern at the popularity of the sweepstake. In 1932 Lord Rothermere's *Daily Mail* began a crusade against it. When the sweepstake began in 1930 the *Mail* had published some unfavourable stories, focusing in particular on the amount of money paid as commission to sellers and the inclusion of free tickets, issued as a reward to sellers, in the draw.[44] In August 1932 the Irish Free State government reacted strongly to the *Mail's* allegations that it was preparing to raid the sweepstake funds for other purposes and to force winners to accept prizes in kind, denying any such intentions.[45]

Spencer Freeman felt that the campaign was not reflective of English public opinion generally to the sweepstake, but merely 'a press stunt in a dead news-period' and an effort by the newspaper to attack the newly elected Fianna Fáil government.[46] Hospitals Trust complained to the government that the delay in releasing the surplus from the 1931 Manchester November Handicap sweepstake to the hospitals appeared to lend credence to the *Mail's* allegations.[47] Count O'Kelly de Gallagh, the Irish Free State Minister Plenipotentiary to France, sought to counter the effect of anti-sweepstake articles published in the continental edition of the *Mail* by rebutting the allegations in an interview with *Paris-Soir*.[48]

Hospitals Trust's counter-offensive against the *Mail* began in September. The company's auditors informed the *Mail* that figures for ticket sales for the 1932 Cesarewitch did not show a decline, as the newspaper had alleged. Joseph McGrath invited the *Mail* to appoint their own auditors to examine the accounts to satisfy themselves of the truth, and promised to pay £10,000 to any British hospital of the newspaper's choice should Hospitals Trust's figures prove to be inaccurate.[49] The challenge does not appear to have been taken up by the *Mail*.

The flood of sweepstake tickets into Britain from 1930 onwards, and the flow of substantial amounts of money in the opposite direction, forced the British government to consider the adoption of new measures to curtail the influx of foreign lottery tickets. In December 1930 Home Secretary Clynes reported to his cabinet colleagues that 'A situation of considerable difficulty is developing in connection with sweepstakes'. Immediate measures were required to prevent the 1931 Grand National sweepstake achieving the same success in Britain that the 1930 Manchester November Handicap sweepstake had. The notion of completely suppressing the sweepstake was impossible, but he believed that 'a great deal can be accomplished by such measures as the stoppage of literature and books of tickets at the Customs and in the post and by the prosecution of the principal distributors of tickets'. He also felt that the Irish Free State government should be requested to discourage the promoters from selling tickets in Britain[50], but the Dominions Office was wary of such an approach: 'The idea that the Government of one country is to take steps to prevent the people of another country committing crimes in that other country would lead to all sorts of absurdities.'[51] Besides, it was considered unlikely that the Free State government would impose any conditions on the sale of tickets.[52] The sweepstake's onslaught on the British market had finally brought the Home Secretary around to the realisation of the need to review and possibly change British lottery law.[53]

In 1931 the Home Office took steps to curtail the use of commercial banks as ticket agents. On receipt of a warning of possible legal action being taken against it by the Director of Public Prosecutions, Lloyds Bank, which had provided application forms for the Calcutta sweep, ceased such activity and also instructed its branches to refer customers seeking Irish sweepstake tickets to Irish banks. By the end of 1931 it was reported that Lloyds, along with the Bank of India, Central Bank of India, Mercantile Bank of India, Grindlay & Company and Cox & Kings had ceased conducting sweepstake transactions.

Under Bank of England rules bank employees were not permitted to take part in any business relating to betting or sweepstakes. As an agent for the Bank of Ireland in Britain, Lloyds was unable to say what use money remitted to Ireland for customers was put to, but guaranteed that no money was sent directly to Hospitals Trust. Staff in other banks – such as Barclays and the Yorkshire Penny Bank – were threatened with disciplinary action if they undertook sweepstake transactions. Clearly, the banks were anxious to avoid prosecution for breaches of the lottery acts. By 1934 the role of banks as sweepstake agents had been greatly reduced: 'It is not likely that many persons in Great Britain obtain or try to obtain their supplies of tickets in Irish sweepstakes through banks in this country.'[54]

Efforts by the government and police to curtail the activities of the sweepstake were hampered by the apparent failure of the judiciary to impose punitive punishments on those convicted of selling tickets.[55] The Deputy Commissioner of the London Metropolitan Police complained that the trivial fines imposed 'indicates the feeling of courts that such proceedings have no practical result beyond the formal vindication of the law'.[56] Minimal fines were also imposed by the Scottish courts.[57] The cases of prosecutions reported in the press illustrate such judicial reluctance to deal harshly with ticket sellers. In the first such prosecution in 1931, John Windsor Stevenson, a Birmingham cinema manager, was fined £5 plus costs for selling Grand National sweepstake tickets. In May of the same year, John More, Harold Crossley, L. P. Joyce and L. Freedman, were each fined 20 shillings, plus costs ranging from £5 to £15.[58] Frederick Andrew Woodhall, a ship's radio operator, was tried in January 1933 on a charge of trying to smuggle 12,900 sweepstake tickets into Liverpool, for subsequent distribution within England and onto Holland, Canada and the USA; the first jury in his case was discharged having failed to agree a verdict but he was convicted by a second jury and fined £25 and five guineas in costs.[59]

Legislative restrictions also prevented the government from taking action against purchasers of tickets; they could not be prosecuted merely for buying tickets and income tax legislation did not cover prizes won in sweepstakes.[60] The difficulty in obtaining convictions, and the relatively small fines imposed in cases where convictions were secured, was further evidence of the inadequacy of contemporary British lottery legislation to deal with the new situation created by the introduction of the Irish sweepstake.

In February 1932, the Home Secretary presented a memorandum to his cabinet colleagues outlining the options available to the government for dealing with the new circumstances, which had arisen regarding lotteries since the establishment of the sweepstake. The simple option of admitting defeat and legislating to legalise lotteries was deemed to be too controversial and likely to lead to considerable opposition and, if adopted, to an undesirable increase in gambling. The reluctance of the judiciary to convict ruled out leaving the current system in place untouched, and made it difficult to introduce a policy of more vigorous prosecution of lottery cases. Approaching the problem from a financial rather than a judicial angle, such as confiscating prizes, or appealing to the patriotism of the British public by encouraging them not to send large sums out of the country, was not suitable either. The final suggestion was to hold an enquiry, in the form of a Royal Commission, into the issue.[61]

THE ROYAL COMMISSION AND THE BETTING AND LOTTERIES ACT

In April 1932 Samuel announced the establishment of a twelve member Royal Commission on Lotteries and Betting, chaired by an eminent judge, Sir Sidney Rowlatt, charged with the task of inquiring 'into the existing law, and the practice thereunder, relating to lotteries, betting, gambling and cognate matters, and report what changes, if any, are desirable and practicable'.[62]

While the Irish sweepstake was an important factor in highlighting the inadequacy of existing British lottery legislation, other developments in betting and gambling in the 1920s contributed to the need for this review, including the use of the totaliser at greyhound-racing tracks, the proliferation of street betting, and the introduction of betting on motor cycle races.[63]

The Royal Commission which sat for just over a year, from April 1932 to June 1933, heard evidence from many of those associated with the betting industry as well as senior civil servants from the Home Office and the police. Sir Ernley Blackwell of the Home Office gave evidence on the substantial sums of money leaving Britain for the Irish sweepstake and the Deputy Commissioner of the Metropolitan Police informed the commission of the difficulty enforcing the law, especially in view of the difference between small private charitable lotteries and enormous public lotteries on the lines of the Irish sweepstake: 'He considers it would be better to authorize lotteries, under proper control within certain limits as to the amount, and for approved objects rather than to continue in a position that has become almost farcical.'[64]

The commission's final report, issued in June 1933, came down heavily against legalising lotteries, domestic or foreign. Recognising that the effectiveness of the existing lottery provisions had been negated by the success of the Irish sweepstake, it considered, but eventually rejected, three options for legalising lotteries in Britain. The commission's members were completely opposed to a state lottery, but felt that the establishment of a statutory board to promote charitable lotteries was 'even less desirable than a state lottery', and they were also against the suggestion of authorising individual charities to run lotteries on their own behalf. Without the situation created by the Irish sweepstake, there would have been no need even to consider such options for legalising lotteries in Britain.[65]

If domestic lotteries were not to be permitted, the ban on foreign ones must also remain, but would have to be made much more effective. The money drain to foreign lotteries was cited as a reason for their continued prohibition. The ineffectiveness of the existing restrictions on foreign lotteries fostered contempt for the law and led to many of the 'evils' associated with unregulated lotteries, especially fraud, of which there was evidence in connection with the sale of Irish sweepstake tickets in Britain.[66]

As the existing situation was no longer sustainable, the members of the Royal Commission considered there to be two alternative courses available to the government; the establishment of large public lotteries to compete with and combat the popularity of the Irish sweepstake, or the introduction of more stringent measures to prevent the sale of lottery tickets in Britain. The first option was never seriously considered. The commission did not believe that there was any 'justification for assuming that there is a sustained or insistent demand in this country for this type of gambling facility', and those who were demanding that lotteries be legalised did not fully appreciate 'the difficulties and disadvantages involved'. Even if lotteries were legalised, the commission did not feel that they would have the desired effect of stopping 'the sale in this country of Irish sweepstake tickets'. Therefore, the commission's overall recommendation was 'that the law against foreign and illegal lotteries should be re-enacted and strengthened', although certain exemptions for small lotteries could be considered.[67]

The government, burdened by a heavy agenda of public business, was unable to give an undertaking 'to introduce legislation in the near future to deal with any part of the wide field covered by the Commission's recommendation', but was anxious to avoid a public perception that the report had been pigeon-holed. Therefore, a representative committee of cabinet was established to examine the report and submit legislative recommendations.[68] The committee reported early in 1934, and recommended that:

> In view of the somewhat limited amount of parliamentary time available and of the contentious nature of the questions at issue, the legislation to be introduced on the subject should deal only with the more urgent aspects of the various questions dealt with in the Report of the Royal Commission.

The cabinet agreed and the Home Secretary, Sir John Gilmour, set about drafting an appropriate bill.[69]

The ensuing Betting and Lotteries Bill was first introduced in the House of Lords at the end of March 1934,[70] where its principal proponent was the former Northern Ireland Education Minister, the Marquess of Londonderry, a hospital governor who was strongly opposed to the idea of funding hospitals with lottery proceeds: 'I am quite convinced that the adoption of the system of public lotteries for the support of our hospitals would be disastrous.'[71]

Explaining the need for new lottery legislation, Sir John Gilmour highlighted the introduction of the Irish sweepstake, the increased popularity of greyhound racing and its attendant betting, and the 'mushroom growth of tote clubs in London and in the other large towns'. The government's principal concern was the effect of gambling on the social life of the country, and as such the bill differentiated between the 'organised provision of betting facilities usually for private gain' and 'private betting between individuals', having no intention to interfere with the latter.[72]

The role of the Irish sweepstake in necessitating the need for new lottery legislation in Britain was highlighted by many of the MPs who spoke on the bill, and some, like Captain F. F. A. Heilgers, were particularly scathing about what they saw as the Irish Free State's exploitation of Britain:

I not only hate the idea of the Irish sweepstake but I hate sending so much money to de Valera by which he is able to make up his balance in trade by the invisible exports we are sending him as a result of the Sweep. But I hate still more the fact, I regard it indeed as an insult, that these sweepstakes are based on the results of races in this country instead of on Irish races, and the fact that there are these great sweepstakes on our races is an inherent danger to racing in this country . . . [73]

Sir William Davison failed to have an amendment adopted which would have allowed for the conducting of a national lottery.[74]

The Betting and Lotteries Act (1934) was composed of two parts, the first dealing with betting and the second with lotteries. The former introduced stricter regulations for on-course betting, particularly in regards to greyhound racing. Under its provisions the totaliser was legalised for greyhound tracks, but strict limits were placed on its use. The number of racecourses for horses and greyhounds, and the number of days racing permitted annually, were also regulated.[75]

The second part of the act, concerning lotteries, raffles and prize draws, modernised the law by repealing the outright ban on all such competitions to permit the holding of small lotteries and raffles, where there were no cash prizes or prizes greater than £10 in value. The principal aim of this section was to clamp down on large public lotteries, in particular the Irish sweepstake. The act aimed to curtail lotteries by limiting their publicity and targeting ticket sellers rather than purchasers. Publication of any other material deemed likely to act as an inducement to participate in a lottery was outlawed. Importing tickets, advertisements and other lottery literature into Britain also became an offence, as did sending money or counterfoils out of the country.[76]

The publication of lists of prizewinners, which in the case of the Irish sweepstake prior to 1934 often occupied three or four pages of a broadsheet newspaper, was prohibited. The government saw this as providing free publicity for the sweepstake and encouraging more people to buy tickets. The Royal Commission on Lotteries and Betting had referred to the detrimental impact of publishing results and recommended that the law be changed to make it illegal. Some newspapers in Britain supported the plan. Harry Pirie Gordon, of *The Times*' foreign department told Home Office officials that he felt the money spent on publishing such lists by his paper was a waste because it did not result in any material advantage by way of increased sales or advertising.[77] However, when the new restrictions were put in place the method of their enforcement was the cause of some press criticism. *The Morning Post* complained that the onus was upon the newsvendors to ensure that references to lotteries in foreign newspapers were obliterated, while the Romeike & Curtis press-cutting agency was informed that it would be liable to prosecution if it distributed items relating to sweepstakes.[78] The Provincial Wholesale Newsagents' Association also complained of the 'very arduous task' imposed upon newspaper wholesalers to ensure there were no references to lotteries and sweepstakes in the publications which they distributed.[79]

While newspapers were the principal target of the Betting and Lotteries Act, efforts were also made to censor references in film which could be deemed as encouraging the sale of sweepstake tickets. A scene depicting the Irish sweepstake draw, was cut from MGM's *The Winning Ticket*, 'a not unamusing comedy concerning the vicissitudes of a winning ticket in the Irish Sweep', by the British Board of Film Censors prior to the film's release in Britain in 1935. The BBFC also persuaded film agents not to book the silent documentary *Dublin of the Welcomes*, made on behalf of Hospitals Trust, essentially a publicity film for the sweepstake, as it contravened the Betting and Lotteries Act.[80]

THE SWEEPSTAKE IN BRITAIN AFTER 1934

Reports from various sources in early 1935 indicated that the Betting and Lotteries Act was having the desired effect of reducing the sale of sweepstake tickets in Britain. According to the *Daily Mail*, 'the restrictions imposed by the Betting and Lotteries Act have had a salutary effect on the Irish sweepstake'.[81] The United Kingdom's Trade Commissioner in Dublin agreed 'that the proportion of money subscribed by United Kingdom residents has considerably decreased'. He estimated that British contributions to the 1935 Grand National sweepstake did not account for much more than 40 per cent of the total.[82] The decline was also noticed by the Irish High Commissioner in London, J. W. Dulanty, who 'expressed the opinion . . . that the number of tickets sold in this country [Britain] had dwindled to a tremendous extent since the Betting and Lotteries legislation was passed'.[83]

This trend is confirmed by an examination of the destination of prizes in the various sweepstakes held after the introduction of the Betting and Lotteries Act. A decline was already perceptible in the last sweepstake prior to its introduction, in which 44.9 per cent of prizes went to British residents, the lowest proportion in any of the sweepstakes held until that date (Table 4.1). Following the introduction of the Betting and Lotteries Act, the sweepstake announcers refused to give the precise address of British prizewinners, using the euphemism 'Europe' instead. 'Europe' accounted for only 41.58 per cent of prizewinners in the 1935 Grand National sweepstake, and in the remaining sweepstakes held until the end of 1939 that figure fluctuated between approximately one-quarter and one-third of the total prizes won (Table 4.3).

This represented a significant decline on figures for the first four years of the sweepstake, when approximately two-thirds of prizes went to Britain.

Table 4.3: Percentage of Irish hospitals sweepstake prizes won by residents of 'Europe' [i.e. Britain], 1935–9

Sweepstake	Percentage of prizes won by residents of 'Europe'
1935 Grand National	41.58
1935 Derby	35.67
1935 Cambridgeshire	36.83
1936 Grand National	35.59
1936 Derby	38.12
1936 Cambridgeshire	33.74
1937 Grand National	30.11
1937 Derby	32.20
1937 Cesarewitch	26.74
1938 Grand National	25.22
1938 Derby	23.79
1938 Cesarewitch	24.00
1939 Grand National	23.27
1939 Derby	26.39
1939 Cesarewitch	13.19

Source: calculated from lists of names and addresses of the prizewinners printed in the Irish daily newspapers after each sweepstake draw.

The decline of contributions from Britain also had the effect of reducing sweepstake income. Proceeds from ticket sales in the 1935 Grand National sweepstake were down by almost £400,000 on the 1934 Cambridgeshire, and the 1935 Derby showed a further reduction, the first time since the 1931 Manchester November Handicap than proceeds were under £2 million. The £2 million figure was regained by the 1936 Cambridgeshire, and proceeds from ticket sales remained steady for the remainder of the 1930s until the threat of war began seriously to affect sales in 1939. The growth of the north American market probably accounts for this recovery, although income never returned to the £3–4 million figures which the sweepstakes enjoyed in the early 1930s (see Appendix). The promoters of the sweepstake were concerned at the drastic restriction of their British market. In September 1935 Joseph McGrath outlined the situation:

Since the passing of the Betting and Lotteries Bill in the British Parliament, the prohibition of all publicity and newspaper references calculated to induce people to buy Irish sweepstake tickets has had a serious effect in lowering the amount of British subscriptions. British subscriptions have amounted to an average of 70% of the total moneys received, whereas in the last sweepstake, the Derby of 1935, the percentage was reduced to 40%, and present indications are that this percentage is further decreasing.[84]

Nevertheless, sweepstake activity in Britain did not cease completely. Between one-quarter and one-third of all prizes, and therefore probably a similar proportion of tickets, made their way across the Irish Sea. The continued flow of tickets to Britain may have been due in part to new measures adopted by Hospitals Trust in an effort to evade detection of its correspondence. It advised customers of new privacy measures which were being introduced on 1 January 1935, coinciding with the coming into effect of the Betting and Lotteries Act. An identification number, rather than a name, would be used for each correspondent; no addresses would be printed on the receipts sent to subscribers; subscribers were advised to send all correspondence through an intermediary in the Irish Free State or to arrange for a business, institution or friend to transmit correspondence on their behalf.[85] The less direct route of transmitting tickets into Britain from France was also used, presumably to avoid the close scrutiny of post between Britain and Ireland.[86]

Seizures of tickets and the prosecution of ticket traffickers also served to indicate the continuation of sweepstake activity in Britain after 1934. In 1937 police apprehended John Witts, of Fulham, 'said to be one of the largest distributors of Irish sweep tickets in England', who distributed 800 books of tickets for each sweepstake and had a number of sub-agents throughout England. He was fined £20.[87] In March 1936 £390,000 worth of tickets for the 1936 Derby sweepstake were reported to have been seized in South Cumberland.[88] Many of these discoveries, however, related to tickets being smuggled into Britain for subsequent transfer to the sweepstake's growing north American market. Tickets seized from the *Aquitania* at Southampton in 1938 were intended for New York.[89]

The Liverpool docks were an important centre of operations for smuggling tickets into Britain, both for distribution there and subsequent transmission to north America. In September 1937, John McDonnell, a labourer at the docks, was fined £15 for distributing tickets and sending counterfoils out of Britain; and in August 1938, Timothy Nesbitt, an assistant superintendent in the Investigating Department of the Canadian Pacific Railway Steamship Services admitted to using his office at Gladstone Dock to distribute sweepstake tickets.[90]

In 1937 one of the largest smuggling rings operating out of Liverpool was uncovered. This case proved seriously embarrassing for the law enforcement authorities as two of the ten defendants convicted were police constables, both of whom received prison sentences of nine months for accepting bribes not to interfere with the activities of the smugglers. Among those also imprisoned and given substantial fines were Frederick Woodhall, a club proprietor from Wallasey, believed to be the conspiracy's ringleader, Thomas Woodhall, a tailor from Cheshire and William Newcombe, a clerk, also from Wallasey, all of whom had previously been convicted and fined for possession of over 1 million sweepstake tickets in June 1936.[91] The operation, believed to have been carried on between January 1935 and August 1937, when it was detected, involved employees on steamships travelling between Dublin and Liverpool, one of whom was believed to be an employee of Hospitals Trust, the two police constables, labourers at Princes Dock and a laundry van driver whose van was used to transport the tickets. The enterprise was finally exposed when the van driver informed the police about it.[92]

Representations made by Britain to the Irish Free State government to take action to prevent the circulation of tickets in Britain also serve as evidence that sweepstake activity continued after the Betting and Lotteries Act. At first Britain considered appealing to the Irish government on the grounds that Hospitals Trust's activities contravened the 1934 Cairo Postal Convention, but this approach was considered problematic 'as it would raise the question of the inter-imperial applicability of International Conventions' and was also likely to be met 'at best with neglect and at worst with the refusal to do anything' by the Irish government.[93]

In February 1935, Dominions Secretary, J. H. Thomas, brought to the attention of J. W. Dulanty, his government's concern at the new policies adopted by Hospitals Trust to evade the restrictions of the new legislation.[94] The principal cause for complaint was a circular issued by Hospitals Trust advising subscribers on the best means of evading detection and promising to pay the fines imposed on anybody convicted of selling tickets.[95] De Valera's government sympathised with the British displeasure:

> The circulars constituted an interference with the administration of justice in Great Britain, and the Government here were obliged to take cognisance of them because they could not remain passive while the laws of a neighbouring State were being contravened by an institution controlled, however remotely, by the State. We were obliged by the Postal Conventions to prevent our services from being used for a contravention of the law in other countries.

The British complaint was relayed to Joseph McGrath who was also warned that continued activity of this nature would lead to more restrictive measures being introduced against the sweepstake in Britain.[96] McGrath replied that the offending circulars had been recalled, the agent responsible for their distribution, Mrs Chapman, 'severely reprimanded', and all agents instructed not to issue similar literature again.[97]

The intervention of the Irish Free State government on this occasion, while it might have resulted in the withdrawal of an offending circular, did little to stop the transmission of Irish sweepstake tickets to Britain,[98] and in mid-1935 British civil servants considered possible representations which could be made to the Irish government to seek their co-operation in curtailing the sale of tickets in Britain. The UK Trade Commissioner in Dublin suggested that:

> An effective undertaking on the part of the Irish Free State authorities that no sales of tickets would be made to residents of the United Kingdom would mean the stoppage of the drain on United Kingdom resources equal to one half of the annual burden of the land annuity payments which have now to be made by the United Kingdom Government.

However, the Home Office was aware that this 'would be to ask the Irish authorities to impose on themselves a very self-denying ordinance'.[99]

The example of British cooperation with the American government to prevent the smuggling of liquor during prohibition was cited but considered difficult to apply in the case of sweepstake tickets, as there was no clearance from bond involved.[100] The Home Office felt that in view of declining ticket sales in Britain and the Irish Free State's desire for better relations with Britain,[101] the Free State government might be more willing to take stronger action against the sweepstake, but the Dominions Office did not agree 'unless there is some prospect of a quid pro quo which could be given to the I.F.S. Government'.[102] The only practical step was to try to convince the Irish government to persuade or compel Hospitals Trust to stop the sale of tickets to Britain,[103] an idea which was, predictably, unenthusiastically received in Ireland: 'I do not think there is any action open to us in the matter. As you know the Government have practically no real control over Hospitals Trust.'[104] No action was taken by the Irish government and the continued activity of the Irish sweepstake in Britain remained a source of concern to the authorities there in the late 1930s.[105]

A BRITISH LOTTERY?

On various occasions during the 1920s the Home Secretary was urged to consider reform of the lottery laws to permit charities and hospitals to run lotteries to raise much needed funds. After 1930 many cash-strapped British hospitals began to examine ways of emulating the Irish example, in the hope that they might reap a similar windfall and keep British money in Britain to assist British hospitals rather than leaving to fund the Irish Free State's hospital building programme. In November 1930, just after the first sweepstake draw had taken place, it was reported that 'London hospitals, inspired by the success of the great Dublin sweepstake, are now considering the possibilities of holding a sweepstake on similar lines – possibly on next year's Derby – and evading the British lottery ban by organising it abroad.'[106] In January 1931 it was revealed that A. F. Shepherd, the Appeals Director of St Bartholomew's Hospital visited Paris to examine the possibility of running a rival hospitals sweepstake from the French capital.[107] However, there appears to have been no further progress with this venture.

Parliamentary demands for a review of the country's lottery laws continued.[108] One of the foremost proponents of a change was the backbench Conservative MP, Sir William Davison. After repeated refusals by the Home Secretary to re-examine the issue, Davison sought to introduce his own bill 'to authorise the raising of money by means of lotteries for the support of hospitals', citing the urgent needs of British hospitals for building, equipment, and maintenance, the Irish example of raising immense sums through the sweepstake, and the favourable reaction to the idea from supporters of St Bartholomew's Hospital.[109]

Urging the Commons not to allow Davison to introduce his bill, the Liberal MP Isaac Foot quoted the findings of the 1908 House of Commons Select Committee on Lotteries which saw in lotteries 'No mode of raising money . . . so burdensome, so pernicious, and so unproductive; no species of adventure is known where the chances are so great against the adventurer; none where the infatuation is more powerful, lasting and destructive.' He also reiterated the standard arguments against the use of lotteries to raise funds for charity: if one group was permitted to use this method of fund-raising others would seek to do likewise; the sources of charity would dry up; the Irish hospitals received only a fraction of the sweepstake's proceeds; hospitals were not in favour of the idea; and it would exacerbate the evils resulting from gambling.[110] The motion to allow Davison leave to introduce the bill was defeated by 181 to 58.[111]

He tried again in March 1932, by which time 130 of those who had voted against his previous attempt had lost their seats in the October 1931 general election. The new parliamentary arithmetic resulted in the passage of the motion to introduce his bill by 176 votes to 123. The second Davison bill envisaged a wider jurisdiction for lotteries 'for charitable, scientific, and artistic purposes, or any public improvement or other public object', not simply hospitals.[112] However, it did not progress any further in parliament.

The failure of Davison's parliamentary efforts led to the revival of the idea of organising a sweepstake in aid of British hospitals from a base outside the country. In October 1932 plans were revealed for a British hospital sweepstake to be run under the auspices of the Casino and International Sporting Club of Monte Carlo and to be known as the 'Principality of Monaco Sweepstakes'. It was to be organised along similar lines to the Irish sweepstake, although fewer proceeds would be expended on expenses, and it was hoped to raise £500,000 for British hospitals and charities.[113] The Archbishop of Canterbury, Dr Lang, expressed his 'distress and concern at the proposal to utilise for English voluntary hospitals a huge sweepstake lottery, organised at Monte Carlo, the Mecca of gambling'.[114] Spencer Freeman, the publicity mastermind of the Irish sweepstake, was involved with the scheme. The prime mover behind it was Sir Arthur Stanley, third son of the sixteenth Earl of Derby and President of the British Hospitals Association, who was noted for his philanthropic work on behalf of medical charities.[115] The plan was eventually abandoned in the face of opposition from the Home Office.[116] Spencer Freeman and his wife continued to be associated with Sir Arthur Stanley and fund-raising for British charities throughout the 1930s.[117]

Another prominent campaigner for the legalisation of hospital sweepstakes in Britain was the Duke of Atholl, a bitter opponent of the Irish Free State and its sweepstake. In a speech delivered at Croydon in September 1933, in which he described the sweepstake as a 'national disgrace', he also complained that:

> Behind the plea of helping charity something like £25,000,000 has gone into Ireland, a very considerable portion of which, according to *The Times*, Mr Halkett, a distinguished London magistrate, said, goes to help Mr de Valera to carry on his disloyal policy against this country.

In his opinion the only 'good defence against the Irish sweepstake would be an organised legalised sweepstake in this country'. He proceeded to allege intimidation by the organisers of the Irish sweepstake against his own sweepstake: 'I have a very able lieutenant, who has received mysterious threats of physical violence if he persists in helping me with my scheme.'[118] Rebutting the duke's allegations, Spencer Freeman challenged him to produce evidence of the threats promising to 'pay £1,000 to any British charity if these charges are substantiated', and Joseph McGrath described the duke's attack as 'regrettable, undignified and unsportsmanlike'.[119]

In 1933 the duke sought unsuccessfully to run a charity sweepstake on the St Leger. In an attempt to evade the letter of the British lottery laws the competition was based on judging the artistic merits of the racing colours of various owners, including the king.[120] By this means it could be claimed that it was a skill-based competition, but the British authorities were not so easily fooled: 'The scheme was obviously an illegal lottery and after warning by the Commissioner of Police it was abandoned.'[121] Tickets for the abortive enterprise were said to have been seized by Irish Free State customs officials.[122]

Undeterred, the duke opened a new fund on behalf of British charities. When the appeal closed at the end of September 1933 the net proceeds were reported at £95,000, £59,000 of which was to be allocated to various charities. In the prize fund of £36,000, prizes varied in value from between £10 and £2,000. Among the 748 prizewinners was Lady Carson (wife of the former Ulster Unionist leader, Sir Edward Carson), who scooped £10.[123] In spite of the duke's prominent position, he was prosecuted and subsequently convicted under the 1823 Lottery Act for selling tickets in a lottery which had not been authorised by an act of parliament. He was fined £25 and ordered to pay 35 guineas in costs.[124] A subsequent appeal was struck out on the grounds of a solicitor's error.[125] In spite of his conviction the duke saw his venture as having a measure of success: 'I think I can lay claim to having had something to do with the fact that the last Irish sweepstake obtained less in contributions from this country than at any time with the exception of the first two efforts.'[126] The results of the 1933 Cambridgeshire sweepstake draw lend legitimacy to the duke's claims: 56 per cent of prizes was won by British residents, the lowest since the sweepstake started, down over 12 per cent from the preceding sweepstake on the 1933 Derby, and proceeds from tickets sales dipped to their lowest figure since the 1931 Grand National sweepstake (Table 4.1 and Appendix).

Public opinion in Britain was far from united on the issue of legalising lotteries. Clearly, the large proportion of the population which subscribed to the Irish sweepstake had few qualms about the use of gambling to raise money for charitable purposes. However, the hospitals upon whose behalf the campaign to legalise lotteries was based, were divided on the issue. At its annual conference in Eastbourne in June 1931, the British Hospitals Association passed a resolution stating that it was 'not in favour of amendment of the law affecting public sweepstakes which purports to be for the benefit of voluntary hospitals'.[127] As was the case with the Anglican clergy in Ireland, the Protestant churches in Britain weighed in against legalising sweepstakes. Where there was support for the idea it was sporadic and usually confined to individual campaigners, like Sir William Davison and the Duke of Atholl. The available evidence would indicate that there was no sentiment in Britain, which was overwhelmingly in favour of the legalisation of lotteries and sweepstakes.

FIVE

THE SWEEPSTAKE IN NORTH AMERICA IN THE 1930s

—

By the time of the Irish sweepstake's arrival, opportunities for legal gambling in the USA, outside of Nevada's casinos, were severely restricted. State lotteries, which had been popular in the USA during the eighteenth century, had been gradually phased out in the early nineteenth. The only survivor was the Louisiana state lottery, which was effectively suppressed by Congress in the 1890s, when a restriction on the sale of tickets outside state boundaries was introduced. The remaining outlets for gambling fell foul of the progressive era of the late nineteenth and early twentieth centuries, so that by 1911 horse racing was permitted in only six states, bookmakers had been banned in many states, and the Western Union Telegraph Company refused to transmit racing news along its wires.[1] Nineteenth-century British lottery restrictions still applied in Canada, although illegal lotteries flourished there during the 1920s and 1930s.[2]

THE POPULARITY OF THE SWEEPSTAKE IN THE USA
AND CANADA

As the economic hardship of the great depression resulted in many turning to illegal gambling as a last resort, the huge prizes on offer in the Irish sweepstake gave it a particular appeal in the eyes of many financially handicapped Americans.[3] An American postal official commented in 1932 that the country had gone 'lottery crazy' during the preceding year, estimating that Americans had spent $100 million on lotteries organised in Canada and Ireland.[4] By 1934 the US Post Office announced that $3 billion had been subscribed to foreign lotteries over a three-year period.[5] Such was the popularity of the Irish sweepstake that American citizens expected their legation in Dublin to 'buy tickets for them and mail the ticket book to the United States'.[6]

In an article entitled 'A lottery craze sweeps the land', in the *New York Times* in September 1932, this new-found popularity of lotteries was attributed to the economic depression: 'The depression has to answer largely for our often pathetic efforts to find the pot of gold.'[7] The Postmaster General Walter Brown also highlighted the role of the newly established Irish sweepstake, and its attendant publicity, in increasing lottery mania by providing an example for other similar enterprises: 'Following the establishment of the Hospitals Trust Ltd., lottery at Dublin and the wide publicity the promoters were able to get for it, numerous other sweepstake lotteries sprung up in a score of other foreign countries.'[8] The Irish sweepstake now became the standard model imitated by other lotteries operating in the USA, such as the British International Association, the Hull (Ontario) Public Maternity Hospital Trust Fund and the Canadian Cancer Hospitals Sweepstake, run from Montréal; the tickets for this latter sweepstake bore a remarkable similarity to those of the Irish sweepstake.[9]

In the early 1930s the USA accounted for only a small percentage of the sweepstake market, which was still most heavily concentrated in Great Britain. The American Consul General in Dublin estimated that slightly over half a million tickets for the 1932 Grand National sweepstake were sold in the USA.[10] Almost seven million tickets were sold in that sweepstake and only 6.47 per cent of prizes were won by Americans. There was a gradual increase in the American market; almost 10 per cent of prizes in the 1932 Cesarewitch went to the USA, rising to 13.85 per cent and 29.39 per cent for the 1933 and 1934 Cambridgeshires respectively (Table 5.1).

The size of the Irish prize money ensured its greater popularity. In 1934, first and second prizes in the Irish sweepstake amounted to US$150,000 and US$75,000 respectively. By contrast, the Canadian Army and Navy Veterans' Sweepstake was only able to offer first and second prizes of US$37,000 and US$12,000.[11]

Even before the Betting and Lotteries Act came into effect in Great Britain, the American market had started to account for a much greater proportion of ticket sales. Nearly one-third of tickets in the 1934 Cambridgeshire sweepstake were sold in the USA, compared to just under 45 per cent in Great Britain. The enforcement of the Betting and Lotteries Act in 1935 and the consequent curtailment of the market for tickets in Great Britain forced the sweepstake promoters to look elsewhere for customers. The growing north American market provided the obvious solution. The 1935 Derby marked the first occasion that a greater number of tickets were sold in the USA than in Great Britain, and the 1937 Grand National draw saw more than half of the tickets sold in the USA for the first time. For the remainder of the 1930s, the majority were sold in the USA.

The continuation of the Irish sweepstake after the introduction of the British restrictions in 1935 was guaranteed by the popularity of sweepstake

Table 5.1: **Geographical distribution of prizewinners, 1930–9 – percentage of prizes won**

Sweepstake	USA	Canada
1930 Manchester Nov. Handicap	5.00	7.59
1931 Grand National	6.50	2.46
1931 Manchester Nov. Handicap	10.85	1.77
1932 Grand National	6.47	2.70
1932 Derby	7.23	1.75
1932 Cesarewitch	9.99	2.66
1933 Grand National	13.10	3.40
1933 Derby	8.90	3.16
1933 Cambridgeshire	13.85	4.70
1934 Grand National	14.59	2.98
1934 Derby	23.05	3.46
1934 Cambridgeshire	29.39	2.17
1935 Grand National	39.82	3.85
1935 Derby	42.41	4.37
1935 Cambridgeshire	43.67	3.22
1936 Grand National	43.77	4.52
1936 Derby	43.92	5.20
1936 Cambridgeshire	47.38	4.80
1937 Grand National	50.81	5.56
1937 Derby	49.75	6.36
1937 Cesarewitch	53.90	6.19
1938 Grand National	53.77	8.13
1938 Derby	57.16	8.82
1938 Cesarewitch	53.86	8.84
1939 Grand National	54.96	7.74
1939 Derby	51.95	8.81
1939 Cesarewitch	61.69	9.34

Source: Collated from results of sweepstake draws published in Irish daily newspapers.

gambling in the USA. However, while the American market helped to compensate for the loss of much of the British one, it did not succeed in replacing the lost revenue entirely. For the latter half of the 1930s proceeds from the sale of tickets remained relatively constant, at over £2 million per draw (see Appendix). These figures never regained the heights of the early 1930s, when well over £3m was contributed to most draws. Therefore, while the American market was crucial in sustaining the Irish sweepstake, it never fully replaced the strong British market of the early 1930s.

An indication of the value of American sweepstake contributions to the Irish economy can by gauged by comparing the estimated amount spent by Americans on Irish sweepstake tickets with the known value of Irish exports to the USA. At a time when Irish exports to the USA were relatively small, the sweepstake was responsible for a vast amount of American currency coming into Ireland. Assuming that the rate of prize-winning corresponded closely to the proportion of tickets bought, American sweepstake customers were contributing over £3 million per year to the sweepstake, well in excess of the amount spent by the USA on Irish imports (Table 5.2).

Table 5.2: Comparison between US contributions to the Irish sweepstake and Irish exports (incl. re-exports, excl. bullion and coin) to the USA in the 1930s

Year	Value of Irish Free State exports to USA (£)	Estimated value of US contributions to sweepstake (£)
1932	106,100	889,881
1933	157,878	1,056,830
1934	124,984	2,041,246
1935	178,338	2,936,339
1936	275,134	3,279,247
1937	238,325	4,202,831
1938	118,386	4,157,958

Source: Irish Free State Statistical Abstract, 1935, p. 75, table 96; 1937, p. 75, table 95; Ireland Statistical Abstract, 1939, p. 91, table 98.

Canadians were among the prizewinners in the sweepstakes organised on behalf of Dublin's Mater Hospital in 1922 and for hospitals in Dublin and Cork in 1923.[12] In 1923, a resident of Ottawa wrote to the Irish Department of Home Affairs seeking to obtain sweepstake tickets and the following year the same department discovered that tickets in a sweepstake organised in aid of a church building fund in Athlone, County Westmeath were on sale in Ontario.[13] In the first hospitals sweepstake in 1930, 6 of the 79 prizes were won by Canadians including second prize of £81,905 won by A. P. Dawe, a garage owner from Vancouver.[14] In order to evade a massive tax liability Dawe invoked a clause in the criminal code whereby lottery winnings were forfeited to the first person to inform on the winner; he was thus sued in a friendly action brought by his brother, a second brother sued their father in case he might have any claim on the ticket, and Arnold Walker, the seller of the winning ticket, was similarly sued by his wife.[15]

The example set by the Dawes was followed by other winners: in 1932 a Winnipeg barrister complained that 'All over the country from time to time these collusive actions are being brought and the situation is rather disgraceful'.[16] The situation led to the criminal code being amended in 1934 whereby 'all prizes won at lotteries are subject to forfeiture to the Crown. The former provision which enabled the individual to sue for lottery prizes has been repealed'.[17] Dawe's windfall did much to boost the popularity of the sweepstake in Canada: 'Because of the publicity surrounding his success, within a year an estimated CAN$250,000 from British Columbia alone was going to Ireland, and by 1938 approximately one-third of Torontonians bought Irish Sweepstakes tickets.'[18]

In the first half of the 1930s Canada's share of prizes fluctuated between two and four per cent. According to official figures produced by the sweepstake organisers, 1,905 prizes of £697,755 were won by Canadians in the first thirteen sweepstakes held between 1930 and 1934.[19] Increased sales of tickets in the USA also led to increased sales in Canada, as seen in Canada's increased share of prize money which climbed to between seven and eight per cent towards the end of the 1930s (Table 5.1). Intermittent efforts by police to crack down on the sale of tickets are also evidence of their popularity:

> . . . in 1936, Vancouver police began a period of careful enforcement of the law against the sale of Irish Sweepstakes tickets, making twenty-five arrests and disrupting the supply of these tickets in the entire region. The cleanup was only temporary, and tolerance was the norm – by March 1938 tickets for the June race at Epsom were 'selling like hotcakes on the streets of Vancouver'.[20]

The amount of money leaving Canada was a cause of much concern. In 1931 a Vancouver resident complained to the Canadian Minister for Justice that 'fully one million dollars has left BC, within this last two years for Ireland and more will go this year'.[21] The situation in Toronto was similar.[22] By 1938, citizens of Toronto were estimated to be spending approximately £3 million a year.[23] The realisation that so much money was flowing out of Canada to support the building and equipping of Irish hospitals in a time of economic depression when hospitals in many parts of Canada were seriously underfunded led to concerted efforts on behalf of some politicians to establish a Canadian equivalent of the Irish sweepstake, but the strength of opposition from Protestant churches prevented it.[24]

THE SWEEPSTAKE OPERATION IN THE USA

The United States criminal code outlawed the importation of lottery material and its distribution through the mail.[25] With a variety of federal and state agencies, including the Customs Bureau, Justice Department and Post Office, endeavouring to prevent trafficking in sweepstake tickets, it was imperative for the promoters to establish a sophisticated underground importation and distribution network.

Initially, they sought out American customers at random, sending out unsolicited publicity material and tickets.[26] Officials in the Post Office Department discovered tickets for the inaugural sweepstake that had been mailed to various regional newspapers, golf clubs and chambers of commerce throughout the USA.[27] As this method of distribution often led to complaints to federal authorities from the recipients, and the subsequent imposition of fraud orders against the senders, it did not prove very effective and was soon replaced by more subtle methods.[28]

Sending counterfoils and money directly to Hospitals Trust in Dublin was problematic. Letters addressed to Hospitals Trust, especially registered letters, which was often the case with letters containing money, would attract the attention of Post Office inspectors on the look out for illegal lottery material passing through the mail. Even if such correspondence eluded the postal authorities, there was then the problem of 'dishonest [postal] employees whose attention is principally attracted to letters addressed to undertakings known to be receiving large quantities of letters containing money'. The solution to both of these difficulties was the establishment of receiving depots, which were usually nondescript post office box addresses in Dublin, such as O. Hanratty, P.O. Box 33k, Pearse Street Post Office, Dublin. Foreign customers were directed to remit their counterfoils and money to such bogus addresses.[29] Another method used to ensure the safe and undetected return of counterfoils and remittances to Dublin was the operation of a system of transit agents: 'Some addresses became well known in the US and Canada as being reliable addresses to send cash and counterfoils for transmission to the Sweep offices.'[30]

The difficulties described above relate to returning counterfoils and money to Ireland. It was equally difficult to get the tickets into the USA in the first place. The vast majority of tickets sold there in the 1930s were smuggled on ships crossing the Atlantic. This was a cumbersome process involving illicit transportation firstly from Dublin to England and onwards to either Canada or the principal ports of the eastern United States. Montréal became a centre for the distribution of tickets throughout north America. For much of the 1930s Hospitals Trust's representative there was Thomas Lee, assisted by Richard Duggan's brother, Joseph.[31]

To facilitate the various legs of the journey numerous bribes had to be paid to customs officials and steamship employees at points of entry and on the journeys themselves.[32] It is impossible to estimate how much of the money received from ticket sales was expended on such under the counter payments because of section 2 of the Public Hospitals Act (p. 33). The going rate for smuggling tickets along the entire journey from Ireland to north America was said to be £10 per thousand books of tickets, £5 to England and a further £5 to the United States.[33] Overall, it was estimated that bribes and protection money paid out by Hospitals Trust to ensure the safe conduct of tickets to the USA amounted to 'well over six figures' each year.[34]

When the tickets had been smuggled successfully into the United States, they were then distributed by means of a hierarchical system of agents. Hospitals Trust employed three different categories of agent: home agents, who sold to the Irish domestic market; English agents, who operated in Britain; and foreign agents, who were based largely in the USA. In turn the larger agents had subagents working within their distribution networks. The commission paid to agents was ten shillings per book of twelve tickets sold, the equivalent of the price of one ticket. Many agents split this commission with their subagents. Agents were not allowed to subtract their commission at source. Rather, all books supplied to a particular agent had that agent's identification number perforated on the counterfoil. This allowed Hospitals Trust to calculate how many of that agent's tickets had been sold and pay out the commission on that basis.[35] Many subagents applied for and were granted agencies in their own right. Initially, many of the tickets sold in America were sold by home agents resident in Ireland who distributed tickets to relatives and friends there, but as the market grew steadily, a US-based agency system was established. All dealings with foreign agents, including the processing of applications to run agencies, were handled by the Foreign Department, under the stewardship of P. J. Fleming.[36]

Hospitals Trust's agents communicated with Dublin using a cipher that included code names for the principal distribution centres in Britain and the United States; the passenger liners on which tickets were smuggled (for example, 'Ashanti' was the code for the *Aquitania*); the names of key people involved in the operation (Connie Neenan, was 'Dollard', and Charles Dalton, 'Chandler'); the office holders to whom bribes had to be paid (policemen were 'underwriters'); and various other terms associated with the sweepstake (the Foreign Department was known as the 'Gresham Trust'). A copy of this cipher surfaced in 2007 and was bought by the National Library of Ireland at Mealys' independence sale in April 2008.[37]

William Kealy, a Dublin fruit merchant, operated an agency in Dublin that distributed tickets in the United States in the 1930s. He secured the agency from P. J. Fleming, a friend of his from their early days in County Laois. In addition to his own agency, he managed one for a New Yorker, John Morton, and also acted as a transit agent, to whose address remittances from the customers of other agents could be sent safely. In return he received the standard commission of ten shillings per book for those sold through his own agency, half of John Morton's commission, and one shilling and sixpence for books returned through the transit agency. The extent of the business thus carried on was sufficient to require the full-time employment of three female clerical staff and the use of a house, 65 St Patrick's Road, Drumcondra.

Kealy adopted a number of ruses to evade the watchful eye of American Post Office officials. The sudden arrival of a consignment of similarly addressed envelopes would arouse suspicion, therefore he got 'as many people as he could to address envelopes so they'd all have different handwriting, and he'd have different sizes of envelopes', which would then be posted in different locations:

> we would go out to Swords and post some of them, and we would go to Dundalk to post some of them and we go down to Abbeyleix to post some of them . . . all over the place, driving around at nights, posting these in different letterboxes, so there wouldn't be a clatter of letters with the same postmark.

Suitcases were among the best receptacles for smuggling tickets into the USA, and Kealy, again through the patronage of Fleming, operated an agency for supplying Hospitals Trust and its agents with suitcases manufactured by Travel Goods Ltd. in Portarlington.[38]

A variety of Irish-American companies operating in the USA during the 1930s were fronts to facilitate the illegal sale of sweepstake tickets. One such firm was the American Travel Exchange, a travel agency with offices in New York and Dublin, which held five agencies, some under the auspices of Hospitals Trust's special agent in America, Joseph McGarrity.[39] The Irish Tourist Association (ITA), which established offices in New York, allegedly paid for by Hospitals Trust, was a similar cover for sweepstake activities.[40] In 1940 the Post Office Department intercepted a copy of the ITA's magazine *Irish Travel*, with tickets for the 1941 Lincolnshire sweepstake pasted to the inside pages.[41] The Ajax Trading Company, based in Dublin, advertised itself in America as 'official intermediaries on behalf of the Irish Hospitals Trust Ltd., in order to facilitate parties interested in the Irish Sweepstakes to obtain tickets'; rather than risk the confiscation of communications addressed to Hospitals Trust, customers could send their contributions through Michael Devlin, the director of the Ajax Trading Company.[42] International exhibitions intended to showcase Ireland abroad were also exploited to the full by Hospitals Trust in an effort to sell tickets in the USA. Joseph Andrews, an employee of the Foreign Department, later claimed that Irish displays were paid for by Hospitals Trust and managed by one of its American agents, Eric Boden. Boden directed the House of Ireland at the California Pacific International Exposition in 1934 and also directed Irish activities at the San Diego exposition in 1935–6.[43]

Hospitals Trust's principal American outlet was its New York office. In the early 1930s this office was run by Dubliner, Paul Moran, his wife Agnes, and Moran's uncle in New York, John Kelly and his family. The Morans emigrated to the USA in 1931 where they were asked to assume the management of the New York office. John Kelly ran a jeweller's shop in Amsterdam Avenue in New York City which doubled as a ticket depot, while his apartment at 364 Central Park West effectively was the sweepstake's New York office.[44] In June 1936 Joseph Andrews resigned from Hospitals Trust to go to the USA. P. J. Fleming asked him to bring some documents on his trip to be delivered to the New York office. These consisted mainly of commission cheques for the American agents. On arrival in New York, Andrews stayed with the Kellys in the apartment at Central Park West. On the morning of 3 July he received a hasty phone call from Kelly ordering him to 'clear everything' from the apartment immediately. Realising that all of the sweepstake's American records were stored in the apartment, Andrews packed all the incriminating documents into suitcases and concealed them in the linen cupboard under a pile of clothing. The police arrived at noon to search the premises but failed to uncover the hiding place. Afterwards the records were removed to Joseph McGarrity's base in Philadelphia. Andrews was 'in no doubt that if the Postal Authorities had captured the records at that time the Sweep would have been finished in the US'.[45]

JOSEPH ANDREWS

The bulk of the evidence on the sweepstake's underground organisation in the USA comes from a former sweepstake employee, Joseph Andrews. This former seminarian 'was within one month of being ordained a priest', when he left intending to join the Royal Air Force but instead acquired a position in the sweepstake through an acquaintance of his father.[46] He worked in the Foreign Department from 1932 to 1938, with the exception of a brief interlude in the USA during 1936. He was responsible for checking the cash sheets drawn up by Hospitals Trust's cashiers to ensure that receipts coincided with the number of counterfoils returned, and also for lodging the department's receipts with the bank.[47] His employment was terminated abruptly in August 1938 when he resigned following an argument with Joseph McGrath. He claimed subsequently that McGrath had engineered the confrontation in order to get 'rid of . . . the only one in the organisation, outside himself and the Directors, who really knew what was going on'.[48]

Disgruntled at his treatment, Andrews sought to use his knowledge of the sweepstake's American organisation to gain both revenge against his erstwhile employers and monetary benefit for himself. He claimed to have written under the pseudonym of P. O'Sullivan, to FBI director, J. Edgar Hoover, in January 1939, informing him of income tax evasion by sweepstake agents.[49] In February 1940 he contacted the American consulate in Dublin offering to provide them with information 'to show the workings of the Irish Sweepstakes and to present evidence which might be of use to officials . . . interested in locating persons guilty of income tax evasion'.[50] The latter reference was to sweepstake agents in the USA who were earning substantial amounts of undeclared income in the form of commission received on the sale of tickets.

He furnished the American Consul General in Dublin with a very detailed report of his experiences in Hospitals Trust, outlining how it operated in the USA, the leading role of IRA and Clan na Gael (the Irish-American republican organisation) leaders Joseph McGarrity and Connie Neenan in it, the details of other principal American agents, allegations of financial irregularities in the accounts of Connie Neenan's New York office, and the instructions issued by the Foreign Department to its American agents on how to avoid detection.[51] This was followed by an offer to obtain and furnish them with a list of 3,000 sweepstake agents operating in the USA in return for a fee of $400 expenses, which would be required in order to obtain the list.[52] Tentative plans were made for Andrews to travel to Boston to meet Post Office officials and hand over this list.[53]

However, at this point Andrews appears to have got cold feet and in April 1940 he informed the American Consul General in Dublin that 'he had decided to "let the whole matter drop"', because he 'had to consider the welfare of [his] family'.[54] The staff at the consulate in Dublin tried to pursue Andrews, but had difficulty doing so, believing that he had gone to London for a time. In spite of Andrews's backtracking the American officials appear to have convinced him to change his mind, and in July 1940 he filled in a detailed questionnaire giving information about the people suspected of being the leading agents in the USA.[55] This was followed in November 1940 by an unsolicited memorandum on the activities of Joseph McGarrity.[56] In 1941 he also furnished the consulate in Dublin with two notebooks 'containing a list of all the agents in the United States selling Irish sweepstake tickets'.[57] These books, containing the names of 1,500 people who acted as agents in the USA between 1934 and 1940, were passed to the Treasury Department's Intelligence Unit.[58] Unfortunately, the archives of this unit no longer appear to be extant.

These notebooks were followed by a batch of letters containing correspondence between Hospitals Trust's Dublin headquarters and some of its agents in the USA, dating from 1937 and 1938, that Andrews obtained when working in the Foreign Department.[59]

The Internal Revenue Bureau at the Treasury Department in Washington DC, eager to pursue sweepstake agents for income tax on undeclared commission, was delighted with Andrews' submissions: 'The material obtained . . . from Mr Andrews is just what this Bureau has been attempting to obtain for a long time.'[60] The correspondence between American officials and Andrews came to an end, in a manner similarly abrupt to his employment with Hospitals Trust, in late 1941, when on requesting further documentation, it was discovered that he had been interned by the Irish authorities.[61]

Andrews's internment resulted from involvement with the IRA and various German agents in Ireland during the Second World War. Soon after the war started he had been refused a commission in the defence forces. Thereafter he sought work in England but was denied a visa. During 1940 and 1941 he became involved in a number of minor pro-German splinter groups in Ireland, including the People's National Party, Coras na Poblachta and the Irish Friends of Germany. About 1941 he came into contact with the German agent in Ireland, Herman Görtz, most likely having been introduced by former sweepstake colleagues Maisie O'Mahony and Helena Kelly, who were also close associates of Görtz. Attaching himself to Görtz, Andrews began to act as his chauffeur, helped him find safe houses, and acted as a courier bringing messages between him and his IRA contacts. He was joined in these activities by his wife who has been described as having 'a special relationship with Görtz'. After ingratiating himself with the German agent he obtained a copy of his secret code and promptly offered to sell it to his former contacts at the American consulate in Dublin, who 'laughed at him and took no further notice of the matter'.[62]

Irish military intelligence also believed that he used the code to obtain money from Germany in return for information about Ireland, for which he appears to have been paid about £100. The information in question referred to allegations that an Irish army officer, Major General Hugo MacNeill, and former Garda Commissioner Eoin O'Duffy were anxious to assist the German war effort.[63] Andrews was initially arrested in October 1941 and released after a day, when a search of his house uncovered nothing incriminating. He was rearrested in November 1941 and interned in the Curragh until the following April. By this stage of the war his activities had come within the purview of British intelligence. In July 1943 they were aware that he was using the Görtz cipher to communicate with the SS in Berlin and were keeping his communications under surveillance.[64] In August 1943 he was rearrested and interned in Mountjoy Jail in Dublin until the end of the war.[65]

All of the intelligence agencies who followed Andrews' activities during the war formed a thoroughly negative impression of him. The Irish army's military intelligence division (G2) described him as 'an astute and plausible rogue without any fixed convictions and mainly actuated by a desire to obtain money rapidly without any due regard as to the honesty of the methods used to secure his ends'.[66] In similar vein, their British counterparts labelled him 'an intelligent, plausible and unscrupulous double-crosser', adding that his wife was 'said to be even more dangerous than he is'.[67] G2 was also of the impression that his departure from Hospitals Trust in 1938 'was a result of some form of dishonesty' and that he had subsequently blackmailed his former employers: 'it is believed that he extracted a large sum of money from the Sweep authorities under the threat of disclosing information concerning agents in countries where the sale of sweep tickets would normally be illegal.'[68]

Andrews sought financial reward for his disclosures. He was informed that if the information he provided led to the collection of unpaid taxes he would be considered for a reward of up to 10 per cent of the amount recovered.[69] As a result of his imprisonment and the termination of his contact with consular officials, it is unclear if any reward was ever forthcoming. However, it is known that he received a reward from the Irish revenue commissioners for furnishing them with similar information about an errant sweepstake agent in Cork. In June 1940 he received a payment of £15 following the successful claim for payment of outstanding taxes from Patrick Collins, College Road, Cork, a brother-in-law of the sweepstake's American supremo, Connie Neenan.[70] Not content with such a reward, he also sought to sell the names and addresses of 1,300 sweep agents to the British Customs and Excise. According to British intelligence, behaviour of this kind came to be known in Dublin as 'doing an Andrews'.[71]

Andrews also brought his vendetta against Hospitals Trust to senior members of the Irish government. In September 1939 he wrote to Minister for Finance Seán MacEntee outlining alleged irregularities in the activities of the sweepstake, including claims that senior civil servants and members of the Oireachtas were evading income tax, presumably in the form of commission on ticket sales, that Hospitals Trust was evading the payment of stamp duty to the government, and violating English currency regulations and international postal regulations. He also applied for a revolver licence, claiming that his life was in danger.[72]

The Irish government was more dubious of Andrews' overtures than its American counterpart. MacEntee categorised the claim that he needed a gun for protection as 'theatrical'.[73] His motive was unclear to them; was he seeking reinstatement in Hospitals Trust or financial reward from the government for his information?[74] MacEntee felt the correspondence was an effort to extort money from the government and should be forwarded to the Attorney General with a view to prosecution; the Attorney General agreed that it was 'a well concealed effort to obtain monetary consideration' but saw no avenue for taking legal proceedings.[75] It was decided to investigate the two allegations which fell within their jurisdiction, those of tax evasion by civil servants and politicians and the violation of postal regulations.[76] In regard to the latter allegation, the Department of Posts and Telegraphs responded that because the sweepstake was established by legislation it was permissible to transmit material relating to it.[77] The Revenue Commissioners investigated the claims thoroughly and were 'satisfied that there has been no deliberate *mala fides* on the part of Hospitals Trust, Ltd.', and only one case of individual tax evasion was discovered, 'a salaried employee of the company who had received considerable payments which the company regarded as expenses', presumably Patrick Collins.[78]

Andrews's activities in hawking his inside knowledge of the sweepstake's American organisation to the authorities in Ireland, Great Britain and the United States, always accompanying his offers with a request for financial remuneration, and his strange relationship with Görtz, provide ample evidence to justify the impression which Irish and British military intelligence had of him as a rogue. It raises the question of the extent to which his account of the sweepstake's American organisation and activities can be believed. The grudge which he clearly bore against Hospitals Trust also leads one to question the veracity of his statements. Yet there is ample reason to believe that his account is largely a true one. In the first place, one of his principal motives was to gain monetary reward from the American government for information on agents who had evaded tax on their commission. If the Internal Revenue Service was unsuccessful in this, there would be no reward. In addition, the level of detail which is contained in his accounts is too intricate to have been fabricated completely, and the documents he supplied to the American authorities appear to be genuine. Finally, there is other independent evidence to corroborate some of the accusations which he made, concerning insider dealing in winning tickets by Hospitals Trust and the activities of Joseph McGarrity's special agents.

JOSEPH MCGARRITY AND CONNIE NEENAN

By the mid-1930s the sweepstake organisation in the USA was increasingly coming under the control of Clan na Gael and the IRA, and especially the personal control of two of the leading figures in those organisations in America at that time, Joseph McGarrity and Connie Neenan. McGarrity was born in Carrickmore, County Tyrone in 1874 and emigrated to Philadelphia in 1892, where he became one of the most senior figures in Clan na Gael, the American counterpart of the Irish Republican Brotherhood. Said to have made a considerable fortune in property dealings in both Philadelphia and New York, he provided much of the funding for the purchase of arms by Irish Volunteers during the revolutionary period. Strongly opposed to the Anglo-Irish Treaty, he drifted further towards hardline republicanism during the 1930s, when he split with long-time friend Eamon de Valera over the latter's attitude to the IRA. Towards the end of the 1930s he was involved in planning the IRA's bombing campaign in Great Britain. Although he died in August 1940, his signature was appended to IRA communiqués for many subsequent decades.

In addition to his subversive activities, McGarrity had considerable business interests in Philadelphia. Initially he ran a wine and spirit business until it was outlawed by prohibition in 1919. In 1930 he was made a member of the New York Curb Exchange but was expelled in 1933 for false bookkeeping entries.[79] Clearly he was in serious financial trouble; Connie Neenan wrote to IRA chief-of-staff Moss Twomey in March 1933:

> Paddy Brennan will get to Dublin about April 12th to 14th. He is going there specifically to get the others to do something for Joe [McGarrity] . . . I saw Joe C. about the case and he has sent a report to DeV[alera]. Mrs McG[arrity] is not well but few know this. Joe C. gave some cash which Paddy gave to Mrs McG[arrity]. Joe McG[arrity] has no idea of this and Mrs McG[arrity] is warned not to say so. Two girls work as waitresses not earning ten dollars between them, that's the entire income. Anything that is being done Joe is unaware of it as otherwise he would kick and spoil the picture.[80]

McGarrity's financial woes were soon alleviated by the acquisition of a sweepstake agency, probably arranged for him by Dr Patrick McCartan, a close friend of both McGarrity and Joseph McGrath. McCartan had previously tried to entice McGarrity to become an agent at the start of the sweepstake in 1930.[81]

Connie Neenan, a native of Croaghtmore, County Cork, emigrated to the USA in the 1920s, having played an active part in the Irish revolution in Cork.[82] In 1927 he was appointed the IRA's full-time representative in the USA. He became the principal link between the IRA leadership in Ireland and Clan na Gael and also had responsibility for recruiting for both organisations, as well as fund-raising and purchasing arms for the IRA.[83] Until his return to Ireland in the early 1970s, Neenan remained one of the most important figures in the sweepstake organisation in the USA. He also became involved in other business ventures which emerged directly from the sweepstake, acting as representative for the McGraths' Waterford Glass Company for many years.[84] During the Second World War he appears to have distanced himself from the IRA and concentrated on sweepstake work. The FBI identified a generational divide: 'it is noted that Neenan represents a leader of the elder Irish Republican Army federation in the United States, which has to a large extent broken away from the present younger IRA leadership' and also believed that 'he was supposedly expelled from the IRA organization because of his association in the Irish sweepstakes'. A legal dispute between Clan na Gael and James McGranery, a Democratic Representative from Philadelphia, over $4,000 bond money for IRA leader Seán Russell (who also worked for the sweepstake in America), contributed to the deterioration of Neenan's relationship with Irish republicanism in the USA.[85] In 1933 Joseph McGrath was reported to have said that Neenan was the sweepstake's 'principal agent in the United States and . . . might make a lot on it'.[86] Evidence of his subsequent wealth suggests that he did. In the late 1960s he was said to reside in a 'plush apartment on the East Side of Manhattan'.[87]

McGarrity was appointed as a special agent, a separate category from the normal foreign agents operating in America. This allowed him to recommend the appointment of his own agents to Hospitals Trust. His agents were designated a special set of identification numbers, between 5001 and 6000, known as the McGarrity series. Among the agents who held numbers in this series were IRA leader Moss Twomey, and Charles Rice, a New York solicitor and senior figure in the city's Clan na Gael organisation, who worked on behalf of Hospitals Trust in the United States, and whose brother Eamonn was a Fianna Fáil TD.[88] Another privilege of this special status was the right to claim commission for both McGarrity and his selling agent. This meant that the sales agent and McGarrity both got a commission of ten shillings on every book.[89] Under this system Joseph Andrews claimed McGarrity profited to the extent of £300,000 in commission between 1933 and 1938, earning £12,000 from the 1936 Derby sweepstake alone, and £20,125 from the 1938 Derby.[90] Following his death in 1940 McGarrity left an estate valued at $20,000. In view of his straitened financial circumstances in the early 1930s, this would suggest that his sweepstake agency had resulted in some financial benefit.[91]

Soon after securing his agency, McGarrity set about muscling in on existing agents in the USA. The Morans were eased out of the New York operation to be replaced by Connie Neenan.[92] Similarly, the manager of the California office, Eric Boden, and Michael O'Kiersey in Chicago, were ousted by Neenan.[93] O'Kiersey subsequently brought an unsuccessful suit against Hospitals Trust for payment that he alleged was still owed to him.[94] McGarrity's agents also appear to have received preferential treatment from Dublin by receiving their books before other agents; when these agents finally received their books and went to sell them to their regular clients they discovered that the McGarrity people had got there before them.[95] As an employee of Hospitals Trust's Foreign Department, Joseph Andrews received complaints from agents whose territory had been taken over by McGarrity. He claimed that Joseph McGrath 'was well aware of what was happening in New York and of how McGarrity was dominating the scene there . . . but he did nothing'.[96]

Andrews also alleged that the expenses of the New York office rose dramatically, from $10,000 to $35,000 per month, after its management was taken over by Connie Neenan, and that serious discrepancies appeared in its accounts.[97] Substantial expenses, in one case amounting to $40,000, were listed in the accounts under the vague heading of 'sundries'. When queried by the auditors, the New York office refused to give an explanation. Noting that the directors of Hospitals Trust appeared to turn a blind eye to the activities of the McGarrity/Neenan Agency, Andrews speculated that McGarrity was rewarding their non-interference:

> It seemed as if the actions with regard to the activities of the McGarrity agents were now also being condoned by the Directors of the Hospitals Trust Ltd. which would point to the fact that, perhaps, McGarrity was sharing his commission with 'some influential person or persons'.[98]

McGarrity's activity on behalf of both the IRA and the Irish sweepstake raises the question of whether or not there was any crossover between them. It certainly appears that the channels used to return sweepstake remittances and counterfoils to Dublin were also used to send arms and funds to the IRA.[99] British intelligence suspected that the sweepstake acted as a cover for routing German money to the IRA via the United States.[100] There were also suspicions that money contributed to the sweepstake was being diverted to funding the IRA.[101] At the least, it would appear that some of the personal profit accruing to McGarrity from his agency was used to fund them in the late 1930s. His diaries document occasions on which he appears to have made personal financial contributions to the IRA.[102]

The American authorities were well aware of McGarrity's and Neenan's association with the sweepstake. In May 1933 the American Vice Consul in Dublin reported back to Washington that 'the principal agency [for trafficking in sweepstake tickets] is an organization known as the Irish Republican Brotherhood'.[103] In 1938 Neenan and McGarrity were indicted in New York, along with Clifford Burgett and the Kellys from the New York office, for 'smuggling into the United States and distributing in interstate commerce tickets purporting to be lottery tickets'. In January 1939 all of the defendants, except Neenan and McGarrity, pleaded guilty; two of the Kellys were fined $1,000 each and given suspended prison sentences. Prosecution of the younger Kellys was abandoned because they were deemed to have been acting under the direction of parents and guardians.[104] Neenan failed to appear in court and a bench warrant was issued for his arrest, which he eluded successfully until 1943, when he eventually appeared to enter a not guilty plea; soon afterwards the case was dropped due to lack of evidence.[105] The prosecution of McGarrity was discharged when the only government witness, a Post Office inspector, failed to identify him.[106] The account of the prosecution in McGarrity's diary illustrates his obvious relief at its failure: 'neither pleaded guilty, nor not guilty. Was asked no questions nor answered any [.] Commissioner said [']discharged['] [.] Thank God! No charge now stands against me. Dear God I thank thee a million million times.' His relief was communicated to Hospitals Trust in the following cryptic cable: 'Papa's operation success [.] Tell little Ann and friends [.] Signed Deirdre.'[107]

DREW PEARSON

One of the most unlikely agents employed by Hospitals Trust in the USA during the 1930s was the journalist Drew Pearson.[108] A relief worker for the British Red Cross in the aftermath of the First World War, Pearson worked briefly as a university instructor in geography in the early 1920s before entering journalism in 1926 as foreign editor of the *United States Daily*. In 1932 he transferred to his more celebrated role as a political columnist, later becoming famous for his behind-the-scenes account of political life in Washington DC in his nationally syndicated 'Washington Merry-Go-Round' column.[109]

According to Pearson's unofficial biographer, Oliver Pilat, he was introduced to the sweepstake promoters by the Irish minister in Washington DC, Michael MacWhite, and at the start of the sweepstakes in 1930 was given a five-year contract to act as the western hemisphere director, for which he was paid an annual salary of $30,000, given use of a chauffeur-driven car, and allowed considerable legal and other expenses.[110] MacWhite and Pearson certainly knew each other and MacWhite was often referred to favourably in the 'Washington Merry-Go-Round', which was not the case with all diplomats based in the American capital.[111] Pearson ran his agency from a solicitor's office in Washington. He made good use of his newspaper contacts to further the cause of Hospitals Trust, using fellow reporters to sell tickets and arranging newspaper criticism of the Postmaster General's attempts to curtail sweepstake activity. Pearson's contacts were also very advantageous to the sweepstake from a publicity point of view, and he was said to have been involved in the

making of MGM's film *The Winning Ticket*, the story of an American
sweepstake winner.[112] Pearson's role in such an illegal enterprise appears
somewhat incongruous in view of his reputation as a 'neo-muckraker' who,
motivated by his Quaker upbringing, exposed corruption in high places and
whose 'call for higher standards of ethical behaviour among American
politicians may have been one of his most significant achievements'.[113]

FRAUD

In addition to the illegality of the sale of tickets, the appearance of the Irish
sweepstake in America in the 1930s fostered the growth of other illicit activities, largely associated with the sale of counterfeit tickets. In August 1930,
when tickets for the inaugural sweepstake draw were being distributed, the
Irish Independent carried a report of fraudulent lottery tickets on sale in New
York which were 'purporting to be issued by the Saorstat Government'.[114]
Similar fraudulent tickets were touted in January 1931 by a non-existent body
calling itself the Irish Free State Association.[115]

A more sophisticated effort to imitate the hospitals sweepstake and con
people into buying what they thought were genuine tickets was discovered by
police in Boston in June 1931. Thomas O. Mahaney, posing as a diplomatic
representative of the Irish government was distributing tickets for a hospital
sweepstake on the 1931 Cambridgeshire. It was clearly a fraudulent operation,
as Hospitals Trust did not run a sweepstake on that year's Cambridgeshire. A
printer, who brought the scheme to the attention of the police, had been
contracted to print one million tickets, at the cost of ten shillings or $2.50
each, some of which had already been distributed in New England and New
York. The *New York Times* believed that if the enterprise had not been
discovered, residents of the USA, Canada and Mexico could have been
defrauded of up to $2,500,000 a week.[116] The sweepstake authorities in
Dublin were aware of a similar 'fraud and forgery scheme' operating out of
Reading, Pennsylvania in late 1931.[117]

The discovery of such schemes did not deter fraudsters eager to capitalise
on the success of the Irish sweepstake. A 'Cork Irish Free State Sweepstake'
claiming falsely to have legislative sanction from the Oireachtas was operating
from Kansas City in 1933.[118] Another such bogus organisation was the Irish
Veterans' Association, Dublin, whose wares were detected in Ohio in 1937.[119]
In 1939 a Boston Post Office investigator claimed that four out of every five
sweepstake tickets sold in the USA were fake.[120] Many of these enterprises
did not confine their activities simply to aping the Irish sweepstake; a fraudu-

lent lottery dealer discovered in Indianapolis in 1941 had fake tickets for Cuban and Jamaican lotteries as well as for the Irish sweepstake.[121]

One of the biggest counterfeiting rackets was uncovered in New Jersey in January 1939. Police discovered over 200,000 fake tickets in the home of Philip Geffen, a bus terminal manager from New Rochelle who had a criminal record for receiving stolen goods. His accomplices, two New York printers, Edward Greenberg and Herman Pflaster, used duplicating equipment to forge serial numbers and watermarks onto bogus receipts that were given to unsuspecting customers in the belief that they were genuine. This was part of a syndicate operating throughout the north-eastern states that was believed to have defrauded the American public of up to $4,500,000 during the preceding three years.[122]

There is also evidence of illegality on the part of sweepstake employees. On arrival in New York in 1936 Joseph Andrews learned from John Kelly that 80,000 books of tickets had disappeared from the New York office. Kelly gave him the impression that this was not a robbery by an external party but that 'other members of the New York office might know something about it'. Andrews went further to hint at possible collusion from sweepstake headquarters in the disappearance of the books: 'It does seem strange that the serial letters and numbers of the "missing" books were never checked upon through the Dublin records to see if they appeared in sales returns.' Around the same time Joseph McGrath sent his henchman and former revolutionary colleague, Liam Tobin, to New York to investigate the circulation of forged tickets and receipts. On his return to Dublin, however, according to Joseph Andrews, McGrath refused to meet with or speak to Tobin, leading to speculation that McGrath preferred not to know the outcome of the investigation.[123]

One employee who caused considerable problems for Hospitals Trust in the USA in the 1930s was a former Irish army officer and Olympic athlete, Gerard Coughlan, who had been recommended for an agency by former Garda Commissioner, Eoin O'Duffy, and former president, W. T. Cosgrave. With his high profile as an athlete who had competed for Ireland at the 1928 Amsterdam Olympics, Coughlan was considered to be an ideal agent. However, he appears to have been too impatient to wait for his business to build up gradually, and began to cream off some of the remittances for himself instead of sending them back to Dublin. Eventually, all remittances to Dublin from Coughlan ceased and letters from ticket buyers complaining about the failure to receive receipts began to arrive at head office in Dublin. Hospitals Trust was forced to issue replacement tickets to some of those who had been defrauded by Coughlan.[124] One New York city customer was assured 'all the counterfoils transmitted to us through Mr Coughlan have been included in the draw for the Grand National Sweepstake'.[125]

The illegality of the sweepstake in America made it impossible to take any action against Coughlan. He remained there where he worked for a chemical firm.[126] A closer inspection of Coughlan's background might have alerted Hospitals Trust to his untrustworthiness. On four occasions during 1931 he was cited in *Stubbs' Gazette* for defaulting on debts totalling over £200, linked to unsuccessful efforts to run a physical education college in Dublin. This financial embarrassment might have been a factor in his removal from the reserve of officers in 1932, onto which he had been placed after his retirement from the army in 1929.[127]

Documents given to the American Consulate in Dublin by Joseph Andrews highlighted another incident of dishonesty on the part of a ticket seller for the American Travel Exchange (ATE). A typist employed by Western Union, named Miss Hannetty, was sent to America in 1938 by an ATE subagent, David Main, who was also a Western Union representative. Hannetty brought over tickets from the American Travel Exchange but, according to Andrews, 'proved untrustworthy and did not return all the money for the tickets she sold'.[128]

In an organisation with as large an underground network as Hospitals Trust it should not be surprising to discover some illegal activities by minor agents. However, there was one clear form of fraud being carried out by a person closely associated with the company's top management. Sidney Freeman, the brother of sweepstake publicity director, Spencer, was involved in systematic insider dealing in regards to the purchase of shares in potential winning tickets. Often referred to as 'Duggie' after the bookmaking firm of Douglas Stuart, in which he partnered his brother-in-law Martin Benson, Sidney Freeman travelled to New York with a considerable amount of cash at the time of each draw. There, from his base in one of the city's most luxurious hotels, he was informed by telegraph of the result of the draw as it took place in Dublin. The telegrams containing this information were sent in code so that nobody else would know the names of the horses drawn. By this method Sidney Freeman was aware of what lucky Americans had drawn the race favourites before they themselves were officially informed. This allowed him to purchase shares in these tickets before his competitors were aware of the draw result.[129]

In 1934 he admitted to the *New York Times* that he bought 'scores' of such tickets; prior to the draw for the 1934 Derby he paid $51,000 for a ticket which had drawn the Derby favourite Colombo, although the horses only finished in third place.[130] Three years later he spoke to the *Times* again, from his established base at the Ritz Carlton, where 'although reticent to discuss his affairs, he has indicated it has been quite profitable'.[131] In 1936 he offered drawers of Reynoldstown, the favourite for that year's Grand National,

$20,000 for their tickets, reminding them 'that no favorite had ever won the race' and that the tickets 'would only be worth $2,500 if the horse ran out of the money'. Eight of those who had drawn Reynoldstown accepted Freeman's offer. Reynoldstown subsequently romped home and Sidney Freeman collected eight first prizes of $150,000 [£30,000].[132] Prior to the 1939 Grand National draw, he was reported to have arrived in New York city with $1 million, and to have disposed of $700,000 soon afterwards, making a total of 200 deals with drawers of tickets, 120 of them in the New York metropolitan area alone. Nine half shares which he bought on tickets that drew the horses that came in the first three positions resulted in gains of $450,000 alone.[133] It was always assumed that Sidney Freeman was working in collaboration with the senior management of Hospitals Trust, who shared in his profits. In the post-war period, journalist Joe MacAnthony claimed that the company was buying up 60 per cent of its own winning tickets in Great Britain in this fashion.[134]

AMERICAN EFFORTS TO CURTAIL THE SWEEPSTAKE

The arms of the federal government principally charged with intercepting illicit sweepstake traffic were the Post Office Department and the Customs Bureau. The incumbent Republican administration of Herbert Hoover took a hard line against the Irish sweepstake at the time of its inception. In October 1930, the Irish minister in Washington, Michael MacWhite, reported that his office

> had many complaints from people who had purchased books of tickets for the Manchester Sweepstake, but had their letters containing remittances, addressed to the Hospitals Trust Ltd., or to individual post office boxes returned to them by order of the Postmaster General marked 'fraudulent'.[135]

In June 1931, the solicitor of the Post Office Department, Horace Donnelly, declared war on all illegal lotteries and sweepstakes operating in the USA, moving to prohibit newspapers carrying advertisements for lotteries from the mails. This action was prompted by the sudden increase in foreign lotteries operating in the USA in the early 1930s.[136] Post Office inspectors also announced that they would try to prevent the delivery of sweepstake prizes by post to American winners.[137]

One of the principal methods by which the Post Office sought to curtail the flow of tickets into its jurisdiction was through the issuing of fraud orders against any person or corporation whose correspondence was discovered to contain lottery-related material. On the issuance of such an order, the Post Office refused to handle mail for the recipient; it was stamped 'Fraudulent' and returned to the sender. Such an order had serious financial consequences as it forbade the certification of postal money orders drawn on the person against whom the order was made.[138] This was soon to pose a serious problem for a number of Irish companies transacting business with the USA.

In order to avoid detection, Hospitals Trust had advised its foreign customers to return their remittances and counterfoils to Ireland using the address of an acquaintance or business in the Irish Free State. They were advised to consult commercial directories, such as *Kelly's Manufacturers and Shippers of the World, vol. II*, and to send their sweepstake correspondence to the address of any Irish business listed therein.[139] The result was that numerous businesses in Dublin, including shops, department stores, publishers and others, received unsolicited mail intended for Hospitals Trust. The assumption was that such mail would be duly forwarded and presumably in many cases it was. However, when the Post Office Department discovered sweepstake material in the post addressed to Irish businesses and issued fraud orders against them, these firms found their legitimate transactions with customers in the USA disrupted. By May 1932, more than four hundred such fraud orders had been issued since the start of the Irish sweepstake two years previously.[140] In February 1932, the Post Office imposed 152 fraud orders, 16 of which were against addressees in Dublin.[141] Anticipating the issuance of such orders, Hospitals Trust frequently issued new lists of addresses to its American customers, in an effort to keep one step ahead of the Post Office inspectors.[142]

Both the Dublin Chamber of Commerce and the Irish Minister in Washington DC, Michael MacWhite, complained to the American authorities about the adverse effect which this was having on legitimate Irish trade with the USA, because of actions which many of the firms involved had neither sanctioned nor encouraged.[143] The Consul General in Dublin was sympathetic to the plight of such firms, warning his superiors in Washington 'that grave damage to American trade interests may quickly result if the United States Postal Department is not very cautious in the matter of intercepting mail'.[144] Among the prominent Irish businesses affected by such orders were sporting goods retailers Elverys, publishers Browne & Nolan, and the sweepstake's auditors, Craig Gardner & Company. Elverys sought to have the order against them lifted, admitting that they had previously acted as a ticket agent but no longer did so.[145] In the case of Browne & Nolan, the order was revoked on receipt of an assurance that the company was not involved in the transfer of correspondence on behalf of Hospitals Trust.[146]

After the Second World War, Craig Gardner sought to revoke the order imposed on them in 1938.[147] They signed a written declaration affirming that 'neither we, nor our employees nor agents, will hereafter participate in the sale or distribution through the mails to residents of the United States of lottery tickets of any character whatsoever'. In addition, any remittances or related material sent to them by American residents would be returned informing the sender of Craig Gardner's inability to furnish them with tickets. Nor would American correspondents be furnished with the names or addresses of those from whom tickets could be obtained.[148] The Postmaster General duly rescinded the fraud order against Craig Gardner in December 1947. However, it was not long until he realised he had been misled by the Hospitals Trust's auditors:

> It was not understood . . . that Craig, Gardner and Company are, in fact, 'pay-off' agents for United States winners in the lottery, nor was it understood that the concern's name is employed by the Hospitals Trust, Ltd. as a means for communicating with prizewinners in the United States . . .

The Postmaster General wanted to reimpose the fraud order, believing it to have been revoked in error.[149] However, the American legation in Dublin cautioned against any action that would disrupt legitimate mail to Ireland or cause embarrassment to either the legation or the Irish government.[150]

Fraud orders appear to have had the effect of forcing Irish banks not to act as intermediaries for sweepstake correspondence. Soon after the establishment of the sweepstake, Hospitals Trust gave the names and addresses of Dublin banks to its American customers. On discovering this the US Post Office contacted the banks involved and received assurances from them that they had informed Hospitals Trust that they would not act in such a role and the letters from the USA 'addressed to them for delivery to the lottery operators would be returned to senders'.[151] Joseph McGrath was thus forced to advise American customers not to send any more correspondence via banks in Ireland.[152]

A change in the US administration after the 1932 presidential election brought a noticeable change in the attitude to sweepstakes and lotteries. Franklin Roosevelt's new Postmaster General, the Irish American Jim Farley, relaxed many of the restrictions imposed by the outgoing regime. In 1934 Farley's Post Office Department announced that while it had 'no intention of nullifying the post laws or regulations with reference to the printing by newspapers of stories and pictures about winners of sweepstakes or lotteries operated in foreign countries', it would in future be guided by a 'liberal interpretation of such laws'.[153] For the remainder of the 1930s newspaper publicity of the sweepstake was very widespread, especially around the time of each draw. The exact nature of Jim Farley's relationship with Hospitals Trust is unclear. Joseph Andrews claimed that 'Farley was a regular visitor to Dublin where he met his friends from the Sweep' and that 'It was widely taken for granted in Hospitals Trust that he received annual "presents" for easing postal regulations to facilitate the passage of tickets'.[154] Farley visited Ireland on one occasion in late 1936, when he had his photograph taken beside the sweep-stake drum, only to receive 'some thousands of letters protesting against' this when he returned home.[155]

In 1937 there appeared to be a reversal of Farley's lenient policy and a return to that of Horace Donnelly. In March the *New York Times* reported that 'Newspapers and other publications having second class mailing privileges are prohibited under the Postal Laws from printing news items about lotteries even if the publications are not sent through the mails'.[156] It also reported surprise in 'congressional circles' at this announcement, and the expression of doubts as to whether the Post Office had the right to so interfere with newspapers not carried in the mail.[157] The Irish embassy in Washington was also taken unawares by the reimposition of the ban on newspaper coverage of lotteries: 'Why it has now been restored it is difficult to say, but it is believed to be mainly due to the huge space devoted by American newspapers to the Irish sweepstake results.'[158] The action was attributed to the very officious Post Office Attorney, Mr Karl A. Crowley who is . . . a Texas Methodist with ambitions to become Governor of that State' and Farley assured the Irish minister that 'he was determined to ignore it'.[159] Judging by the continued coverage of sweepstake draws in the mainstream American newspapers the policy reversal had little practical application.

While Jim Farley may have been prepared to adopt a softer policy towards the Irish sweepstake the same did not apply to other government agencies. The Treasury sought to locate those agents who were receiving considerable commissions in order to tax such undisclosed profits. Customs continued to detect tickets being smuggled into America, and had some noticeable successes. One million tickets for the 1931 Derby sweepstake were reported to have been seized in New York from a passenger travelling on the *Aquitania*; Joseph McGrath admitted that some tickets had been confiscated, but claimed that it was only one or two books.[160] In 1935 $1.5 million worth of tickets was confiscated in Philadelphia. In the same year New York customs officers were said to have 'seized a huge bundle labeled "Rags made in Belgium"', that was found to contain 50,000 books of tickets. On the eve of the 1936 Grand National sweepstake, $100,000 worth of tickets was taken from the office of a Baltimore insurance broker who was also the prin-cipal ticket distributor in the city.[161] In 1938, 'a small truck load' of 46,000 books of tickets, valued at $2.5 million, was discovered on the SS *Capulin* at Philadelphia, and the ship's captain, E. W. Hickey, was fined $1,000 by the Washington DC Commissioner of Customs for failing to declare his illicit cargo.[162]

The Justice Department pursued agents responsible for the distribution of those tickets which successfully eluded either the Customs or Post Office officials. In one notable case in 1936, father and son sweepstake agents, Oscar and Lincoln Stevenson from New York were convicted of using the mails to receive and deliver sweepstake tickets. Believed to be among the chief distribution agents for tickets in the USA, they operated out of a four-room suite at the Belleclaire Hotel on West 77th Street and from an office at 147 West 42nd Street that masqueraded as a beauty parlour.[163] Although they received very light penalties, fines of $200 and $350 respectively, greater damage was done to the sweepstake organisation in New York by the discovery of their operation, including the names of thousands of selling agents.[164] The Stevenson trial highlighted the popularity of the sweepstake in New York at the time; it took a number of days to empanel a jury because it proved so difficult to find twelve people none of whom had ever purchased an Irish sweepstake ticket. Having 'exhausted two panels' of potential jurors, a jury was not empanelled successfully 'until three Deputy United States Marshals . . . went out into the streets and hailed pedestrians into the new Federal Building for jury service'.[165] In 1939 a Los Angeles district attorney subpoenaed 72 sweepstake prizewinners to appear before a grand jury in an effort to smash the ticket distribution network on the west coast and eliminate counterfeit lotteries.[166]

In addition to trying to frustrate the sweepstake operation from within the USA, the State Department undertook moves to convince the Irish government to pressurise Hospitals Trust to desist from its more egregious violations of American law. As early as 1931 the Postmaster General's office asked the State Department to obtain an assurance from the Irish authorities 'that appropriate action would be taken by them with a view to having the Hospitals Trust, Ltd . . . refrain from mailing their lottery matter into this country and otherwise violating our postal laws'.[167] The following year the State Department considered inviting the Irish minister in Washington DC, Michael MacWhite, to the State Department 'to point out to him that there ought to be something which the Irish Free State Government could do toward diminishing or preventing entirely the flooding of this country with sweepstake tickets in violation of our laws', but it was considered that there was very little which could be done to ask the Irish government 'to take steps to prevent the importation of lottery tickets into the US . . . because of the lack of control in any country over the content of the mails'.[168] In 1936 the Post Office Department reiterated these calls to bring pressure on the Irish Free State government to take action against the circulation of illegal sweepstake tickets in America.[169]

Finally in 1937, the consul in Dublin, John Cudahy, raised the objections of his government to the activities of Hospitals Trust and its agents in the USA directly with the Irish government. With Irish-American ancestry, Cudahy was deemed more sympathetic to Ireland 'than his more anglophile predecessors'.[170] The issue was initially brought to the attention of the Secretary of the Department of External Affairs, Joseph Walshe, who agreed that soliciting ticket sales in the USA in violation of criminal law 'was not consistent with the amity between friendly nations', and promised to raise the matter with Hospitals Trust, discouraging them from such activity.[171] Walshe's representations did not have the desired effect; late in 1937 the State Department still had evidence that sweepstake material was being posted into the USA.[172]

Cudahy was instructed to revisit the issue with Walshe in 1938 'to ascertain whether the Irish Government intends to take some action which would prevent the solicitation in this country of the purchase of these tickets'. Instances were cited of assistance given to the USA by foreign governments during the prohibition era which could act as useful examples of how the Éire government might be able to act in relation to the illegal distribution of sweepstake tickets in the USA.[173] Cudahy's representations received a sympathetic hearing from Taoiseach and Minister for External Affairs, Eamon de Valera, who was never a strong advocate of the sweepstake, and as Minister for External Affairs was well aware of the damage which they did to Éire's reputation abroad. In spite of this shared feeling, however, de Valera was unable to produce any solution for Cudahy and his government. The sweepstake was legal in Éire, thus by asking the government to take measures to prevent Hospitals Trust violating American laws, the USA was effectively asking Éire to be responsible for the enforcement of American criminal law. The only commitment which the Taoiseach was able to offer the American consul was 'to take the matter very seriously under advisement and . . . try to find some method whereby closer cooperation with the American authorities might be found, but at the present time no feasible method occurred to him'.[174]

Cudahy also lobbied those responsible for the relationship between the hospitals and the sweepstakes, aware that they would be sensitive to any adverse publicity. In a meeting with Sir Joseph Glynn, of the Associated Hospitals Sweepstake Committee, and Joseph McGrath, he predicted that the continued exponential growth of the sweepstake's popularity in America would eventually be self-defeating: 'It would become a wholesome scandal . . . and measures would be demanded in Congress for its suppression.' He received assurances that Hospitals Trust would instruct its agents no longer to 'engage in advertising or wholesale methods of distribution'. McGrath also promised that neither tickets nor lottery related material would be sent through the mails.[175] Arising from this agreement, Hospitals Trust appears to have toned down its activities in the US for a period; in May 1939, P. J. Fleming informed agents that: 'Indiscriminate circularising on the part of some Distributors forced us to take drastic action in the interests of the organisation and all concerned. However, we are now reverting to the old arrangement, but on very strict conditions.' Agents were no longer to solicit indiscriminately for business: 'If it is discovered that you are circularising, your appointment shall be immediately cancelled and no credit shall be given for any commission that may have accrued.'[176] John Cudahy's exhortations may not have put a stop to sweepstake activity in the USA, but they forced Hospitals Trust to curtail the egregiousness with which its agents flouted the law.

In spite of Cudahy's efforts, there was a limit to how far the American government was prepared to push the matter. Following Cudahy's efforts, the Post Office Department indicated that it was 'not disposed to press the matter to a point where it might cause a rift in good relations between the United States and the Irish Government'. It appears to have been satisfied with McGrath's promises and by the fact that the American government's displeasure had been communicated officially to its Irish counterpart.[177]

While most arms of the federal government sought to prevent the sale and distribution of sweepstake tickets, the Treasury actually benefited from this. The Internal Revenue Service (IRS) was interested in claiming substantial income tax on the commission paid to agents. The coffers of the federal government were also augmented with the tax levied on prizewinners. Winners of first prize ($150,000) were forced to surrender almost $65,000, while winners of second ($75,000) and third ($50,000) prizes had to part with just under $20,000 and $10,000 respectively.[178]

In an effort to discover the identity of American prizewinners, the IRS sought assistance from within Ireland. In 1938 the revenue collector at Detroit refused to allow Bello Stefanoff, a Serbian-born resident of St Louis, to travel to Dublin to collect his winnings for fear he would not return and thus evade his tax payment. On the authority of Stefanoff, the American consul in Dublin was delegated to collect the prize money and deduct the income tax due on it.[179] The IRS was still dissatisfied with the extent to which it was able to discover the identity of prizewinners. In August 1939, an official from the Treasury Department sought the assistance of the Irish government in getting access to Hospitals Trust's records, a request that was considered to be naïve and not of concern to the Irish government.[180]

AMERICAN ATTITUDES TO THE SWEEPSTAKE

By the mid-1930s the Irish sweepstake had clearly captured the imagination of many Americans. Journalists were especially interested in this new enterprise. Writing in the *New York Times Magazine* at the time of the 1934 Derby sweepstake, Clair Price compared the sweepstake draw to 'a kind of Mardi Gras, minus only the confetti and the false noses'.[181] In 1937 Hugh Smith wrote in the *New York Times* of its importance to Irish commerce: 'running the sweeps has become one of the Free State's most important industries.'[182] *Good Housekeeping* suggested a themed 'Irish Sweepstakes Party' for St Patrick's Day in 1934.[183] The F Street and Soroptimist Clubs in Washington DC held Irish sweepstake parties in 1934, and Mrs Nina Cunningham also hosted one at the Tryangle Club in Bloomington, Indiana in 1938.[184] In the 1950s the *Washington Post* printed a recipe for 'sweepstakes bread', a variation on Irish soda bread that included caraway seeds and raisins.[185]

American newspapers were especially interested in reporting human-interest stories concerning the fortunes of sweepstake winners. The death of Rolland C. Steele, who won $40,000 in 1935 and was stabbed while celebrating his good fortune in New Orleans, was widely reported.[186] Eleanor Hanley of Hoboken, New Jersey, suffered a physical breakdown and told a number of newspapers that 'My winnings have brought me nothing but misery'.[187] By 1938, the $150,000 that Amos Stout won when Reynoldstown won the 1936 Derby had been whittled away to just over $3,000.[188] Philanthropic gestures by sweepstake winners were frequently reported: Herbert Walton gave most of his $3,800 prize to the Overlook Hospital in New Jersey, while Pearl and Benjamin Mason used their $150,000 windfall to redevelop a block of slums into low-rent housing for fellow black Americans in south Philadelphia.[189] Dramatic scenarios, such as the loss of a prize-winning ticket or the feared kidnap of a couple *en route* to Ireland to collect their winnings also gave added fame to the sweepstake.[190] The good fortune of O. P. Nelson of St Paul, Minnesota, who won three prizes between 1936 and 1937, made it into the syndicated 'Ripley's Believe it or Not' column.[191]

Current affairs periodicals also took an interest in the sweepstake. In 1934 *Harper's Magazine* dispatched John McCarthy to Dublin to research an in-depth article about all aspects of sweepstake activity. The result was one of the first detailed accounts of the entire enterprise, highlighting the size and operating methods of Hospitals Trust, the extent to which the draw had become a tourist attraction, the use of the Irish diaspora as a ticket distribution network, and the difficulties posed by fraudulent sweepstake imitators in America.[192] The article was implicitly critical of many aspects of the sweepstake. McCarthy calculated that the percentage of those winning prizes in the 1934 Derby Sweepstake was only .0035 per cent of ticket buyers. He also raised the issue of American and British 'banking institutions with the loftiest reputations' carrying out financial transactions related to the sweepstake, in spite of its illegality in their jurisdictions: 'The banks' commissions for handling such big-money transactions are too sweet to refuse.'[193] McCarthy's most stringent criticism was reserved for the promoters. Richard Duggan was described as 'a quiet, retiring chap' who was 'Once a bookie', but now 'rides to the hounds with the swankiest of the swank Irish gentry'. He was also well aware of the growing concern being voiced at the substantial profits accruing to the promoters, as the following sardonic comment indicates:

> Considering the huge organization necessary to handle an Irish Sweep, the profit percentage for the promoters is fairly reasonable, especially as the juicy, private profit melon from the Irish sweeps is not cut many ways. Messrs Duggan and McGrath comprise in the main the entire body of the deserving stockholders. Furthermore, the owners of the Sweeps are not faced with sharing profits with politicians or other usual 'We-Boys' who declare themselves in on such sporting enterprises in America and elsewhere. Graft is unknown in Ireland.[194]

The syndicated columnist Westbrook Pegler, noted for his conservative opinions and aggressive journalistic style, was a harsh critic of the sweep.[195] In his 'Fair enough' column in March 1936 he criticised the mis-allocation of funds. The sheer amount of money entering the Irish Free State should have produced massive medical benefits for its population:

> considering that they are supposed to have had the benefit of more than $40,000,000 worth of medical attention since the lottery began . . . There are not quite 3,000,000 souls in the Irish Free State and unless the majority of the population has been enjoying very poor health the dividends from the great international gamble should have been sufficient to relieve the sick of every ill money can cure.

However, on making enquiries of his 'kinfolk in Connemara and elsewhere', he discovered that they 'have not been getting their medicine on time and very little medicine at all', although '[t]here is plenty of money for advertising and salaries and for the wine with which to reduce to a state of coma the journalists of the wide world who can be induced to accept free transportation to Ireland to ballyhoo the promotion'. He went on to predict that the sweep would eventually fall victim to its own success: 'The hospitals' share is too big to be spent usefully in a short time and the British boycott was imposed only because the lottery outgrew its philanthropic character and became a serious parasitic growth on the body of England.'[196] The following month his focus shifted to Hospitals Trust's violation of American law to sell tickets illegally, criticising the Irish government for its failure to prevent such activity.[197] In a similar vein, he was opposed to the more lenient policy adopted after the appointment of Jim Farley as Postmaster General.[198]

The piece which did most damage to the reputation of the sweepstake in the USA was the publication of 'Not a clean sweep: The inside workings of the Irish lottery', in *Collier's* magazine on 4 June 1938, an account of the inner workings of the sweep by one of its American agents writing under the pseudonym of Fred McDonald, in collaboration with *Collier's* Bob Considine.[199] McDonald had been staying with family in Dublin at the time of the Wall Street Crash, which resulted in the loss of considerable investments for him. Rather than return home to a bleak future, he stayed in Ireland and attended the first sweepstake draw in November 1930. Seeing a new business opportunity he offered his services to Hospitals Trust as an agent. Following instant success in selling tickets, he rose to the level of distributor by the time of the 1932 Derby sweepstake.

The most damaging aspect of McDonald's account was the allegation of the level of fraud involved in the sweepstake operation in America. Readers were warned that if they were in possession of a ticket they did not have 'the faintest idea whether [their] ticket is genuine' and that the odds were two-to-one against being able to buy a genuine one. Boiling the ticket in 'three parts water and one part common household tea' would prove whether or not a ticket was genuine as the watermark on the real ones would still be visible afterwards. Sweepstake customers were also warned that the mere possession of a receipt was no guarantee either, as counterfeiters had proven adept at forging those also. Between the activities of counterfeiters and the authorities who tried to stop the sale of tickets in America, McDonald estimated that Hospitals Trust was outmanoeuvred to the tune of 'a quarter of a billion dollars in paper profits each year'. Due to the large number of fake tickets in circulation, the chance of winning a prize was said to 'correspond roughly to your chance of being named emperor of Japan'. For those who succeeded in buying the genuine article there was a lesson in what actually became of their $2.50 contribution. They were disabused of any notions that the majority of this money went to help Irish hospitals:

> the man who sells it to you takes a commission of 42 cents. In time the distributor who supplies the agent with the ticket gets 21 cents, and the wholesaler who supplies the distributor gets another 21 cents, reducing your $2.50 to $1.66. About fifty more cents are taken out at the Dublin office for 'expenses,' a word that covers a multitude of abuses. Out of the remaining dollar, give or take a few cents, now comes the twenty-five per cent cut given to the fifty-two beneficiary Irish hospitals ... So by the time your $2.50 is ready to go into the winners' pool it has shriveled to about 75 cents.

Many of the allegations made by McDonald correspond with other accounts of the sweepstake's activities in the USA in the 1930s, including those of Joseph Andrews. However, McDonald also made the unusual accusation that the draw was fixed to ensure a good geographical distribution of tickets:

> the operators of the Sweep definitely fix the Draw so that no section of this betting-mad globe is left out of the prize distribution? . . . 'Of course we spread the prizes around,' one of them told me in Dublin. 'We've got to. If we didn't there would be millions of protests from the sections that were left out.'

This was the allegation to which Hospitals Trust chose to respond. In a letter to the *Washington Post*, which had published extracts from the *Collier's* article, publicity director, Jack O'Sheehan, promised to give $50,000 to any charity in the USA if the claim of draw fixing could be substantiated.[200] There is very little evidence that the sweepstake draw was fixed. On the contrary, there is ample evidence that Hospitals Trust went to great lengths to ensure a fair mixing of counterfoils. What is most interesting about O'Sheehan's response is that he chose the accusation which is most likely to have been untrue, while studiously ignoring the more plausible allegations concerning the circulation of fraudulent tickets and payment of handsome commissions to agents. The critical nature of much of the American coverage of the sweepstake, especially the articles in *Harper's* and *Collier's* lends much credence to Marion Casey's argument that the sweepstake created an adverse impression of Ireland: 'Clothed in an aura of respectability, wherein pretty Dublin nurses drew winning tickets from a huge drum in Dublin . . . the Irish Hospitals' Sweepstakes nevertheless contributed to an image of the Irish as not being completely honest.'[201]

Winning the Irish sweepstake was a popular theme in many American films of the 1930s, such as the 1935 production *Sweepstakes Annie* (known in the UK as *Annie doesn't live here anymore*), in which the eponymous heroine, Annie Foster, won $150,000 in the Irish sweepstake, only to be exploited by all those around her.[202] In *Sweepstakes Winner* (1939), waitress Jennie Jones used her $150,000 to exact revenge on con men who swindled her out of her inheritance.[203] Well-known cartoon characters were also seen to gamble on the Irish sweepstake on screen. In a 1938 episode of *Captain and the Kids*, entitled 'The winning ticket', the characters successfully foiled the efforts of the evil John Silver to steal their winning sweepstake ticket, and in a 1941 episode entitled 'Olive's $weep$take', Popeye's girlfriend, Olive Oyl, won first prize but could not find her ticket. The sweepstake theme continued in post-war American cartoons; in 'The Sweepstake ticket' episode of the *Flintstones'* first season in 1960, Fred Flintstone and Barney Rubble purchased a ticket unbeknown to their wives, Wilma and Betty, unaware that the women had done likewise.[204] Winning the Irish sweepstake also formed part of the plot in contemporary popular novels that drew on the Irish immigrant experience in America, such as Doran Hurley's *Herself, Mrs Patrick Crowley: A romantical tale* (1939).

Another stratum of American public opinion with an interest in the fortunes of the Irish sweepstake was the lobby that promoted the legalisation of gambling. The dire financial situation prevailing in depression-era America was part of the motivation behind this campaign. A correspondent to the *New York Times* writing in 1933 under the pseudonym 'Fix It' proposed that the solution 'to end the depression and obtain a vast amount of much needed revenue is ... to legalize hospital sweepstakes, and thus help a great charitable work all over the country'.[205] Even President Franklin D. Roosevelt was believed to favour the introduction of a national lottery for charitable purposes.[206] New York Mayor, Fiorello LaGuardia, preferred introducing a lottery to raising new taxes to alleviate New York City's depression-hit finances and his city council passed a motion in favour of such a move in 1938.[207]

Edward A. Kenney, a Democratic Congressman from New Jersey, was the most prominent political advocate of repealing the prohibition on lotteries. In June 1933 he introduced a bill to Congress seeking to repeal the ban on the use of mails for transmitting lottery material in an effort to promote a lottery for the benefit of war veterans. The following January he introduced a further lottery bill 'to authorize the raising of funds by lottery for the purpose of providing additional means of defraying the cost of government, including expenditures authorized for veterans and their dependents, and for other purposes'. The bill sought to authorise the Veterans' Administration, on the president's approval, to conduct a lottery to raise funds not exceeding $1 billion in any one year.[208] Under the bill's provisions, the government would sell lottery tickets at the cost of $2 each. Forty per cent of the proceeds would be retained for distribution to the VA and 60 per cent allocated as prizes, ranging in value from $500 to $120,000.[209] In support of the bill, the substantial amounts of money leaving for foreign lotteries, in particular the Irish sweepstake, was noted.[210]

The issue of providing financial aid to veterans of the First World War was a thorny one in the USA during the great depression; Herbert Hoover's use of the armed forces to clear the 'bonus army' of 15,000 veterans and their families demanding the early payment of bonuses, due to them in 1945, from Washington DC in 1932 contributed to his defeat in the presidential election later that year. The Irish minister in Washington, Michael MacWhite, reported back to Iveagh House that Kenney's bill was initially regarded as a joke, but that sentiment in its favour had grown 'like a snowball'. However, his conclusion that it was unlikely to become law for a very long time, if at all, because of religious opposition to legalised gambling proved correct. Kenney's bill reached the House Ways and Means Committee, where it provoked considerable debate, but made no further progress.[211]

Outside of Congress political pressure for the legalisation of lotteries was also growing at state level; bills for the promotion of state lotteries were introduced in New York, Kansas and Ohio.[212] An extra-parliamentary lobby was also emerging. Edward Kenney was a strong supporter of the National Conference for Legalizing Lotteries, formed in New York in 1935 and presided over by Grace Harriman.[213] A similar organisation formed in Boston – the Massachusetts Council for Legalizing Lotteries – included among its officials Sheila O'Donovan Rossa, daughter of the old Fenian leader, Jeremiah O'Donovan Rossa.[214] Although such efforts to legalise lotteries in interwar America were ultimately unsuccessful, they indicated that American public opinion was beginning to soften on the issue, a trend which would continue in the post-war period, paving the way for the eventual introduction of state lotteries in the 1960s.

SIX

SURVIVAL AND RECOVERY
1939–61

—

THE SWEEPSTAKE IN WARTIME

The hospitals sweepstake achieved phenomenal success during its first decade, surviving the threat posed to it by the British Betting and Lotteries Act. However, as the end of the 1930s approached, an even greater threat beckoned in the shape of world war. The gross proceeds of the sweepstakes on the 1939 Derby and Cesarewitch – the latter held after the start of the war in spite of the actual race being cancelled – were considerably lower, at £1,670,839 and £1,353,719 respectively (see Appendix). Restriction of postal services and the curtailment of racing in Great Britain now raised the serious question of whether the sweepstake could continue during the war.

Comparing the gross proceeds from tickets sales for the war years with the foregoing decade indicates how perilous the sweepstake's existence became in the early 1940s. Proceeds from each sweepstake from late 1940 until 1942 were well under £100,000. Even at the highest points, early in 1940 and after the end of the war in 1945, they only reached £333,000 (see Appendix). There were a number of reasons for this decline. Postal restrictions and increased postal censorship reduced foreign contributions significantly. Rumours that the sweepstake had closed affected American subscriptions badly in 1940, as did the decline in value of sterling relative to the US dollar, which had the effect of reducing the dollar value of sweepstake prizes by 28 per cent.[1] The curtailment of racing in Britain led to most wartime sweepstakes being run on less well-known Irish races. In order to maximise the number of customers, the price of tickets for most wartime sweepstakes was halved from ten to five shillings. Reduced proceeds inevitably meant less money was available for prizes; first prize in most of the sweepstakes during the war was £10,000, one third of the pre-war sum. This much less lucrative reward now attracted fewer customers.

News of the sweepstake's declining fortunes led competitors to encroach on its territory; Canada was reported to be flooded with Cuban lottery tickets in 1940 and in 1941 and a South African newspaper commented that 'Éire's loss in the famous Irish sweepstakes, due to the war making them impracticable, is Rhodesia's gain. Recent lists of winners in the Rhodesian Sweep

144

made clear the growing popularity of the Colony's enterprise in this "easy way to wealth" scheme'.[2]

HOSPITALS TRUST (1940) LIMITED

In late 1939 and early 1940 rumours circulated widely both in Ireland and abroad that the sweepstake was going to close down for the duration of the conflict. In January 1940 a number of British regional newspapers asserted confidently that 'The Irish Hospitals' Sweep is to close down after the next sweep on the Grand National'.[3] A similar story was reported in Canada, the USA and Australia.[4] To counter the adverse effect of these false stories Hospitals Trust distributed leaflets denying them and reminding foreign customers that 'Ireland is not at war . . . As a neutral country it is desirous and capable of maintaining its industries and institutions. The sweepstakes will, therefore, be continued.'[5]

The war did not force Hospitals Trust to close down completely but it did cause a serious curtailment of its business and a complete overhaul of the company. In October 1939 a memo from the directors warned staff that the war would have an adverse effect on the company. The first lay-offs came in February 1940 when 900 staff were made redundant, including 'men . . . [who had been] with the sweep for several years and having distinguished records in the national struggle'.[6] The remaining 1,300 permanent staff were given one week's notice on 1 April 1940, with a promise of assistance in helping them seek other employment.[7]

In July 1940, 500 of the women who had been laid off held a meeting in Dublin to draw attention to the distress caused by their dismissal. Most of them had been entirely dependent on their employment at Hospitals Trust. They demanded that the government 'devise a scheme for providing work for the recently dismissed employees of Hospitals Trust', and that if plans for a Red Cross factory were realised they be given first preference in seeking jobs there.[8] As the sweepstake continued on a much reduced scale during the war, some of the staff were retained on a temporary basis, but their pay and conditions were criticised in the Dáil by Labour's James Everett, who labelled the weekly wage of £3 10s per week, often including Saturday and Sunday work, a 'scandal', while there were 'well-off people in the Government service, friends of the directors and friends of the promoters, receiving fabulous salaries for excuses of jobs [in Hospitals Trust]'.[9] By December 1940, 700 had been re-employed, at least temporarily.[10]

On 4 April 1940 Joseph McGrath announced that Hospitals Trust had gone into voluntary liquidation 'owing to it being considered uneconomical and impracticable to continue an organisation designed for international business when war conditions so greatly limit the scope of its operations'.[11] A new company was duly formed, named Hospitals Trust (1940) Limited, with Joseph McGrath and the late Richard Duggan's sons, Patrick and Richard, as directors. Shareholders in the new enterprise were McGrath, Spencer Freeman, the two Duggans, and Hospitals Trust's solicitor, Philip O'Reilly and his wife.[12]

Although Spencer Freeman was listed as one of the directors of the new company he had very little involvement during the war. Instead he returned to British government service with Lord Beaverbrook's Emergency Services Organisation in the Ministry of Aircraft Production. He also served on the Radio Board and towards the end of the war was seconded to the Board of Trade to assist in restoring British industry to peacetime production. After the war he returned to his old position with Hospitals Trust. In recognition of his service he was awarded a CBE in the King's birthday honours in 1942.[13]

The draw for the Grand National sweepstake was held on 2 April 1940. The liquidation of the original Hospitals Trust and dismissal of its staff immediately afterwards left the future of the sweepstake in doubt. Opening the draw Sir Joseph Glynn of the Associated Hospitals Sweepstake Committee called on the government 'to alter the law so as to prevent any heavy loss falling on either the Associated Hospitals' Committee or on Hospitals Trust'.[14] The future of the sweepstake now appeared to be in the hands of the government.

THE PUBLIC HOSPITALS (AMENDMENT) ACTS, 1939 AND 1940

The passage of legislation to protect Hospitals Trust during the war was largely responsible for the survival of the sweepstake. Early in 1939, aware of the potentially drastic consequences of the looming war, Hospitals Trust had convinced the government to introduce amending legislation to the 1933 Public Hospitals Act that would have the effect of indemnifying it against any losses that the sweepstake might suffer. The first Public Hospitals (Amendment) Act of 1939, passed in July, established a reserve fund, separate from the Hospitals Trust Fund and capped at £250,000 'to meet expenses that would not be fully covered by the percentage of receipts from sale of tickets fixed by the Act of 1933'.[15] Under section 5 of the act, in a case where the Minister for Local Government and Public Health was

> Satisfied . . . that, owing to an emergency which could not reasonably have been foreseen by the sweepstake committee managing such sweepstake and which was not occasioned or contributed to by any act or default of such sweepstake

committee . . . the Minister may direct the [Hospitals Trust] Board to pay to such sweepstake committee such sum as may be necessary to discharge the amount by which the said expenses exceed the said total amount so lawfully applicable for the payment thereof.[16]

The legislation resulted from lobbying by the Associated Hospitals Sweepstake Committee who warned that the future of the sweepstake was in doubt if such a provision was not introduced: 'the risk now involved in proceeding with further sweepstakes is too great unless provision is made to secure the Committee against loss.'[17] Fine Gael offered no opposition to the legislation, believing that 'It simply makes a working arrangement for matters that might arise, and that were unforeseen in the ordinary way'.[18] The lone voice of complaint belonged to Labour's James Everett, who used the debate on the bill to criticise working conditions in Hospitals Trust.[19] Seanad Éireann did not object either and the bill was enacted in July 1939 to take effect regarding sweepstakes from 1940 Grand National onwards.

With minimal opposition the Oireachtas had legislated to ensure that, in the event of war affecting adversely the income from sweepstakes, the promoters would not suffer a financial loss. The practical effect of this became clear after the 1940 Grand National sweepstake, when a payment of £61,628 was made from the reserve fund to Hospitals Trust to compensate them for the fact that the sum allowed for expenses had not been sufficient to cover the running costs of the sweepstake which brought in just over £500,000. The Hospitals Trust Board's share of the proceeds was £102,718 (see Appendix). Effectively, 60 per cent of the hospitals' share of the 1940 Grand National sweepstake was returned to compensate the promoters for the loss they had incurred in running the sweepstake.

Realising the practical impact of the 1939 act, the government acted quickly to introduce legislation that would prevent a recurrence of this embarrassing situation. The act was not considered to be applicable to future sweepstakes because it had been introduced to deal with an 'emergency which . . . could not reasonably be foreseen when starting the sweepstake'. However, by 1940, with the war in progress in Europe, it 'could not be relied upon to cover a second emergency, as in the present conditions an emergency could reasonably be anticipated'. With the 1939 amending act no longer applicable, Hospitals Trust demanded 'fresh safeguards against loss in conducting sweepstakes'. To satisfy this demand, the Sweepstake Committee requested that in circumstances where 'the expenses of the sweepstake exceed 30% of the monies received from the sale of tickets, the excess shall be paid out of monies in the control of the Hospitals Trust Board' and that the Minister for Local Government and Public Health be given 'absolute power . . . to allocate monies in the control of the Hospitals Trust Board for hospital purposes towards meeting the expenses of a sweepstake'. This would require the enactment of yet another amendment to the Public Hospitals Act. Civil servants were anxious at extending the precedent set in the 1939 act of subsidising 'future sweepstakes out of the proceeds of past sweepstakes' and felt that 'it would be difficult to justify' giving the minister *carte blanche* to disseminate the Hospitals Trust Fund money in the manner suggested by Hospitals Trust and the Sweepstakes Committee, recommending instead that the Minister for Justice be permitted to increase the proportion of proceeds allocated for expenses by up to 10 per cent.[20]

Agreement was eventually reached whereby 'A definite percentage, equivalent to thirty per cent of the proceeds from the sale of tickets on each sweepstake [was] to be fixed to cover all expenses of promoting a sweepstake . . . including promoter's fee'. To ensure an adequate amount was available to pay this figure, the Sweepstake Committee accepted a temporary reduction, for the duration of the war, of 5 per cent in the sum allocated to the hospitals. Hospitals Trust was thus guaranteed an income of 30 per cent of the gross proceeds from ticket sales. In cases where the expenses of running the sweepstake did not amount to thirty per cent the balance would constitute Hospitals Trust's promoter's fee.[21]

The Public Hospitals (Amendment) Act of 1940, which was principally concerned with establishing the bed bureau, also legalised this new method of paying expenses. In practice for the remaining sweepstakes between its enactment and the end of the war, the proportion of proceeds given to the Hospitals Trust Board was reduced from 25 to 20 per cent, from which stamp duty also had to be deducted. The 1940 Phoenix Plate and Irish Cesarewitch were the only sweepstakes held after the passing of this act in which expenses exceeded 30 per cent and Hospitals Trust was forced to repay £2,874 to the Hospitals Trust Board. In the remaining 23 sweepstakes, until the end of 1945, expenses never exceeded 30 per cent so the balance making up 30 per cent was paid by the Hospitals Trust Board to Hospitals Trust. In short, hospitals had to endure a reduction of 5 per cent in the already meagre amount accruing to them during the wartime sweepstakes to ensure that the promoters were not at a loss financially.

Aside from some TDs and Senators who questioned the incongruity of including provisions to alter the payment of promoters' fees in a bill primarily concerned with establishing the bed bureau, the only note of concern in the Oireachtas came once again from James Everett, the only TD who noticed, or perhaps the only one willing to state publicly, that the proposed amendment would have the effect of empowering Hospitals Trust 'to receive more in respect of expenses and to give less to the hospitals'.[22]

In addition to the passage of legislation to protect Hospitals Trust, other actions were taken by the government to facilitate the sweepstake during the war, especially in the area of posts and telegraphs, where the operation of wartime censorship had the potential to obstruct Hospitals Trust's communications with its customers. A reciprocal arrangement was put in place whereby a member of the postal censorship staff was based in Hospitals Trust's headquarters in Ballsbridge to screen outgoing mail and Hospitals Trust employees were allowed into the postal censorship rooms to seal sweepstake mail after it had been examined by the censors. To avoid foreign postal authorities noticing that the Irish censors were passing sweepstake mail, illegal in most of its destinations, Hospitals Trust supplied fresh envelopes and stamps so that mail passed by the censor could be re-packaged. An exception was also made in the use of foreign language telegrams. Officially foreign languages were prohibited, to get around the problem of telegrams in German, but Hospitals Trust was allowed to send telegrams in French and Spanish, if accompanied by an English translation.[23]

HORSE RACING IN NEUTRAL IRELAND

The continuation of horse racing in neutral Éire was another reason for the survival of the sweepstake during the war. The curtailment of racing in Britain had the potential to destroy the sweepstake, had an alternative, albeit a much less glamorous one, not been available in Ireland. By the 1940s Joseph McGrath had emerged as one of the leading figures in Irish horse racing and in this role was extremely influential in the continuation of the sport. McGrath's involvement in racing began in the mid-1930s; following the death of Richard Duggan he bought his deceased partner's star mare, Smokeless. In 1939 he became a serious racing man with the purchase of the Brownstown Stud in the Curragh, County Kildare, eventually turning it into 'one of the greatest thoroughbred centres anywhere in the world'.[24] Also, in 1939 he bought Windsor Slipper from Martin Benson, Sidney Freeman's partner in Douglas Stuart. This colt became one of his most successful race horses.[25]

A serious outbreak of foot and mouth disease in the early months of 1941, combined with the introduction of stringent petrol rationing that effectively brought motorised transport to a standstill in 1942, had a drastic impact on racing, leading to the abandonment of many meetings and making it very difficult to transport both horses and spectators to those meetings that were held. 1941 saw the fewest race meetings held in Ireland since 1918 and only about half of the usual number of meetings took place in the second half of 1942. To balance the demands of racing with the exigencies of the wartime restrictions, the government established a Central Racing Advisory Committee to draw up a list of fixtures. This committee was chaired by the former Fianna Fáil minister Patrick Ruttledge, who had been the leading race-horse owner in Ireland in 1939 and was one of McGrath's closest racing allies. McGrath was also a member representing the Bloodstock Breeders' and Horse Owners' Association. This committee was able to ensure the survival of wartime racing on a scaled-down basis.[26]

The continuation of Irish racing in wartime was a major boost to McGrath's position within the sport; the undefeated Windsor Slipper became only the second ever winner of the Irish Triple Crown (Two Thousand Guineas, Derby and St Leger) in 1942. From 1942 to 1946 inclusive he was the champion owner in Ireland, with his horses winning the most money. In 1944 he was also the leading owner, as his horses won more races than those of any other owner. His cumulative winnings in this period amounted to £31,401.[27]

THE RED CROSS SWEEPSTAKES

Another factor that contributed to the survival of the sweepstakes during the war was the decision to run some of them in aid of the newly established Irish Red Cross Society. This decision was probably the result of the crossover of personnel between the Associated Hospitals Sweepstake Committee and the Red Cross; Viscountess Powerscourt, whose husband had served as chairman of the Associated Hospital Sweepstake Committee, was a member of the Red Cross Executive Committee, along with Dublin surgeon Robert Rowlette, who was also involved with the Sweepstake Committee. The relationship between the Red Cross and the sweepstake was cemented by the appointment of Joseph McGrath to the society's Central Council in December 1943.[28]

In October 1939 the Oireachtas passed another amending act to the Public Hospitals Act 'to enable the Irish Red Cross to raise funds by means of sweepstakes and drawings of prizes held under the Public Hospitals Acts, 1933 to 1939'. A clause that allowed the Irish Red Cross to donate portions of the proceeds to foreign Red Cross societies was a significant departure from one of the guiding principles of the sweepstake up to that time, that the money raised was to be used only within the Irish state.[29] The portions to be allocated in this way were decided by the ticket buyers themselves, who would nominate the society of their choice, to which the Irish Red Cross would subsequently make the appropriate grant.[30] Under this scheme £30,846 was donated to the British Red Cross and £1,748 to the Red Cross in Northern Ireland, out of the proceeds of the 1940 Red Cross Steeplechase sweepstake.[31]

This provision was probably designed to encourage continued foreign participation in the wartime sweepstakes. The philanthropic nature of the gesture even softened the hearts of some English magistrates faced with offenders under the Betting and Lotteries Act. Two Southampton defendants charged with selling sweepstake tickets had the charges dismissed in February 1940 having argued that their actions were of assistance to the British Red Cross.[32] Northern Ireland magistrates were less easily swayed; James Rice, a Belfast commission agent, employed a similar defence when charged with publishing proposals to sell sweepstake tickets, but was convicted and fined £5.[33]

The first Red Cross sweepstake was held in January 1940 on a specially organised Irish Red Cross Steeplechase run at Leopardstown. To attract as much interest as possible from owners and punters a prize fund of £3,000 was offered by the Red Cross and Hospitals Trust.[34] This was considered the biggest prize ever offered for a horse race in Ireland and had the desired effect of attracting leading English and Irish horses, including Workman and Kilstar which had been placed first and third respectively in the 1939 Aintree Grand National.[35] With the 1940 English Grand National scheduled to be run on a more modest scale at Gatwick, rather than its traditional Aintree home, an English periodical predicted that the Red Cross Steeplechase 'is going to knock spots off our substitute Grand National'.[36] An initial entry of 52, subsequently whittled down to 22, forced alterations to be made to the Leopardstown course to accommodate the large field.[37] Initially scheduled to be run on 20 January 1940, the race was postponed for a week and was won by the Irish-trained Jack Chaucer.[38]

Hospitals Trust declined a promoters' fee and the Irish Red Cross Society garnered £61,401.[39] When pledges to foreign Red Cross societies had been honoured, £27,250 remained for the Irish Red Cross.[40] However, this sweepstake represented the high point of sweepstakes for the Irish Red Cross. Contributions to Red Cross sweepstakes dipped significantly, in line with the overall reduction in sweepstake proceeds, until 1943 when they began to make a noticeable recovery. The ten wartime sweepstakes run for the benefit of the Red Cross raised over £218,000. For the period from September 1939 to the end of 1944, income from sweepstakes was the largest single source of revenue for the Irish Red Cross Society, representing 41 per cent of its entire income.[41]

Although Justice Conor Maguire, Chairman of the Irish Red Cross Society, was disappointed that the December 1940 Irish Red Cross Chase sweepstake raised only £11,640, rather than the projected £20,000, he recognised 'But for the sums made available as the result of sweepstakes our doors would be closed'.[42] Income from sweepstakes allowed the society to establish a reserve fund of £20,000 in 1942, to subsidise the purchase of uniforms, provide grants to local branches, and fund its larger projects such as the Irish Red Cross Hospital at St Lô in France.[43] After the war a request from the Red Cross to continue sweepstakes on its behalf was rejected by the government and the sweepstake reverted to its original purpose of funding hospitals.[44]

Linking the sweepstake to the Red Cross allowed Hospitals Trust to represent it as an even more philanthropic venture than funding hospitals. Permission was given to Hospitals Trust to use the Red Cross logo on tickets and Red Cross sweepstakes were advertised as 'Ireland's Great Humanitarian and Sporting Gesture'.[45] To capitalise on the wartime relevance of these sweepstakes, advertising space was bought on the roofs of overground air-raid shelters in Dublin, although these proved very tempting to vandals.[46] Another effort was made to convince President Douglas Hyde to lend his support to the sweepstake by inviting him to purchase the first ticket in the first Red Cross sweepstake in 1940, a ceremony which Hospitals Trust hoped to film and no doubt use for propaganda purposes. This approach was rejected by both the President, who had refused similar invitations to attend previous hospital sweepstake draws, and the Taoiseach, who felt the proposal was 'scarcely in keeping with the dignity of the Presidential post'.[47]

The Red Cross, with its countrywide network of branches and dedicated volunteers, provided a ready-made sweepstake agency; in 1941 Joseph McGrath 'requested that a circular letter should be sent to all Branch Secretaries asking them to give a list of active workers in their areas to push the sale of tickets'.[48] The relationship between the Irish Red Cross and Hospitals Trust was mutually beneficial. The former raised nearly half of its entire wartime income through sweepstakes, while the latter found a cause to help sell tickets in the depressed wartime market. However, the Red Cross needed to be wary not to encroach too much on its partner's territory; in 1941 when the society considered running a race meeting at Baldoyle to raise funds, Joseph McGrath warned that 'Hospitals' Trust will take a serious view of the Baldoyle Meeting and that it would adversely affect the Sweepstake'. His demand to have it called off was acceded to.[49]

The recovery of the market for tickets in Britain by 1943 was a fourth factor sustaining the sweepstakes. In the first two sweepstakes of 1940 the largest proportion of prizes went to British citizens, with the USA's share being reduced very significantly. Fifty per cent of the Red Cross proceeds from the 1940 Red Cross Steeplechase sweepstake was allocated to the British Red Cross, in line with the wishes of ticket buyers, an indication of the strength of ticket sales in Britain. When sweepstakes were switched to Irish races from the 1940 Phoenix Plate sweepstake in August, a very noticeable downturn in foreign contributions occurred. From then until late 1943 the overwhelming majority of prizes stayed in Éire, indicating that the majority of tickets were sold on the home market. The recovery of the British market in 1944 and 1945 resulted in a significant boost to proceeds (Table 6.1). The small Irish market had sustained the sweepstake through the leanest years of 1941 and 1942 and with the return of a significant number of British customers it had successfully seen off the challenge to its existence posed by the war.

Table 6.1: Destination of prizes in selected sweepstake draws, 1940–5

	Éire	NI	'Europe'/GB	USA
1940 Red Cross Steeplechase	30.62		68.07	
1940 Grand National	18.75		38.85	29.34
1940 Phoenix Plate	53.38		27.03	14.86
1940 Irish Cesarewitch	75.27		19.56	3.32
1940 Irish Red Cross Chase	71.15		28.85	
1941 Irish Red Cross Chase	85.71	4.08	10.20	
1941 Irish Lincolnshire	75.44	10.5	14.03	
1941 Galway Plate	85.45	3.64	9.09	
1941 Irish Cesarewitch	79.37	7.93	11.11	
1942 Irish Red Cross Chase	67.85	13.39	16.96	
1942 Irish Lincolnshire	75.97	7.75	16.26	
1942 Irish Derby	65.88	15.08	18.25	
1942 Naas Chase	65.73	12.92	20.79	0.56
1943 Hospital Chase	61.17	22.35	16.47	
1943 Leopardstown Chase	37.86	9.46	49.70	0.29
1944 Baldoyle Chase	31.41	13.48	55.00	
1944 Phoenix Nursery Handicap	37.58	11.74	49.32	
1945 Baldoyle Chase	35.14	9.65	51.98	0.99
1945 Curragh Nursery Handicap	13.57	4.95	79.00	0.64

Source: Collated from results of sweepstake draws in Irish daily newspapers. As newspapers did not always carry full results for all draws it was not possible to compile a comprehensive table.

POST-WAR SWEEPSTAKES

In 1946 Hospitals Trust formed a post-war reorganisation committee, chaired by Freeman and including Patrick Duggan, Joseph Griffin, Eamon Martin and Frank Saurin, to help restore the sweepstake's fortunes.[50] The 1946 Derby sweepstake was the first occasion since the 1939 Cesarewitch when proceeds exceeded £1 million. Subscriptions continued to rise throughout the 1950s, due in part to a doubling in the price of tickets from 10 shillings to £1 in 1951.[51] Ticket sales peaked at just over £6 million for the 1961 Cambridgeshire (see Appendix).

The sweepstake's imminent return to its pre-war status was seen by the civil service as an opportunity to re-examine the entire enterprise; in late 1945 the Department of Justice expressed the opinion that 'if the Sweeps are given time to increase to anything like their pre-war proportions, it will be more difficult to abolish or restrict them, than it would be at the present time'. This suggests that serious unease existed in government circles about the way in which the sweepstake operated. It represented the first occasion that serious official consideration was given to whether or not it should continue.

In revisiting the position of the sweepstake, the Department of Justice considered its social effects in terms of increased gambling and its desirability 'from the point of view of our international relations and our national reputation abroad', feeling that the attitude to these two issues should determine whether or not they should 'be discontinued or restricted' and, if allowed to continue, whether the promoters' profits would be restricted. While there was not sufficient evidence 'to justify either the closing of cash betting offices or the abolition of the Sweeps', it was definitely felt that the underground activities employed to facilitate foreign ticket sales were an embarrassment to the government. The Department of Justice was especially sensitive to this as its minister had to approve the scheme for each sweepstake: 'it seems questionable whether it is proper for the Minister to sanction a scheme which contains provisions designed to promote the sale of tickets in countries in which their sale is unlawful.'[52]

Yet, Justice was aware that its reservations had to be balanced against the material advantages that the sweepstake brought to the Irish economy, including funding for hospital construction, employment, and the influx of considerable sums of foreign currency, especially US dollars. While it continued to benefit the economy to such a great extent, there could not realistically be any question of abolishing it. A possible compromise, that would retain the financial benefits but possibly reduce some of the more embarrassing and discreditable aspects of the sweepstake, was to reduce the promoters' profits. The Minister for Justice had already taken a small step in this direction by reducing the percentage of proceeds allocated for expenses and fees from the wartime figure of 30 per cent to 25 per cent. Nonetheless, it was estimated that since 1930 Hospitals Trust had profited to the extent of almost £2 million. In addition to this figure, which only represented the fee for promoting the sweepstake, Hospitals Trust's directors were paid fees and shareholders' dividends, including an annual salary of £3,000 paid to managing director Joseph McGrath. Civil servants were also aware of other methods by which the promoters benefited financially: 'It is possible that some of the shareholders have made big additional profits by way of commissions on the sale of tickets, profits on purchase of winning tickets, etc.' The Minister for Justice's overall assessment was that Hospitals Trust had 'already been rewarded very handsomely' and if the sweepstake was to continue in its present form 'the rate of profit of the promoters should be cut drastically'.[53] Whether or not his opinion was shared by his cabinet colleagues is not known because his proposals were never considered by them.[54]

THE SWEEPSTAKE IN POST-WAR BRITAIN

By the late 1940s there were signs of the sweepstake's revival in Britain. During the war the British Post Office had suspended the practice of using Home Office warrants to intercept mail suspected of containing lottery-related material. When the practice resumed in March 1947 'a heavy traffic' in Irish sweepstake tickets was revealed, which led to a number of prosecutions.[55] In London, between May 1947 and May 1948, the Metropolitan Police investigated 804 cases relating to the sweepstake under the 1934 Betting and Lotteries Act, resulting in 500 prosecutions, a massive increase on the annual wartime average of 30 cases and pre-war average of 100.[56] As a result of this the sweepstake authorities sought alternative methods of smuggling tickets into Britain. The 'growth of a messenger service between Great Britain and Ireland' was noticed. While a decline occurred in the amount of sweepstake-related correspondence seized by the Post Office, the value of sterling postal orders cashed in Ireland in the months coinciding with sweepstake draws remained very high.[57]

A second royal commission on gambling, which sat from 1949 until 1951, was informed by a number of witnesses that the Irish sweepstake was the principal foreign lottery causing concern in Britain. The Commissioner of the Metropolitan Police, Sir Harold Scott, told the commission that the Betting and Lotteries Act had 'notably failed to stop the traffic in Irish Hospitals Sweepstake tickets'. It was also his understanding that it was 'not too difficult to get a ticket for the Irish sweep if you want to'.[58] Similar evidence was given by police chiefs in other parts of England and in Wales and Scotland.[59] Nevertheless, the commission concluded that the significant drop in the annual income of the Irish sweepstake, from over £11 million before the enactment of the Betting and Lotteries Act, to approximately £5 million in the immediate post-war years, 'would appear to show that the activities of the promoters in this country have been severely restricted', and it did not recommend any new measures to deal with it.[60]

The trend of declining sweepstake activity in post-war Britain, identified by the royal commission, was accurate. From the 1950s onwards it ceased to be as much of a problem for the legal authorities in Britain. This may in part be due to the greater availability of alternative forms of gambling. The immediate post-war period saw a massive increase in annual sales figures for the football pools, from £17.5 million in 1945–6, to £42 million in 1946–7, and £65 million in 1948–9.[61] In 1956, Conservative Chancellor of the Exchequer, Harold Macmillan, introduced a premium bonds scheme, under which the interest accruing from the bonds was allocated to bond holders by means of a lottery.[62] Finally, various measures introduced during the 1950s and 1960s liberalised British betting and lottery laws to permit off-course cash betting, the broadcast of betting odds by the BBC, the licensing of bingo halls, the establishment of casinos, and the holding of small public lotteries for charitable and sporting purposes.[63] In 1978, when the British government established yet another royal commission on gambling, under the chairmanship of Lord Rothschild, the Irish sweepstake, which forty years previously had been the principal cause for establishing such a commission, barely merited a mention.[64]

THE SWEEPSTAKE IN AMERICA

The war of attrition between the sweepstake and the various branches of the American federal government resumed as the sweepstake revived after 1945. A number of high profile seizures of tickets from ships arriving in American ports indicated that illicit sweepstake traffic had resumed on a scale similar to the pre-war years. In July 1948 82 cartons of tickets, valued at US$7 million, hidden in a cargo of food loaded at Cobh, were accidentally discovered by food checkers aboard the passenger liner *America* at New York.[65] The following year Philadelphia's vice squad seized 50,000 books of Grand National tickets, worth in excess of US$1.5 million.[66]

The establishment of the state-owned merchant fleet Irish Shipping Limited in 1941 provided a new conduit for smuggling tickets directly from Ireland to the USA. Two of the most high-profile ticket seizures of the post-war years involved liners belonging to the company. In September 1953 a taxi driver, waitress and labourer were arrested for possessing tickets valued at almost US$2 million, unloaded from the *Irish Hazel* at Wilmington, North Carolina. Irish Shipping was subsequently fined US$10,000, and there was speculation that this was paid by Hospitals Trust.[67] A similar haul was seized by Customs and Coast Guard officers from the *Irish Elm* at Newport News, Virginia, in June 1961, following a year-long surveillance operation. Two men arrested on this occasion were eventually freed after a jury was unable to agree a verdict.[68] The development of transatlantic air traffic also facilitated the transfer of tickets to north America; in 1949 the FBI was reported to have broken a five-man ring that had been smuggling tickets aboard aeroplanes.[69]

Vigilant Post Office inspectors also continued to hamper correspondence between Hospitals Trust and its American customers. In 1949 the manager of the Western Union telegraph office in Dublin sought assistance from the Department of Posts and Telegraphs in overcoming 'the difficulty Hospitals' Trust has in getting prize money to the United States owing to seizures of postal remittances by the United States authorities'. Permission was sought either to increase the limit of telegraph money orders from £20 to £40, which would allow the Western Union to send prizes in the form of such orders, or to allow a bulk sum to be sent to the Western Union headquarters in the US for subsequent distribution to prize winners. This latter provision would enable Hospitals Trust and the Western Union to evade the restriction on sending lottery remittances through US mails, which did not extend to sending them via telegraph. Posts and Telegraphs was unwilling to grant either request, fearing that 'we would be running a risk on having our Money Order Convention with the United States suspended', and seeing 'no reason why we should be a party to evade the spirit of the United States legislation for the sake of gaining additional traffic for the Western Union'.[70]

The American legation in Dublin continued to lobby both the Irish government and Hospitals Trust to force the latter to curtail its violations of American lottery and postal regulations. The company continued to resist such pressure, denying 'that it had used the United States mails for the distribution of tickets', which was clearly a false statement given that US postal officials continued to detect such packages in the mail. The American Postmaster General was especially annoyed by a leaflet distributed by Hospitals Trust claiming that mail relating to prize money did not violate postal laws and as such should be passed by postmasters, which he considered 'a bold attempt to mislead and deceive postmasters'. A suggestion that Hospitals Trust 'refuse to accept remittances from the United States' or that the Irish government legislate to prohibit their acceptance, was understandably rejected by both Hospitals Trust and the government, who pointed out that the promoters were legally obliged to accept remittances and that such a regulation would create even greater problems as it would 'result in the purchase of tickets by persons abroad in the names of persons in Ireland'. In response to the American representations Hospitals Trust claimed it was putting measures in place to ensure that 'the organized sale of its tickets in the United States will be discontinued after the current Sweepstakes on the Grand National of 1948'.[71]

In 1948 Hospitals Trust entered into negotiations with the Mexican National Lottery. Representatives from Dublin travelled to Mexico and a mock-up of a Mexican lottery ticket, based closely on those of the Irish sweepstake was produced.[72] Following complaints from the State Department that 'the Irish lottery operators are now endeavouring to enter into an arrangement with a Mexican lottery to exploit lottery ticket sales' in the US, assurances were received from the Department of External Affairs that the arrangement between Hospitals Trust and the Mexican government had been 'terminated'. Diplomatic pressure from the USA, and the consequent embarrassment for the Irish government, appear to have been instrumental in this.[73]

In spite of some high-profile ticket seizures, the distribution of tickets in the USA in the 1950s remained widespread. An investigation into sweepstake activity in California, carried out in 1960 by state Attorney General, Stanley Mosk, at the behest of Governor Pat Brown, revealed how a network of small-time and not easily detectable distributors had been built up gradually during the preceding three decades:

> A few of the sellers . . . had at one time lived in Ireland or had relatives there now. These sellers simply continued a practice begun over there or were sent their tickets by the relative. More frequently, however, the sellers were people who had originally been purchasers of tickets and then, either dissatisfied with the slowness of getting their receipts back, or wanting the prestige which they felt could be obtained from being the person to see for a Sweepstakes ticket, had decided to sell tickets themselves.

None of them had been engaged directly as agents by Hospitals Trust, and they were not wholesale distributors along the lines of the McGarrity-Neenan agents on the east coast, selling only three or four books for each sweepstake to personal acquaintances. Nor were they seriously involved in criminal activity; most were 'engaged in socially accepted occupations' and selling sweepstake tickets was 'their only illegal activity'. As the tickets bought in California were usually posted from New York or New Jersey, and also within the state, Mosk's investigation provides a good insight into how the tickets filtered down through the domestic distribution network after they had been smuggled into the United States.

Mosk concentrated on the money trail to Ireland in an effort to ascertain the extent of California's subscriptions to the sweepstake. An examination of bank drafts from Bank of America branches in the state to Ireland during September 1959, a month before the Cambridgeshire sweepstake draw, revealed that drafts amounting to £26,158 and $115,087.36 had been sent to Ireland (there was a noticeable rise in the number of drafts sent to Ireland in the run-up to sweepstake draws). It was estimated that approximately

$52,000 of the latter figure comprised sweepstake contributions as it was made up of multiples of $2.85, the US dollar equivalent of the £1 ticket price. This figure accounted for only one bank and one form of payment from the state, leading Mosk to conclude that overall sweepstake contributions from California ran 'into millions' each year.

The main purpose of the investigation was to suggest possible action to curtail the violation of state and federal anti-lottery laws and the loss of large sums of revenue to the sweepstake. One option was to warn the local ticket distributors 'that they are violating California law', a time-consuming exercise that would require the employment of a team of full-time investigators to trawl through bank draft records searching for the names of sweepstake subscribers. This information could then be turned over to the Post Office which had the ability to 'put a considerable crimp in the sweepstakes business simply by holding up the receipts sent back to sellers'; the failure to issue receipts in a timely manner would do great damage to the reputation of the sweepstake and its agents.

Approaching Hospitals Trust directly was also suggested, in an effort to see what use Californian subscriptions were being put to and to ascertain who was running the American distribution network. The likelihood that Hospitals Trust 'might refuse to provide the information' was considered, and Mosk's belief that such a 'public refusal would tend to discredit the enterprise and discourage the support given to it' indicated how little he know about the promoters; if they were prepared to tell blatant lies to the Irish Department of External Affairs, the American Legation in Dublin and the State Department in Washington, they would have treated the Attorney General of California with even greater disdain. In the end Governor Brown appears not to have taken any action against the operation of the sweepstake in California.[74]

When federal government officers discovered illicit sweepstake traffic, it was often difficult to secure a conviction of the suspected smugglers, as seen in the instance of the *Irish Elm*. The burden of proof lay with the government and was often difficult to achieve, a problem illustrated when the Justice Department prosecuted Jeremiah Dunne for selling tickets in Philadelphia. In May 1949 Dunne's post was stopped by a local postmaster who suspected it to contain prohibited matter, which turned out to be the following somewhat cryptic typewritten letter:

Ref: 9–1/408/KN

59, Rathdown Road,
N. C. Road,
Dublin.
22nd April 1949

Dear Sir,

Your request for extra supplies has been received and we are endeavoring to fulfil, but would inform you that you have received more than your full quota based on returns.

Assuring . . . our best attention at all times,

Yours faithfully,
T. A. Grogan.

The prosecution case claimed that this referred to the supply of sweepstake tickets, but failed to identify T. A. Grogan, produce evidence of who resided at the address in Dublin, show that Dunne was continuing to sell tickets, or produce the original communication from him to which this was believed to be a reply, and Dunne was duly acquitted.[75]

ISAAC WUNDER

In 1961 Isaac Wunder, a 64-year-old New Yorker, initiated proceedings in the Irish High Court against Hospitals Trust, claiming to hold twenty different winning sweepstake tickets dating back to the 1948 Cambridgeshire. Over the course of the next thirteen years, a total of ten judgements were issued against him in both the High and Supreme Courts. While some of these actions were in progress, Wunder made further claims to hold winning tickets in sweepstake draws held in 1963 and 1966. In all cases Hospitals Trust was able to provide detailed documentary evidence that the tickets had in fact been held by others. Chief Justice Cearbhall Ó Dálaigh's only explanation for Wunder's insistence that his claims were legitimate was that 'he has imagined them and now believes what he imagined'. He was unable to find 'even a shadow of substance' in the claims. The Irish judiciary felt a mixture of sympathy and frustration at these proceedings. Justice Murnaghan felt he was 'more to be pitied than anything else' and Ó Dálaigh urged him 'to place his affairs in the hands of some friend or relative before he renders himself penniless by this pointless action', while Declan Costello described the claims as 'frivolous and vexatious'. The episode gave rise to a new term in Irish law, Isaac Wunder Order, the description given to a case deemed 'frivolous, vexatious and an abuse of process of the court'.[76]

THE GAMING AND LOTTERIES ACT (1956)

In 1950 the government initiated a process to reform the law on gaming and lotteries. Apart from off-course betting and the sweepstake, gaming and lotteries in Ireland were still largely governed by nineteenth-century British legislation, which was no longer appropriate for the mid-twentieth century. As the British had found in the early 1930s, these laws were no longer enforceable; often they were ignored by the Gardaí and when prosecutions were brought the offenders were dealt with lightly by the courts. The Minister for Justice, Seán MacEoin, also felt that Irish public opinion did not support the extent of the restrictions on lotteries and gaming, and while he did not favour removing them entirely, he wanted to examine the possibility of relaxing them to permit the holding of small competitions under District Court licence.[77]

MacEoin's transfer to Defence and the fall of the inter-party government in 1951 delayed progress, but did not bring about any major change in policy. In 1952 Fianna Fáil Justice Minister Gerald Boland announced his intention to submit proposals to the government similar to those considered in 1950. The need for new legislation was now greater because of the proliferation of illegal pools to raise funds for schools and hospitals and the growing popularity of gaming machines.[78] By the early 1950s small lotteries organised by the Irish language promoter Gael Linn, the Sports Federation of Ireland, the Bon Secours Hospital in Glasnevin, and the Mater Hospital in Belfast had become quite popular in Dublin.[79] Boland was 'very doubtful whether it was wise to legalise the Hospitals' Sweepstakes, and he would not favour legislation which would permit the growth of other big gambling institutions'.[80] While the proposals were being formulated the existing laws prohibiting lotteries would be enforced strictly.[81] At this time Hospitals Trust made the first of a number of applications to run a weekly lottery. The Department of Justice refused the request, recognising that:

> the real object of the scheme is not so much to increase substantially the funds available for the hospitals as deliberately to destroy the small weekly lotteries in aid of Church-building etc. which are said by Hospitals Trust (1940) Ltd., to interfere to some extent with the volume of Irish subscriptions to the Sweepstakes.[82]

The Gaming and Lotteries Act was eventually passed in 1956 by the second inter-party government.[83] Although it relaxed the prohibitions on small prize competitions, the conditions under which they could operate were still very restrictive. The promotion of a lottery, as well as the importation, printing, sale, and distribution of lottery tickets, was prohibited. Such unlawful lotteries could not be advertised in newspapers or on radios or cinema screens in the state. Lawful lotteries were defined as those 'promoted as part of a dance, concert or other like event' where the organisers 'derive no personal profit from the event or the lottery', and where the prize fund did not exceed £25. It was also permissible for circuses and travelling shows to run small lotteries within their confines, where the price of tickets would not exceed six pence and the maximum prize one person could win was ten shillings.

A third category of lawful lottery was that given a permit by a local Garda Superintendent where the organiser received no personal profit, the prize fund did not exceed £300, and the value of prizes was printed on each ticket. This convoluted and often confusing piece of legislation also permitted a fourth type of lottery, licensed by a District Court for 'some charitable or philanthropic purpose', where once again there was no personal profit accruing to the organisers, the total prize fund was limited to £500' and up to 40 per cent of the gross proceeds could be allocated to cover the expenses of promoting the lottery. These were raised from the original bill's figures of £300 and 25 per cent as a result of successful lobbying by lottery promoters who argued that the limits were not sufficient.[84] The sweepstake was exempted from all of these provisions.

YOUNG PHILANTHROPISTS (YP) POOLS

In formulating the Gaming and Lotteries Act, the Oireachtas had to deal with the dilemma of what to do with the Young Philanthropists Pools. These football pools had been established in Northern Ireland during the 1950s to raise funds for Belfast's Mater Infirmorum Hospital, a Roman Catholic voluntary hospital that had refused to participate in the National Health Service and consequently had its state grants withdrawn. Unlike the rest of the United Kingdom, voluntary hospitals in Northern Ireland were not allowed to opt out and still retain their grants. The governors of the Mater feared the loss of its religious character if it participated in the NHS.[85] The withdrawal of state grants had a serious adverse effect on the Mater's finances; according to one source payments for insured workers were less than a quarter of their pre-NHS levels: 'The Workers' Maintenance Committee contributions have fallen considerably. Before the Health Act they averaged £22,000 per year, but now they amount to less that £5,000.'[86] The YP Pools subsequently became the single most valuable source of income for the Mater until it eventually agreed a favourable compromise to join the NHS in 1972; in 1958, £66,111 of the hospital's total income of £111,282 came from the pools.[87]

In 1949 both Bishop Mageean of Down and Connor and Archbishop D'Alton of Armagh sought financial support from the Irish government; Mageean wondered if hospital sweepstake funds might be made available to the Mater to avert the possibility of its closure. Taoiseach John A. Costello replied that the legislation governing the sweepstake would not allow for this but undertook to examine the question of running a special sweepstake for the Mater. However, his government concluded 'that it would not be feasible to arrange for the organisation of a sweepstake to provide funds in this connection'.[88] The compromise offered was effectively to allow the YP Pools to operate in the Republic in breach of the prohibition there against large lotteries other than the sweepstake. When YP agents were prosecuted the courts adopted a very lenient attitude in view of the object of their lottery. In February 1954, after the government had agreed on a stricter enforcement of the existing law in advance of the introduction of new legislation, Frank Doherty had his prosecution for selling YP Pools in contravention of the 1823 Lottery Act dismissed by Mr Justice O'Sullivan who was concerned that the restriction of the pools would lead to the Mater's closure.[89]

In 1952 Taoiseach Eamon de Valera regretfully informed Bishop Mageean that the 'action which we are finding it necessary to take in regard to pools generally' would have an adverse effect on the YP Pools.[90] His Fine Gael successor, John A. Costello, appears to have been more willing to find some compromise that would permit the pools to continue operating. In 1954 he instructed the Department of Justice 'to give further careful consideration to those provisions of the Bill that affect pools such as the pool which is operated for the benefit of the Mater Hospital, Belfast, with a view to seeing how these provisions might be modified so as to mitigate their adverse effect on such pools'.[91] One possible solution was to insert a '"Mater clause" in the proposed Bill or by a separate statute', but this was considered likely to lead to too many objections from both the Republic and Northern Ireland. There was opposition to the existence of these pools in the south, even from 'a high ecclesiastical authority' who complained to the Department of Justice that they 'were permitted to operate to the detriment of local charities'.[92] The Department of Justice had little sympathy for their fate: 'our view is that charity begins at home and that the Mater Hospital has scandalously abused the toleration extended to it and made it impossible for us to enforce the law against the promoters of illegal lotteries of the same type.'[93]

During the debate on the bill in the Seanad the case for the YP Pools was made by Senators Arthur Cox and Louis Walsh, the latter arguing that 'Considering the substantial amount contributed by the nationalists there towards the Hospitals Trust Fund here, it is only fair that we should reciprocate by permitting the YP Pools, which circulate here at the moment, to continue'.[94] Cox attempted unsuccessfully to move a number of amendments that would have exempted the pools from the restrictions of the new legislation.[95] Eventually, the increase of the prize money limit for charitable lotteries from £300 to £500 and the provision that permitted lotteries 'conducted wholly within the State in accordance with a permit or a licence' were considered sufficient to allow the YP Pools to evade the restrictions of the new act. Under the latter provision a licence was subsequently given to the YP Lotteries Society Limited, based in Parnell Square, Dublin, to run the Republic of Ireland section of the pools.[96]

INDUSTRIAL RELATIONS IN HOSPITALS TRUST

The hostile relations between Hospitals Trust's management and the trade union movement were heightened in the post-war years when the Workers' Union of Ireland (WUI) began a battle to seek recognition to negotiate on behalf of its members in the sweepstake. Under the stewardship of James Larkin Junior, the WUI expanded rapidly in Dublin after 1947, attracting workers in semi-state companies including Aer Lingus and the Electricity Supply Board. In 1949 the union boasted that its banner 'is today proudly flying at full mast' in the Guinness brewery and Hospitals Trust, where their membership included 'some hundreds of the 1,400 workers'.[97] The introduction of the WUI appears to have been initiated by a group of workers dissatisfied at being forced to work 'excessive overtime'.[98]

The union's elation at gaining a foothold in two of the city's biggest employers was soon quelled by the realisation that it was powerless to force Hospitals Trust to recognise its right to represent its members there. Apparently in direct response to the introduction of the WUI, a house association was established in opposition to it in February 1949, allegedly at the instigation of management. 'Virtually the whole eligible staff' joined the house association, in contrast to approximately 380, less than one-third of the workforce, who were in the WUI.[99] The nature of the sweepstake's work made it impossible to resort to industrial action in the face of Hospitals Trust's recalcitrance: 'The Union is reluctant to open a form of struggle against the Trust which might adversely affect the finances available for hospitalisation.'[100]

Instead the WUI resorted to the newly-established mechanism for resolving industrial disputes, the Labour Court, claiming that Hospitals Trust's refusal to negotiate with it concerning its members pay and conditions of employment was tantamount to denying sweepstake employees the right to organise, an assertion rejected by the court, pointing to the existence of the house association: 'employees are entitled to decide for themselves what form of organisation they want.' The court did not feel that the union had succeeded in showing that its members were disadvantaged and did not feel that Hospitals Trust's management was under any obligation to negotiate twice on behalf of employees who were members of both the house association and the union branch. Nevertheless, the blanket refusal to negotiate with the WUI contravened 'the right of an employee to be represented by the organisation of his own choice', and the court recommended that Hospitals Trust recognise and negotiate with the WUI 'on condition that the Union shows that a substantial proportion of the staff desire to be represented by it and not by the [House] Association'.[101]

Labour Court recommendations were not binding, however, and Hospitals Trust management simply refused to implement this one. The WUI claimed further that the company's influence with the media, as one of the country's leading advertisers, limited newspaper publicity of the ruling, alleging that the labour correspondent of one daily newspaper was 'severely reprimanded' by his general manager for reporting it.[102] For the remainder of the 1950s resolutions supporting the recognition of WUI members in Hospitals Trust were passed at annual conferences of the union, but failed to move the management.[103] In the meantime the WUI had some minor successes on behalf of its sweepstake members. A pay rise in 1951 was attributed to the management's fear of the union, and two female employees, dismissed for attending a wedding while supposedly on sick leave (they had the misfortune of being involved in a car accident that was reported in the newspapers), were reinstated by Joseph McGrath after an appeal on their behalf by the union's national organiser, Christy Ferguson.[104]

RADIO AND TELEVISION ADVERTISING

Hospitals Trust's sponsored programme resumed on Radio Éireann in 1945, running daily from 1.45 to 2.15 p.m. In October 1945 it returned to a night-time slot and from September 1948 became a half-hour programme broadcast between 10.30 and 11 p.m., comprising twenty minutes of music and ten minutes of racing results, including the 'three best' tips for the following day's racing.[105] Relations between Hospitals Trust and the Department of Posts and Telegraphs remained strained. Spencer Freeman continued to complain about the poor reception of Radio Éireann in Britain and the adverse affect this had on sales of tickets there. Even in Newry, close to the border between the Republic and Northern Ireland, reception of the programme was 'sometimes uncertain'.[106] In 1949 Hospitals Trust conducted a radio listenership survey in Britain and found the responses to it quite disappointing in the important population centres of London and the midlands.[107] The Department of Posts and Telegraphs attributed this to interference with the Athlone frequency from a station based in East Germany, but also suggested that Hospitals Trust might wish to consider 'whether the poor response was due to dislike of the programmes'.[108]

T. J. Monaghan, Radio Éireann's chief engineer, became exasperated with Freeman's persistent complaints and demands that something be done to improve reception in Britain. He did not feel Radio Éireann was under any obligation to the sweepstake: 'at no time has any promise been given by the Department to the Hospitals Trust that reception in any territory outside Ireland will be good', and rejected once again the idea of moving the transmitter from Athlone to the east coast.[109] Nonetheless, Freeman continued to bully the department, threatening to move the sponsored programme to Radio Luxembourg and trying to cajole it with promises of increased revenue from a longer programme if better reception could be achieved, behaviour dismissed by civil servants as 'facile' and 'special pleading'.[110]

To placate Freeman, he was permitted to engage French engineers to examine whether the use of new aerials would improve matters. Engineers at Posts and Telegraphs were not impressed with this slight to their expertise – 'We are quite conversant here with the up-to-date development of aerial systems and feel that we do not really require any technical advice on the matter' – and the department refused to fund it, 'we shall not be involved in any expense whatsoever in connection with their enquiries'.[111] The French consultants' subsequent findings were disputed, with Freeman claiming that new aerials would improve Radio Éireann's reception by 60 per cent in all directions, and Posts and Telegraphs' engineers that there was no evidence for this assertion.[112]

His aggressiveness having gained little other than the enmity of the department, Freeman switched to a policy of trying to convince it that increasing the power of Radio Éireann's transmitter was in the interests not just of Hospitals Trust but of the nation; improved reception in Britain would benefit tourism, provide a link to emigrants, enhance the revenue of the department, and, conscious of the state's balance of trade crisis, 'enable demonstration of enterprise, ability and efficiency to an extent that would create a desire for our products'. He also enlisted support from other organisations seeking to enhance their profile in Britain, especially Bord Fáilte.[113] Posts and Telegraphs continued to resist all such overtures, insisting that tampering with Radio Éireann would be a breach of the 1948 Copenhagen Plan that assigned frequencies; this would trigger 'similar breaches by other countries and the general result would be chaos in broadcasting reception throughout Europe'.[114]

By the late 1950s Hospitals Trust was losing patience with the department's failure to accede to its requests. The company was also becoming increasingly interested in television broadcasting as an alternative. In these circumstances Joseph McGrath indicated that Hospitals Trust was quite prepared to end its relationship with Radio Éireann: 'Mr McGrath said that for a long time he had personally resisted the pressure within the Trust to discontinue the Radio Éireann programme but felt he could no longer do so.'[115] Posts and Telegraphs appear to have taken the threat more seriously on this occasion for fear of losing the £36,000 brought in annually by the sponsored programme. Hospitals Trust was still undoubtedly the most valuable sponsor on Radio Éireann, paying £90 for its half-hourly programme on weekdays and £125 for its Sunday slot, compared to other firms that were charged £40 (Irish firms) and £60 (non-Irish firms) per half hour.[116] An approach was made to Senders Fries Berlin asking it to either move off the 566 kc/s frequency or reduce its power after 10.30pm to avoid interfering with Radio Éireann's signal, and it was planned to seek an exclusive wavelength for Athlone and to make greater use of the very high frequency band.[117]

A minor compromise was agreed in 1957 when Hospitals Trust's programme was moved to 11 p.m. to avoid the worst of the night-time interference from competing stations; this led to better reception but was offset by the disadvantage of its lateness.[118] In 1959 a request to revert to the 10.30 p.m. slot was rejected, as 'popular programmes' such as *City Newsreel*, *Job of Work* and *Céilí House* were being broadcast at that time.[119] The refusal to allow Hospitals Trust to return to its 10.30 p.m. slot was the issue on which its often-fractious relationship between both organisations was sundered. Joseph McGrath refused to renew the contract in 1959 and, although the programme continued on a day-to-day basis for a few months, the last Hospitals Trust sponsored programme was broadcast on 31 March 1960, by which time it had already begun broadcasting on Radio Luxembourg.[120]

The termination of Hospitals Trust's relationship with Radio Éireann stemmed both from its frustration with the failure to strengthen the signal and the company's growing interest in television as a more favourable method of advertising. Since 1950 the Department of Posts and Telegraphs had been investigating the establishment of an indigenous television station.[121] The government received two offers to establish a commercial station, one of which was from a Romanian expatriate, Charles Michelson. His proposal was to establish and run public service and commercial stations alongside each other. The government would retain control of content and would not incur a financial risk. However, in return Michelson sought permission to base high-powered commercial radio stations in Ireland that could broadcast and advertise to British and European audiences, similar to the earlier proposals of George Shanks.

Support for Michelson's proposal came from Hospitals Trust, Córas Tráchtála Teoranta (CTT – Irish Export Board), Bord Fáilte, Aer Lingus, and the Vatican. In 1957 the Minister for Posts and Telegraphs came 'under considerable pressure from Hospitals Trust, Bórd Failte [*sic*], CTT and Aer Lingus' to accept Michelson's proposal, which suited Hospitals Trust '100%'; Joseph McGrath 'personally . . . intervened in emphatic terms' on Michelson's behalf.[122] The inclusion of the proposal for commercial radio broadcasting appears to have endeared him to the Michelson plan, because it offered an opportunity to circumvent the restrictions on sweepstake publicity in Britain; McGrath believed that 'Michelson's proposals for Short Wave broadcasting . . . would enable us to keep the Sweepstakes in front of people in the distant countries of the world'.[123] In the post-war period the worldwide press publicity given to the sweepstake was negligible compared to the 1930s. This decline, combined with fears that advertising restrictions similar to those in Britain would be introduced in Canada and the USA, and the growing popularity of the British football pools, underpinned Hospitals Trust's advocacy of the Michelson plan.[124]

A Television Commission set up by the government reported in 1959 recommending the establishment of a commercial station that would be run by a private monopoly while remaining under the control of a public authority, but this was rejected by the government which chose to establish a public service station. This decision was in line with the traditional support of the Department of Posts and Telegraphs for retaining government control of broadcasting, as seen in its various dealings with Hospitals Trust in the preceding thirty years. The rejection of the Michelson proposal and the decision to retain the state's broadcasting monopoly was a defeat for Hospitals Trust, but was fully in accordance with the policy of the broadcasting section of the Department of Post and Telegraphs towards the sweepstake since the 1930s in not submitting to the demands of Hospitals Trust.

WATERFORD GLASS

During the 1930s the directors of Hospitals Trust began to reinvest their substantial profits into indigenous Irish industry. One of the first companies into which sweepstake proceeds were invested was the Irish Glass Bottle

Company (IGB) in Ringsend, Dublin, bought by Joseph McGrath and Richard Duggan in 1932, which 'quickly became the largest supplier of glass jars and milk bottles in Ireland'.[125] In the 1950s McGrath used IGB to take over the newly re-established Waterford Glass.

In 1947 the glass manufacturer Charles Bačik left his native Czechoslovakia, where he feared that his factories would be taken over by the resurgent communists, and, along with Miroslav Havel and the Dublin jeweller Bernard Fitzpatrick, revived the tradition of glass manufacture in Waterford. In 1950 Bačik sought capital investment from Joseph McGrath to expand Waterford's activities. Rather than joining Bačik's venture, McGrath ended up buying him out, possibly with the intention of merging Waterford with IGB. It would appear that McGrath used some shrewd tactics to convince Bačik to sell his stake, undermining Waterford's sales of beverage glasses by importing cheap glasses from the continent and convincing IGB customers not to deal with Waterford: 'One prominent Limerick publican and beer franchise . . . had invested some money in the Bačik operation and was reportedly warned by IGB that if he continued doing business with Waterford Glass he would be cut off as an IGB customer.' The decision to sell to McGrath was one that 'Bačik probably regretted . . . for the rest of his life'.[126]

Most of the day-to-day running of Waterford was left to McGrath's partner, Joseph Griffin and his son, Noel, under whose direction a new factory was opened in Johnstown in October 1951, an event which marked 'Joe McGrath's first and only visit to Waterford Glass' and at which he expressed the controversial 'hope that "only Irish workers" would eventually comprise the company's employees', remarks for which he had to apologise to the company's Czech workforce.[127]

McGrath soon realised that Waterford could be turned into a specialist company manufacturing luxury crystal products for the lucrative American market. The existing sweepstake distribution network was used to sell Waterford's products. For the best part of twenty years from the 1950s until his return to Ireland in the 1970s, Connie Neenan doubled as the principal agent in the USA for both the sweepstakes and Waterford Glass. The development of popular lines such as Lismore, Deirdre, Eileen, and Colleen and the establishment of links with Altman's Department Store in New York City and with a number of American sporting organisations that commissioned Waterford Glass trophies transformed Waterford into a world-renowned brand name by the 1960s. In 1966 Waterford separated from IGB and floated on the Irish stock exchange, reducing the share holding of the McGraths.[128] Patrick McGrath, who would later succeed his father as head of the family's various business interests, began his business career in IGB and often deputised for his father as chairman of Waterford, before succeeding him following his death in 1966. He considered Waterford to be one of the most important components of his family's business empire: 'Waterford paid a tremendous amount of bills for us.'[129] It would remain so until the early 1980s.

SPORTS SPONSORSHIP

Hospitals Trust was a pioneer of sports sponsorship in Ireland. In 1958, at the request of Bord Fáilte, the company promoted the first of five Irish Hospitals golf tournaments at Woodbrook Golf Club in Dublin, with a prize fund of £5,000. This tournament helped to fill a gap created by the suspension of the Irish Open between 1953 and 1975. It served as an opportunity to advertise the McGraths' two leading enterprises, the sweepstake and Waterford Glass, as the winner received a Waterford Glass bowl, in addition to £1,000 prize money.[130] Between 1958 and 1962 the event attracted some of the world's leading golfers, including the Australian Ken Nagle and Britain's Peter Allis, who came first and second in respectively in 1961. The leading Irish golfer of the time, Christy O'Connor Senior, claimed first prize in 1960 and 1962.[131]

During the post-war years the company also provided valuable sponsorship for many of the major English races, especially those upon which its sweepstakes were run. Between 1958 and 1963 it contributed £5,000 to the prize money for the Aintree Grand National.[132] Fears for the future of both the Aintree racecourse and the race itself led to the withdrawal of this sponsorship and the decision from 1966 to run the spring sweepstake on the Lincolnshire instead, before reverting to the Grand National in 1980.[133] In the 1970s it offered between £5,000 and £7,500 to the Cambridgeshire.[134]

In 1962 Hospitals Trust withdrew its golf sponsorship in order to concentrate on horse racing. That same year it began to sponsor the Irish Derby, and switched the sweepstake from the Epsom to the Irish Derby, marking the first occasion since the war that a sweepstake was run on an Irish race. The purse of £30,000 put up by Hospitals Trust, combined with entrance and forfeit dues and a contribution from the Irish Racing Board (of which Joseph McGrath was Chairman), brought the value of the Irish Derby to £60,000, making it most valuable race in Europe at the time, ahead of the Epsom Derby which was valued at about £33,000. Prior to the involvement of Hospitals Trust the Irish Derby was worth only £7,000.[135]

In Britain the elevated status of the Irish Derby was seen as a threat to the Epsom classic and other prestigious English races; the *Sunday Despatch* complained of a 'Big Irish Menace to our Derby', an extra 10,000 guineas was added to the prize fund of the English 2,000 guineas in 1962, and the timing of the race in June was expected to reduce the field for the King George VI and Queen Elizabeth stakes at Ascot three weeks later.[136] The new-found status of the Irish Derby resulted in a much larger field after 1962, attracting many notable foreign owners, trainers, and jockeys, although there was some disappointment when Sir Winston Churchill's Kemal withdrew from the inaugural Sweeps Derby.[137] Another measure of the race's prestige was the decision of the BBC to televise it.[138] The sponsorship of the Derby was also seen as giving a major boost to Irish bloodstock breeding and to the popularity of Irish racing among spectators.[139]

Sponsorship of the Derby heightened further Joseph McGrath's dominance of Irish racing. In the twenty years after the war he was frequently leading owner (1947, 1954–7, 1964–5) and champion owner (1955, 1957, 1959) in Ireland, winning almost £100,000.[140] His greatest successes in these years were the victories of Arctic Prince, a horse he had bred at Brownstown, in the 1951 Epsom Derby, and Panslipper, trained by his son Séamus, in the 1955 Irish Derby. His reputation as a breeder was enhanced with the sale of Nasrullah, a colt he had purchased from the Aga Khan for 19,000 guineas in 1941, to an American syndicate for £132,857 in 1949. Closely related to Northern Dancer, Nasrullah sired fifteen champions in the USA and was grandsire to Secretariat, winner of the American Triple Crown (Kentucky Derby, Preakness Stakes and Belmont Stakes) in 1973.[141]

McGrath was also the most important administrator in post-war Irish racing, aptly described by Fergus D'Arcy as 'the Napoleon of Irish racing'. In 1945 he was influential in the establishment of the Racing Board, of which he remained a member until his death in 1966, serving as Chairman from 1956 until 1962. He was also President of the Bloodstock Breeders Association of Ireland and a steward of the Irish Turf Club. From the late 1940s most of his horses were trained by his son, Séamus, at Glencairn in Dublin. After his death the family interest in racing was maintained by his three sons, Joseph Junior, Patrick, and Séamus. The family's close association with the Irish Derby was epitomised by the victory of Weaver's Hall in the 1973 race; this horse, owned by Patrick McGrath and trained by Séamus, won a race sponsored by the family's business on which they also ran a sweepstake.[142] Hospitals Trust's sponsorship of the Irish Derby continued until 1986, by which time the sweepstake's closure was imminent.

SEVEN

DECLINE AND CLOSURE
1961–87

—

A major change in the administration of Hospitals Trust took place during the 1960s with the replacement of many of the original managers. Frank Saurin died rather suddenly from cancer in 1957 and Joseph McGrath's son, Patrick (Paddy), was fast-tracked into the business in his stead. Paddy McGrath graduated to managing director when his father died on 25 March 1966, having suffered a heart attack at the sweepstake's office in Ballsbridge the previous day. Joseph McGrath had continued to run the sweepstake, even though he was in his late seventies, and his death was a big loss to the company. His son inherited an enterprise that was starting its decline and he would oversee the demise of the sweepstake and with it the business empire his father had built up during the preceding thirty years.[1]

Gross proceeds from sweepstake ticket sales peaked in 1961; the return of £6.1 million for that year's Cambridgeshire draw was the highest ever achieved. However, the dramatic slump to just under £4.5 million for the following year's Cambridgeshire was the first sign that a sustained decline had begun. Proceeds remained relatively steady for the remainder of the 1960s at between £4 million and £5 million, but the decline became more precipitate during the 1970s. At the start of that decade each draw was still taking in £4 million, but this had reduced dramatically to £1.8 million by 1979. When the increase in ticket prices from £1 to £2 in 1975 is taken into account the decrease becomes more pronounced; £4 million represented a similar figure for ticket sales, whereas £1.8 million indicated that only 900,000 tickets had been sold (see Appendix).

THE LEGALISATION OF LOTTERIES IN THE USA AND CANADA

The principal cause of this decline was the legalisation of state lotteries in north America. Religious and social objections to gambling in the USA declined significantly in the post-war years and support for the use of lotteries to raise revenue resulted in the establishment of the first state lottery in New

Hampshire in 1963.[2] Paul A. Fino, a Republican congressman from New York, was the strongest political proponent of municipal lotteries in the USA during the 1960s. In 1966 New Yorkers approved a constitutional amendment in favour of a lottery which was established the following year. Massachusetts, New Jersey and Illinois, states that were traditionally strongholds of the sweepstake because of their large Irish populations, also legalised lotteries during the 1970s.[3]

The debate on legalising sweepstakes in Canada was rekindled in the late 1950s and early 1960s; between 1959 and 1963 eleven bills seeking to legalise lotteries were introduced in the federal parliament.[4] A Joint Parliamentary Committee on Capital Punishment, Corporal Punishment, and Lotteries was established in 1953 it recommended that small lotteries in aid of charitable, religious, and community groups be permitted, but opposed the introduction of state lotteries, pools, and sweepstakes.[5] Advocates of lotteries continued their campaign during the 1960s until state lotteries were legalised under the Criminal Law Amendment Act, 1968–9.[6] The first lottery under the new provisions was held in Montréal in 1968 to clear the debt incurred from holding Expo '67. The first national lottery was held in 1974 to finance the 1976 Montréal Olympics, and in 1976 the federal government introduced Loto-Canada.[7]

The United Kingdom remained one of the few countries not to have a national lottery, due largely to residual opposition to the use of lotteries to raise revenue and the existence of the football pools.[8] There were some unsuccessful efforts to introduce a British lottery during the 1960s. In 1965 Lord Jessel hoped to establish a hospital sweepstake, primarily aimed at saving Aintree racecourse from destruction by property developers, and a national sweepstakes bill was debated in Parliament in 1967. The following year Labour's Chancellor of the Exchequer, Roy Jenkins, considered introducing a lottery. Much to the relief of Hospitals Trust none of these materialised. Eventually, in 1992, the UK became the last country in the European Union to introduce a national lottery.[9]

HOSPITALS TRUST'S CAMPAIGN FOR EXPANDED SWEEPSTAKES

As income from the sweepstakes began to decline Hospitals Trust made a number of requests to the government to increase the number of sweepstakes held annually. In 1966 Patrick McGrath requested permission to double the number of sweepstakes from three to six. The proposal sought to bring the sweepstake closer to a weekly-style lottery by including provisions for an 'interim weekly distribution of prizes'.[10] Draws would take place in three cycles during the year, each cycle having 17 or 18 weekly draws, during which

90 per cent of the prize fund would be distributed. The remaining 10 per cent would be pooled into the final draw at the end of each cycle, which would be held in conjunction with a horse race. The additional sweepstakes would be run on Irish races, the 2,000 Guineas, St Leger, and Leopardstown Chase. First prize in the weekly draw would be £15,000 and for the draw at the end of the cycle first, second, and third prizes would be £41,000, £20,500, and £13,500 respectively.[11] The new American state lotteries were largely weekly competitions, as were the British football pools, allowing for an element of continuity absent from the sweepstake.

McGrath's proposal was supported by the Fianna Fáil Minister for Health, Donogh O'Malley, who was 'seriously concerned with the insufficiency of the moneys available in the [Hospitals Trust] Fund'.[12] The outstanding construction work amounted to £17 million, but there was only £5.5 million then available in the Hospitals Trust Fund, so McGrath's estimate that the additional sweepstakes would gross £2 million annually was attractive to O'Malley and to his successor, Seán Flanagan.[13]

Other government departments were less enthusiastic about the plan. The Department of Finance, though not in principle opposed to the idea of running additional sweepstakes, questioned the 'unrealistic' estimate of £2 million additional income; to achieve this amount weekly subscriptions would need to be close to 1.5 million, the equivalent to each household in the Republic of Ireland buying two tickets every week.[14] The Department of Justice had serious reservations about the additional profit that would accrue to Hospitals Trust; it was felt that the promoters had done a good job concealing the fact that they were likely to make a sales commission of nearly £900,000 per year under the proposed new scheme, in addition to payment for promotion expenses, office expenses, and directors' salaries.[15] In spite of these reservations, the government gave its approval in principle to the scheme in December 1966.[16]

The Department of Justice had also raised the issue of the possible adverse effects that the expanded sweepstake might have on the smaller local and charitable lotteries that had proliferated since the relaxation of lottery restrictions in 1956.[17] The organisations running such competitions now came together to lobby against the proposal. The Federation of Voluntary Charitable Organisations (FVCO), representing 28 'cultural, social, sporting, medical, health, rehabilitation and missionary groups', including the GAA, Polio Fellowship of Ireland, YP Lotteries Society, Irish Wheelchair Association, Central Remedial Clinic, and Gael Linn, was formed as a single-issue group to oppose the scheme.[18] The extent and organised nature of opposition from such influential organisations in Irish society, and the failure of Hospitals Trust to give adequate assurances that these smaller charitable lotteries would not suffer, was successful in forcing the government not to proceed any further with the plan to expand the sweepstake at this stage.[19]

Instead, Hospitals Trust was allowed to make a number of small changes. A fourth sweepstake was introduced in 1969, run on a specially organised Irish Sweeps Hurdle at Cheltenham. In the short term this appears to have been successful in increasing sweepstake revenue; by 1974 it was estimated that the 'total annual proceeds from the sweepstakes are now approximately one sixth greater than in 1968'.[20] In 1970 a super-prize of £200,000 was introduced to 'counteract the New York $1m lottery which has eaten into Sweepstake ticket sales in New York'. The doubling of ticket prices from £1 to £2 in 1975 allowed for the super-prize to be increased to £400,000 and the regular prize units from £120,000 to £140,000, with first prize rising from £50,000 to £70,000, the first major change in the price of tickets and size of prizes since 1951.[21]

The case for the increases cited higher administration costs due to inflation and the need to compete with American and Canadian lotteries which offered larger prizes.[22] Payment of the £400,000 prize was staggered, rather than being paid in a single lump sum, so that the winner would avoid a substantial income tax bill; £75,000 was paid initially and the remainder as an annuity plus interest.[23] In 1977 the super-prize was pruned to £250,000 and abandoned in 1979.[24] An analysis of the destination of super-prizes indicates that the USA and Canada were still the largest markets for sweepstake tickets, with Canada being especially so in the early 1970s; of the 36 super-prizes awarded between 1970 and 1979, 15 went to both the USA and Canada and 3 each to England and Ireland.[25]

The government was unwilling to permit these changes without some *quid pro quo* from Hospitals Trust. The perennially thorny issue of its profits was important: 'There is no information from the Sweeps as to how much of the "Organisation and Management Fee" goes into McGrath's pocket.' In the end the request for the increases was granted, but on condition that Hospitals Trust furnish the Minister for Justice with 'detailed particulars of all costs, commissions, expenses and outlay in relation to the selling of sweepstake tickets and the conduct of the sweepstakes generally', and that the share of proceeds allocated to the Hospitals Trust Fund be increased to 30 per cent; from the 1975 Cambridgeshire the prize fund was reduced from 45 to 40 per cent and the Hospitals Trust Fund share augmented from 25 to 30 per cent.[26]

In 1975 Hospitals Trust made yet another attempt to turn the sweepstake into a weekly lottery, arguing that 'the project is not viable as operated at present'; subscriptions had been declining steadily since the 1960s and in the preceding three sweepstakes – the 1974 Derby, Cambridgeshire and Sweeps Hurdle – expenses had exceeded the permitted 30 per cent limit. Hospitals Trust might have felt that the contemporary political situation was more conducive on this occasion; a Fine Gael–Labour coalition had been formed in March 1973 and Patrick McGrath was now a member of Seanad Éireann nominated by the Fine Gael Taoiseach, Liam Cosgrave. Under the new proposal, the traditional sweepstake draws would continue, alongside a series of weekly draws to be staged in conjunction with greyhound races, run on eighteen different tracks around the country, for which tickets costing 25p would be sold each week. It was hoped that these additional sweepstakes would increase annual proceeds by £10 million.[27]

Patrick McGrath warned that if the new scheme was not up and running by 1 January 1975 the sweepstake would have to close, making its 900 staff redundant.[28] McGrath also had to counter growing calls for the replacement of the sweepstake with a government-run national lottery; Denis Larkin of the Workers' Union of Ireland urged the Taoiseach to give 'serious considera-tion' to 'the complete abolition of this Organisation and its substitution by a scheme of a National Sweepstake'.[29] McGrath defended his ability to run the proposed new lottery arguing that Hospitals Trust was the only enterprise with the experience and status to operate it; central government could not do so effectively because sweepstake organisers 'had often to overcome difficul-ties which could be highly embarrassing to a Government or State agency here', while local authorities did not have the experience, lacked Hospitals Trust's international network of agents, and competition between local councils would produce chaos.[30]

Aware that its previous bid had been scuppered by the opposition of the FVCO, Hospitals Trust sought to head off another similar challenge by offering these organisations the prospect of benefiting from their new scheme: 'The various charitable institutions in this country devoted to rehabilitation, and other ailments outside the normal scope of the hospitals, will be able to benefit by the weekly Sweepstakes through the sale of tickets by their organ-isations.'[31] The organisations comprising the FVCO refused to be placated; in August 1975 they expressed concern to the Taoiseach at the weekly greyhound lottery scheme.[32] The extent of opposition from this powerful lobby group once again proved successful in preventing the government acceding to Hospitals Trust's request. The Department of Justice shared the concern that 'Weekly sweepstakes of the magnitude proposed could have a serious adverse effect on promoters of periodical [*sic*] lotteries', and also feared that one of the larger groups running these competitions, such as Gael Linn, might mount a challenge to the constitutionality of the sweepstake's exclusion from the provisions of the 1956 Gaming and Lotteries Act.

Concerns were also raised about the source of the additional income that Hospitals Trust aimed to raise. To generate the estimated additional £10 million annually by selling tickets in the Republic of Ireland alone 'every man

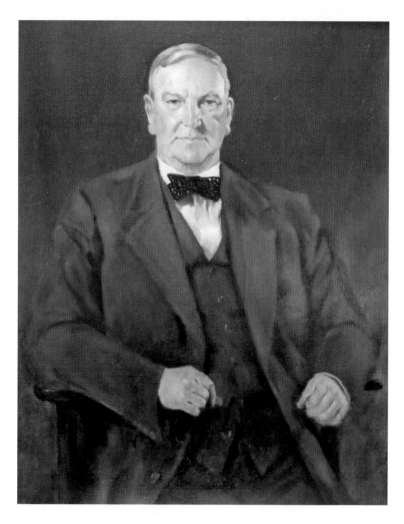

1 Joseph McGrath. Portrait by William (Liam) Belton, RHA, and Michael Brett (1969),
based on an original by Leo Whelan, RHA

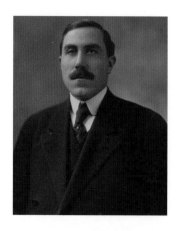

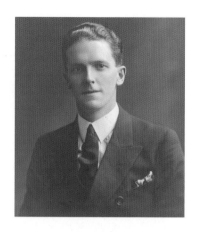

2 Joseph McGarrity

3 Connie Neenan

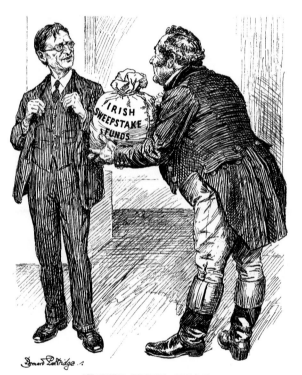

CHARITY BEGINS ABROAD.

Mr. DE VALERA (*relaxing a little of his customary austerity*). "THANK YOU ONCE AGAIN FOR BEING MORE KIND TO OUR HOSPITALS THAN YOU ARE TO YOUR OWN."

4 Bernard Partridge, 'Charity begins abroad', *Punch*, 28 March 1934

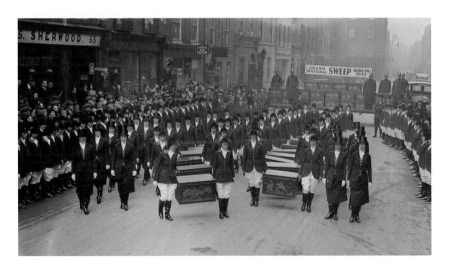

5 The parade of tickets counterfoils through Dublin for the Grand National Sweepstake Draw,
March 1933

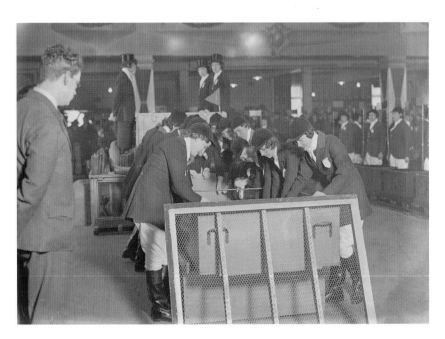

6 Hospitals Trust staff mixing counterfoils for the Grand National Sweepstake Draw, March 1933

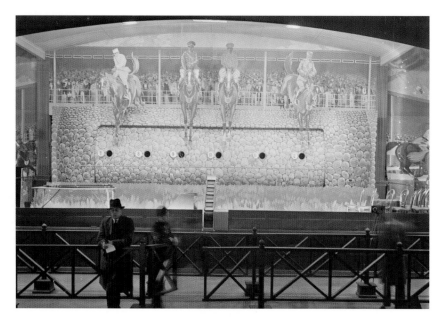

7 The sweepstake drum decorated for the Grand National Sweepstake Draw, March 1933

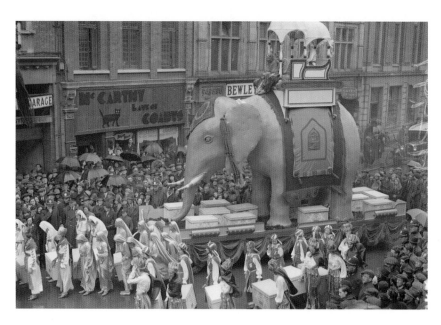

8 The parade of counterfoils through Dublin for the Grand National Sweepstake Draw, March 1935

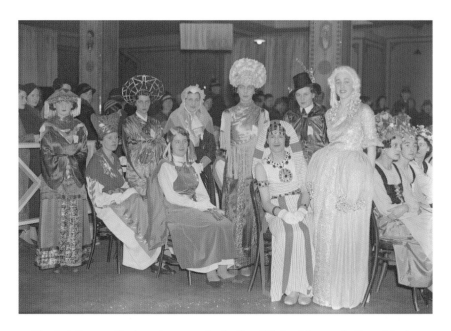

9 Hospitals Trust staff in themed costumes for the Grand National Sweepstake Draw, March 1935

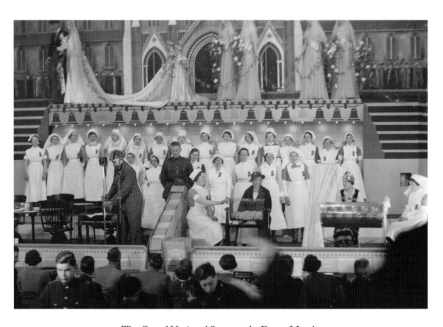

10 The Grand National Sweepstake Draw, March 1935

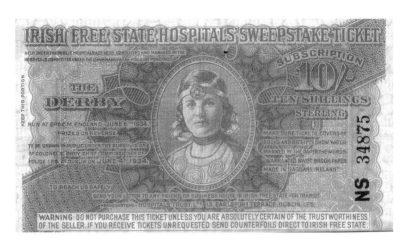

11 1934 Derby Sweepstake Ticket: Grania, daughter of Cormac MacArt

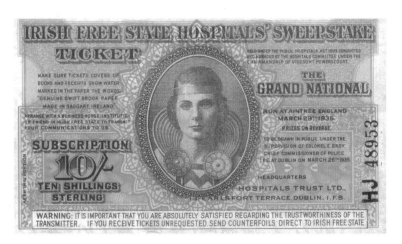

12 1935 Grand National Sweepstake Ticket: Granuaile (Grace O'Malley)

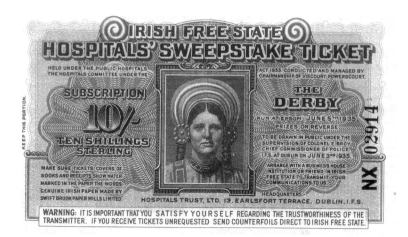

13 1935 Derby Sweepstake Ticket: Deirdre

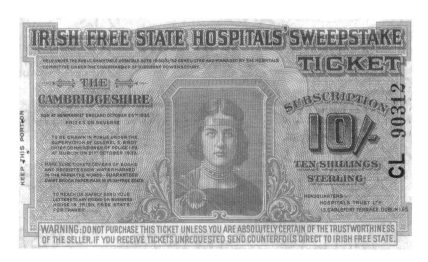

14 1935 Cambridgeshire Sweepstake Ticket: Fionnuala, one of the children of Lir

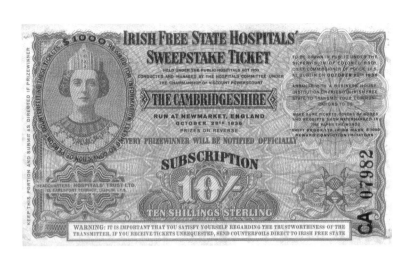

15 1936 Cambridgeshire Sweepstake Ticket: King Laoghaire's wife

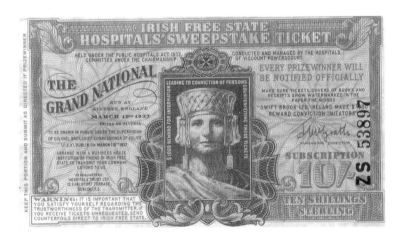

16 1937 Grand National Sweepstake Ticket: Brighid, Goddess of Wisdom

and woman gainfully employed would have to buy a ticket each week', which was not considered likely by Justice. Therefore:

> there will be a strong temptation for the promoters to seek a market abroad and in the context of a weekly lottery, this confines 'abroad' to the United Kingdom. Such sales would have to be surreptitious for they would be illegal in the UK. If tolerated they would lead inevitably to increased sales in this country of English Football Pools coupons. If not tolerated they would result in prosecutions which could embarrass the Government because of the special statutory position of the Sweeps Organisation.

The Department of Foreign Affairs supported Justice's reservations about permitting the weekly sweepstakes, envisaging considerable difficulties should weekly sweepstake tickets be sold abroad. Irish governments in the 1970s were less prepared to tolerate Hospitals Trust's flouting of British law than their predecessors had been forty years previously, especially as the sweepstake revenue now constituted a much less valuable portion of the health budget.

The case against weekly sweepstakes was strengthened by the embarrassment at Hospitals Trust's directors' large personal wealth: 'a further monopoly would be given to a group who have allegedly made many millions in profits'; the possible undesirable social effects of increasing gambling opportunities; and the fact that the Department of Finance was not convinced that there was a need for them. Support for the proposal came, unsurprisingly, from the Departments of Health, which was in favour of anything that 'would ensure that the income of the Hospitals Trust Fund is sustained and improved', and Agriculture, which felt the scheme would benefit the greyhound industry.[33]

The strength of opposition within government, and the influence of the FVCO, resulted in the government once again refusing the request for weekly sweepstakes. However, some reform of the existing scheme was required. Subscriptions continued to decline; from the 1975 Sweeps Hurdle onwards ticket sales never grossed £3 million again. As tickets now cost £2 this meant that only between 1 and 1.5 million tickets were being sold for each sweepstake, less than half the figure for the early 1970s.[34] This resulted in Hospitals Trust placing its staff on a two-day week in January 1976, a move it blamed on the government's procrastination over the weekly greyhound sweepstakes. The eventual compromise agreed was to increase the portion allowed for expenses to 40 per cent, facilitated by a reduction in the prize fund of 10 per cent.[35] The Public Hospitals (Amendment) Act, passed in June 1976, legislated for these changes, and also confirmed the provision in force since

1975 for hospitals to receive at least 30 per cent of the proceeds.[36] This compromise merely postponed a decision on the eventual future of the sweepstake. The sustained decline in subscriptions meant it could not survive long and demands were increasing for its replacement with a new national lottery that would benefit a wider array of social and cultural organisations.[37]

IRISH FOOTBALL POOLS

The influence of the organisations running small charitable lotteries was also a crucial factor in the decision of the government to refuse a request from Vernon's Pools to establish a base in the Republic of Ireland. In March 1976 Vernon's requested an exclusive licence to promote football pools in the state, promising the Taoiseach that the proceeds 'could be disbursed for sporting, cultural, or other social purposes; or as your Government so chooses'. Half of the proceeds would be allocated as prizes, a quarter retained to cover operation and management, and the remaining quarter, forecast to be approximately £2 million annually, distributed among the beneficiaries. A lotto was offered as an alternative as 'Some of the elements required for the success of a football competition may be absent in Eire'. Football pools were illegal in the Republic of Ireland since the betting acts of the 1920s and no serious effort had been made to establish them there, no doubt because of the success of the sweepstake. However, Vernon's were clearly well aware of the difficulties being experienced by Hospitals Trust in the mid-1970s and sought to capitalise upon it.[38]

The Minister for Justice, Patrick Cooney, gave a lukewarm response to the proposals, which would have required amendments to existing betting and gaming legislation, could have an adverse effect on the small charitable lotteries, and might lead to increased gambling.[39] The Taoiseach's own department agreed that 'the voluntary charitable organisations must . . . be protected', thought the request for an exclusive licence was unconstitutional, and felt that the economic climate was not appropriate for the introduction of an extensive gambling scheme.[40]

Surprisingly little attention was paid to the potential impact on the sweepstake of legalising pools or on the reaction of Hospitals Trust, an indication that government policy on lotteries was increasingly conditioned by the role of the smaller charitable lotteries than by the increasingly inefficient sweepstake. The Minister for Justice felt that the impact on the sweepstake 'would be unlikely to be crippling since information supplied by Hospitals Trust about a year ago indicated that about 85% of their income comes from overseas countries'.[41] However, in view of the contemporaneous plan to increase the proportion of expenses allowed to Hospitals Trust for promoting the sweepstake, civil servants warned that 'If the Government were to allow Vernons to proceed, a further approach seeking relief could be expected from Hospitals Trust'.[42]

Another proposal was that of Dublin County Council, which was seeking approval to run weekly lotteries to relieve rates. Although this was expected to be rejected because its prize fund exceeded the limits allowed by the Gaming and Lotteries Act, the Department of Local Government was considering a wider scheme that would allow 'local authorities to run weekly lotteries'. The enactment of the Public Hospitals (Amendment) Act and the growing pressure to widen lottery provision brought the question of establishing a state-run national lottery to the forefront. The Department of An Taoiseach felt the question of 'a State-run lottery is probably worthy of further examination'. However, it was adamant that the government would not repeat the mistake of 1930 in granting a monopoly to a private company:

> The establishment of State-run lottery might not be considered desirable but would be preferable to granting a monopoly to a private firm. Hospitals Trust is a firm which has made large profits under State protection. This privilege should not be granted to another firm.[43]

CRITICISM OF THE SWEEPSTAKE

As long as the sweepstake remained essential to financing Irish hospitals very little criticism of it was voiced, in spite of the existence of much unease about its underground activities and the state of industrial relations in Hospitals Trust. However, by the 1970s the lustre was clearly wearing off and critics felt they could now voice their opinions without endangering Irish hospitals. Occasionally foreign journalists would delve into the murkier aspects of the sweepstake, like *Collier's* in 1939. In 1966 an Irish-born journalist, Thomas O'Hanlon, wrote a piece for the American business periodical *Fortune*, outlining the profits earned by the promoters and US-based agents, the efforts of the US and Canadian government officials to stop the sweepstake's activities in their jurisdictions, and the covert distribution methods employed.[44]

One of the first public criticisms of the sweepstake in the Irish media was contained in an episode of the current affairs series *7 Days*, which examined the failure of Hospitals Trust to recognise the WUI: 'The picture that emerged was that of a successful company using methods illegal in other countries, yielding fat profits to a limited group of families, the whole stamped with the symbol of charity.'[45] However, the most sensational investigation of the sweepstake was the article by Joe MacAnthony published in the *Sunday Independent* on 21 January 1973, which remains one of the best pieces written on the sweepstake and a landmark in Irish investigative journalism. The original intention was to run the 8,000-word article in two parts over consecutive Sundays, but Conor O'Brien, editor of the *Sunday Independent*, 'realised . . . that if the first half was published, the second half would in all probability never see the light of day.'[46]

MacAnthony's investigation focused initially on the money trail, revealing how little of the actual money contributed to the sweepstake made its way to the hospitals; the substantial fortunes, estimated at £100m, amassed by the three founding families; and the existence of a partnership between some people in Hospitals Trust and a well-known bookmaker to buy up shares in winning tickets, similar to the activities of Sidney Freeman in the 1930s. The legislative anomalies that benefited Hospitals Trust, including section 2 of the Public Hospitals Act and the Public Hospitals Amendment Act (1939), were also explained. Joseph Andrews appears to have been an important source for the article, especially the accounts of events from the 1930s, including the McGarrity agency, the Stanhope case, Sidney Freeman's ticket buying schemes, and allegations that Hospitals Trust breached international postal regulations. MacAnthony also used details from an article that appeared in the April 1959 American edition of *Readers' Digest* that condemned the sweepstake as 'the greatest "bleeding heart" racket in the world'.[47]

By 1973, the contraction of its American market meant that much of Hospitals Trust's foreign activities were centred on Canada and MacAnthony's article gave a very detailed account of how tickets were smuggled there and of the suspicions of Canadian police that much of the money contributed was simply pocketed by extremely wealthy local agents. Closer to home, the failure to recognise the WUI and the poor pay and conditions, especially the paltry pensions paid by Hospitals Trust to its retired staff, were also probed. Finally, criticism was levelled at the Associated Hospitals Sweepstake Committee for failing to impose any regulation on the activities of Hospitals Trust.[48]

While most attention was focused on MacAnthony's article in this particular edition of the *Sunday Independent*, the acerbic editorial is also worthy of analysis. The declining 'revenue brought in by illegal Sweeps activities abroad' no longer justified 'a Government involvement which clearly brings its own name into disrepute'. It was time for the replacement of the sweepstake with a national lottery. The embarrassing image of the begging bowl associated with the sweepstake was no longer suitable for a modern country that had just joined the EEC three weeks earlier:

The Government must also have regard to its own pride and image abroad. We are rapidly developing into a modern industrial nation with all the prestige that such a position endows on a people in the world today. Yet . . . we still persist in seeking the world's charity to maintain our health services. And we are prepared to countenance illegalities in order to do so.

This simply will not do. It is about time that our representatives in Government decided that we are an independent nation, depending on ourselves for sustenance and not on other people's sympathy. The poor mouth is no longer representative of the new Ireland.[49]

MacAnthony's revelations would not have been widely known outside the circles of those employed in the sweepstake and some government departments like Justice and Posts and Telegraphs. There was incredulity in some quarters that an Irish journalist, and an Irish newspaper, would publish something so potentially damaging to what was still regarded as a vital Irish enterprise. Sweepstake employees were surprised 'that somebody would deliberately go out to sabotage the sweep', especially at a time when it was coming under pressure from competing north American lotteries: 'We were having tough times because of the Canadian lottery [for the Montréal Olympics], why would somebody do this on one of their own?'[50] The controversy reached the USA, where *Newsweek* opined that 'the sacrosanct image acquired by the sweeps over the years was badly tarnished'.[51]

The fall out from the publication of MacAnthony's *exposé* was wide-ranging, justifying the decision to publish it in its entirety. Lucrative advertising from the various companies under the McGraths' control was withdrawn from the newspaper for two months; a plan by the McGraths to purchase the Independent group was abandoned; and MacAnthony was effectively forced to resign and pursue his career in Canada.[52]

The official response to MacAnthony came from the Associated Hospitals Sweepstake Committee, which published a pamphlet entitled 'Irish Hospitals' Sweepstakes: The facts' that also appeared in all Irish national newspapers on 16 June 1973. This was little more than a summary of the legislation governing the sweepstake. Emphasis was placed on the role of the auditors in certifying the receipts and disbursements, but the omission of certain disbursements allowed by section 2 of the Public Hospitals Act was not properly addressed. Finally, readers were reminded of the financial boon resulting from the 137 sweepstakes which had been held until then and had raised over £79 million.[53]

The publication of MacAnthony's article was a watershed in the public attitude to the sweepstake. Henceforth critics were more willing to attack it publicly and, as a result of the detailed information on the workings of the sweepstake revealed by him, had the ammunition to do so. The Oireachtas debate on the 1976 Public Hospitals (Amendment) Act, which increased Hospitals Trust's expenses ratio to 40 per cent, is particularly revealing in this regard. In previous parliamentary debates concerning the sweepstake there had occasionally been a lone voice of dissent, usually from the Labour Party. By contrast, the 1976 debate represented the most serious public criticism from legislators to date, with serious reservations being expressed by members of the opposition Fianna Fáil party but also by some members of the junior partner in the coalition government, Labour.

The former Fianna Fáil Justice Minister, Desmond O'Malley, who had tried unsuccessfully to raise objections to the expenses paid to Hospitals Trust when sweepstake schemes came to him for approval, attacked the sweepstake basing many of his objections on issues raised by MacAnthony.[54] He criticised the problematic nature of section 2 of the Public Hospitals Act for leaving both the auditors and the Minister for Justice in the dark about how much money was spent in easing foreign ticket sales: 'My experience as Minister for Justice was that that information was not forthcoming.' He highlighted the contrast between the high fees earned by the promoters and the negligible contribution sweepstake income was now making to overall health spending, which he estimated to be just 'a little over 1 per cent' and called attention to the activities of the promoters in buying back shares in winning tickets.[55]

O'Malley's highlighting of the evasive nature of section 2 raised the issue of the lack of accountability in the operation of the sweepstake, a theme taken up by his party colleague, P. J. Lalor, and Labour's Dr John O'Connell, both of whom were dissatisfied that it was not subject to scrutiny by the Comptroller and Auditor General.[56] The Minister for Justice, Patrick Cooney, responded to such requests for greater scrutiny by pointing out that it was 'not realistic' to impose 'public accountability over a private company'.[57] This response highlighted a convenient excuse that had enabled successive Irish governments to distance themselves from the illicit and embarrassing foreign activities of sweepstake agents; while the sweepstake had been established by the legislature it was promoted by a private company, thus allowing the state a convenient level of distance and non-responsibility.

In spite of the fact that the legislation under discussion was a government measure, Labour Party members were among its strongest critics. In the Dáil Dr John O'Connell made the sensational allegation that he had

> been intimidated by people in the last few months in regard to the Hospitals Sweepstake telling me that unless I voted for this there would be serious repercussions . . . I have been intimidated by people – not in the House – that there would be serious repercussions if I did not vote for this Bill; I would be smeared in my constituency – this was conveyed to me just two weeks ago, last

Sunday week – that I would be smeared in my constituency and everything done to get me out.

He complained further that 'the Hospitals Sweepstake . . . has damaged our good name abroad'.[58] His party colleague in the Seanad, John Horgan, a close friend of Joe MacAnthony and a colleague on the government side in the upper house of Senator Patrick McGrath, found 'the whole sweepstake operation . . . abhorrent' and called for a 'substantial rethink of the whole sweepstake operation . . . by the Government'.[59] Fellow university senators, Patrick Quinlan of the National University and Mary Robinson of Trinity College, agreed that a 'full-scale, independent examination of its operation' was needed.[60] Robinson also highlighted the plight of those in the media who had the temerity to examine the underbelly of the sweepstake, although she did not mention Joe MacAnthony by name:

> We know that those journalists who have sought further information and who have investigated the operation of the Irish Hospitals Sweepstakes have not furthered their careers in doing so. Indeed, if anything, they have either changed their immediate employment or left the country entirely.[61]

Another arm of the Irish media to feel the dissatisfaction of the sweepstake in 1973 was *Profile* magazine. The original edition for July 1973 included a review by Thomas O'Hanlon of Oliver Pilat's unauthorised biography of Drew Pearson, which revealed Pearson's identity as a sweepstake agent in the USA during the 1930s, and the front cover pictured the late Joseph McGrath, with his customary hat, bow tie, and cigarette, along with the caption 'Joe McGrath – "Mr Sweep"'. This edition was withdrawn very soon after its appearance and replaced with an alternative issue that did not contain either the review or the picture of McGrath on the cover.[62]

The influence still wielded by Hospitals Trust against journalists perceived as hostile meant that no media outlet would venture to explore its workings again for some time. In 1978 RTÉ's *Politics Programme* took a 'brave decision' to film a documentary similar in content to the MacAnthony article. Extensive interviews took place in Canada with both sweepstake agents and police officers, and the smuggling of sweepstake tickets out of Dublin port was filmed secretly. Donal Ó Moráin, a former chairman of the RTÉ authority furnished the researchers, Charlie Bird and Michael Heney, with a Department of Justice memorandum highly critical of the sweepstake, although some within the national broadcaster felt that 'it would be unpatriotic' to make use of it. A very comprehensive picture of the activities of Hospitals Trust in selling its tickets abroad illegally was compiled; according to Michael Heney: 'We had the lists; we had the names; we had the addresses; we had the places; we had the events; we had the smuggling; we had the pay-backs, the kick-backs, the money paid to the hauliers; we had chapter and verse.'[63]

Concerned at the damage these revelations would cause to its already declining sales, Hospitals Trust wrote directly to the Director General of RTÉ to express its concern at the plan to show the programme and it was initially postponed and eventually shelved, although extracts were broadcast as part of a *Today Tonight Special* in 1992, five years after the sweep had closed and the impact of the revelations was greatly lessened. Media commentators and those involved in the programme have criticised its suppression as representing a major failure on the part of the national broadcaster, but the episode also indicates how influential the directors of Hospitals Trust remained during the late 1970s. In spite of declining sweepstake ticket sales and the negligible portion of the proceeds allocated to hospitals they still wielded substantial commercial power, through the advertising associated not alone with the sweepstake but with their associated businesses like Waterford Glass.[64]

It was not until 2003 that RTÉ was prepared to broadcast a detailed historical documentary on the sweepstake, as part of its inaugural *Hidden History* series. The film-maker, Liam Wylie, had been trying for some time to interest the national broadcaster in this project. This comprehensive analysis examined the sweepstake's historical origins, interviewed former employees, and examined the murkier elements of the operation in considerable detail.[65] It proved extremely popular, attracting a viewing audience of 330,000, and its revelations still surprised some commentators.[66] It resulted in a number of newspaper features on the sweepstake and on Joe MacAnthony's famous *exposé*, as well as an effort to rehabilitate the McGrath's (ironically published in the *Sunday Independent*) by highlighting their investments in Irish industry.[67]

INDUSTRIAL RELATIONS

The difficulties experienced by Hospitals Trust with declining sweepstake income and growing public unease at its activities, made the early 1970s a timely occasion for the Workers' Union of Ireland to renew its campaign for recognition. The issue had lain dormant for most of the 1960s, after an unsuccessful ten-year battle to hold Hospitals Trust to the terms of the 1950 Labour Court decision. The union returned to the Labour Court in 1967, claiming the right to negotiate on behalf of seven male night cleaners. Of 59 night cleaners employed by the trust, 52 were represented by the House Association. Nevertheless, the Labour Court reiterated its 1950 finding, recommending 'that the Company should concede to the Union the right to negotiate on behalf of its members in the Company's employment'.[68] Once again Hospitals Trust simply ignored the proceedings, refusing to attend the hearing or to act upon the recommendation.[69] The union did not follow through on its threat of strike action that might have disrupted the Cambridgeshire draw[70] because of the vulnerable position of employees and the desire not to damage further the already declining proceeds.[71] A further Labour Court recommendation advising recognition, issued in 1971, was similarly disregarded by Hospitals Trust.[72]

The task of the WUI was undoubtedly made more difficult by the fact that it lacked support among the overwhelming majority of sweepstake staff. Less than a quarter of the clerical staff were in the WUI and some of these were also in the House Association.[73] Industrial relations remained governed by the old-fashioned paternalistic methods adopted by Joseph McGrath during the 1930s. Yet, there is very little evidence that the majority of the staff were dissatisfied with this, although the WUI argued that this was because they were afraid to voice any such feelings 'for fear of victimisation' by management.[74] By the 1970s the realisation that declining contributions could lead to the closure of the sweepstake, with little prospect of alternative employment, contributed to the passivity of the workforce.[75] The attitude of the directors to unionisation in the sweepstake contrasted markedly with the policies pursued in their other businesses, in particular Waterford Glass, where unions were strong and industrial relations generally good.[76] Glass-blowers in Waterford were skilled craftsmen who the management could not afford to alienate. By contrast, the vulnerable widows, elderly women, and disabled people employed in the sweepstake were entirely dependent on Hospitals Trust for their livelihoods.

The challenge facing the WUI from a largely unsympathetic workforce became clear when the union attacked Hospitals Trust's pay scales and the absence of a formal pension scheme. Claims that wage rates were as low as £9 per week were rejected vehemently by Nora Stephen, the Honorary Secretary of the House Association, who stated that the basic wage had risen to £12 per week.[77] Her position was supported by Betty Ray, who defended Hospitals Trust as 'very good employers', and criticised the WUI for trying to 'cause dissension amongst the staff'.[78] Underlying these views appears to be a fear that the interference of the WUI might actually make things worse for the employees; if the union's campaign damaged the sweepstake it could have an adverse effect on jobs there. A strong camaraderie existed among the Hospitals Trust staff. Outside of the building in Ballsbridge they socialised frequently, including organising an annual pilgrimage to the Marian shrine at Knock.[79] The WUI's campaign appears to have caused some fracturing among the staff, another reason for the hostility to it: 'The inter-union thing soured a certain cohort of the staff, and there was always that "them and us" bit, even on a day-to-day working basis.'[80]

Representations by the House Association, and perhaps the need for management to show that its employees did not require trade union representation, produced some improvements in working conditions during the 1970s. A proper pension scheme was introduced. Previously retiring employees received a gratuity on leaving: 'it was a contribution, a percentage that was paid into your personal account every sweepstake and when you were leaving it would be several hundred pounds, or maybe if you were really long there it could be £1,000.' The prohibition on women continuing to work after marriage was also lifted.[81]

The continued intransigence of Hospitals Trust and the growing public criticism of the sweepstake hardened the resolve of the WUI to win its battle for recognition. It widened its attack beyond the limits of the powerless Labour Court, referring the dispute to the International Labour Organisation (ILO), threatening further strike action, and making an official complaint to the Employer–Labour Conference (ELC) that Hospitals Trust had broken national wage agreements.[82] Hospitals Trust's attitude to the ELC was similar to its response to the Labour Court, refusing to attend hearings or act upon the conference's finding that it had broken the 1972 national wage agreement and was 'in breach of obligations fundamental to the operation of national pay agreements' through its continued non-recognition of the WUI. This ruling, and the argument that the failure to recognise the WUI breached ILO conventions ratified by Ireland, embarrassed the government, especially the Labour Party's Minister for Labour and former trade union official, Michael O'Leary.[83] It was hoped that the formation of a coalition government containing the Labour Party would help the cause of the WUI, although the appointment of Patrick McGrath to the Seanad seemed to indicate that Fine Gael Taoiseach Liam Cosgrave 'did not have strong feelings about the union's grievance.'[84]

The decline in proceeds which resulted in a deficit in the expenses allowed to Hospitals Trust resulted in the introduction of a three-day week at the end of 1974, to cover the traditional lean period between the Sweeps Hurdle in December and the following year's Lincoln sweepstake. Social welfare payments then covered a six-day week, so the employees were able to draw an allowance for the three days that they did not work. The three-day week was reinstated intermittently during the 1970s.[85] This was a serious sign that jobs in Hospitals Trust were under threat and it appears to have lessened the hostility of the workforce to the WUI and given a boost to the union's demand for recognition:

It was easy to make hay once the short-time started because then the staff had a gripe, they were suffering, so those that were in awe of the directors or the management or fearful of losing their jobs, that fear was dissipating by the fact that 'now they are starting to treat us like a real boss and they're saying we haven't the work so we're not going to pay you'.[86]

Hospitals Trust's failure to consult the WUI about the introduction of short-time led to the union serving strike notice in February 1975. This time it was determined to proceed with the industrial action, which was supported fully by the ICTU and was to include workers at Hospitals Trust who belonged other congress-affiliated unions.[87] The seriousness of the union's intentions, and the potential damage that such a widespread strike could do to the up-coming Lincoln sweepstake, led to an eleventh-hour capitulation by Hospitals Trust and the end of its 28-year refusal to recognise the right of the WUI to negotiate on behalf of its members employed in the sweepstake. Under the settlement, brokered by Tom McGrath, the industrial relations officer of the ICTU, the WUI agreed not to seek a closed shop while Hospitals Trust undertook to negotiate separately with the WUI and the House Association on behalf of their respective members.[88]

This conclusion to one of the longest-running battles for trade union recognition in independent Ireland did not usher in a period of harmonious industrial relations in the sweepstake. While Hospitals Trust negotiated with the WUI (the Federated Workers' Union of Ireland from 1978), the union was often at odds with the company over redundancies and the implementation of wage increases. On three further occasions, in 1977 and 1983, such disputes ended up in the Labour Court.[89] In May 1977 an official strike took place at Hospitals Trust, when 200 WUI members picketed the Ballsbridge headquarters in a dispute over retrospective payment of national wage agreement increases. The strike was not supported by non-WUI members, leading to some tension between both sides: 'The building labourers emptied a bucket of water over the head of a maintenance man who went into work. "And they told him it wasn't all spring water."' The strike lasted for over a month before a settlement was brokered by the ICTU.[90]

A redundancy scheme that would reduce the staff from 900 to fewer than 200 over the next ten years was introduced in September 1975. Initially 200 staff aged between 60 and 66, some with fewer than fifteen years' service, were offered voluntary redundancy following negotiations between the management, the WUI and the House Association.[91] This was followed by 200 more redundancies in 1978.[92] Short-time and temporary lay-offs continued periodically during the late 1970s and early 1980s.

The most serious threat to the sweepstake workers' jobs was a post office strike in 1979 that resulted in the cancellation of two sweepstake draws; during this period 250 of the remaining 300 staff were laid off temporarily.[93] Hospitals Trust had never before been forced to cancel a draw, even during the crisis at the start of the Second World War. Patrick McGrath commented subsequently on the lasting damage caused by the strike: 'What really began to kill the Sweep was the prolonged postal strike of 1979. We lost forty per cent of our overseas business, because the local post offices would send the tickets back – they were not accepting anything for Ireland. We never recovered from that.'[94]

In an effort to sustain employment after the postal strike, the government sanctioned the introduction of three yearly Shamrock sweeps, smaller competitions with a first prize of £20,000 in which tickets (costing £1) were only sold in Ireland. These were held on races that took place in the lean periods between the bigger draws and the proceeds were only between £200,000 and £400,000 for each draw. Shamrock sweeps were introduced to provide work for underemployed Hospitals Trust workers and made virtually no contribution to the Hospitals Trust Fund.[95]

THE McGRATH EMPIRE IN DECLINE

Even though the sweepstake was encountering difficulties during the 1970s, the McGrath business portfolio that had been built upon its early success remained profitable. The McGraths were still one of the richest families in the state: 'They had so much money they were able to leave the father's estate untouched for years.' Apart from some indulgences – 'Paddy McGrath cruised around town in a Rolls Phantom VI, the only one in Ireland at the time', they lived relatively private and unobtrusive lives in Dublin and Kildare.[96]

An investment company, initially called Dodder Investments, but renamed Avenue Investments to avoid confusion with Dodder Properties, one of the biggest property developers in Dublin, was formed to manage the financial interests of the three sweepstake families.[97] The majority share-holding in Avenue – 60 per cent – belonged to the McGraths, with the Duggans and Freemans commanding 16 per cent each. The remaining 8 per cent was in external hands.[98] Alan Jeffers, the Assistant Managing Director of the Jefferson Smurfit Group, was recruited to build up the company's investment portfolio.[99]

The jewel in Avenue's crown during the 1970s was undoubtedly Waterford Glass. Throughout the 1960s, while still a subsidiary of the Irish Glass Bottle Company, Waterford became highly profitable on the basis of demand for luxury hand-cut glass in the USA. Net profits increased rapidly from £51,000 in 1958 to £86,000 in 1961 and £156,000 in 1963.[100] This trend continued throughout the 1960s and into the 1970s, with demand for Waterford's products always increasing, resulting in a significant expansion of production capacity.[101] By 1977 the company employed nearly 3,000 people in its glass production facilities alone and was said to be 'the largest producer of high-quality crystal in the world'.[102] In recognition of their contribution to the local economy, Patrick McGrath and Noel Griffin, the Managing Director of Waterford Glass, were both awarded the freedom of Waterford city.[103]

Waterford's profitability resulted in a significant expansion of Avenue's commercial portfolio. By 1980 it had six subsidiary companies: Waltham Holdings, manufacturers of audio equipment; Fannin Holdings, manufacturers and distributors of health-care products; Danfay Distributors, an importer of Yamaha motor parts; bed manufacturers Odearest; Squash Ireland; and Watson and Jameson sail-makers. In addition, it controlled significant proportions of Memory Computer; bloodstock sales company R. J. Goff; Ergas, suppliers of bottled gas; Irish International Biochemicals; the Irish Credit Bank; Hibernian Insurance; and airline company Avair. With an estimated annual turnover of £40 million, Avenue was one of the twenty largest companies in Ireland.[104]

Companies under the Avenue umbrella also began to diversify. In the early 1970s the Waterford Group acquired Aynsley China, Switzer's – a Dublin department store that distributed Waterford Glass, and the postcard company John Hinde.[105] These acquisitions made commercial sense as the companies were involved in similar lines of business to Waterford: luxury tableware and products aimed at the tourist market. However, financial commentators began to raise eyebrows when Waterford started to expand beyond the boundaries of its traditional activities. Surprise was expressed at the purchase of a controlling interest in the Renault car distributor, the Smith Group for £4.6 million in 1974: 'it is less clear what sense the move makes to Waterford . . . there appears to be little relationship between its existing activities and those of Smith apart from the fact that both could be described as concerned with distribution.'[106]

Stretching its investments beyond its traditional business interests, combined with the onset of a recession in the early 1980s, began to cause difficulties for Avenue; 1980 saw a decline in profits at Waterford Glass for the first time in 26 years.[107] A further drain on the company came in the form of the third generation of the founding families. The grandchildren of the founders were now coming of age and looking for their share of the families' accumulated fortune. As Patrick McGrath noted in 1986, 'What started off as a shareholding split between three people is now split between sixty or seventy of the Duggan, Freeman and McGrath families.'[108] The fact that the sweepstake was no longer a source of finance for the families' wider business interests also added to the financial pressure on Avenue. As a result a sustained programme of divestment was undertaken in the early 1980s, starting with the sale of a portion of Waterford in 1980. This was followed by the offloading of Fannin for £1.8 million in 1981 and 20 per cent of Hibernian Insurance for £5.3 million in 1982.[109]

The apogee of this disinvestment programme was the disposal of the entire remaining shareholding in Waterford in 1984. Financial crises in both Avenue, which reputedly owed £7 million to Bank of Ireland, and Waterford – where borrowing was reported to be out of control – resulted in Avenue seeking a purchaser for its most important company.[110] Initial estimates suggested that Avenue could make up to £22.5 million from the sale. However, difficulty in attracting a suitable buyer resulted in the eventual sale to Globe Investments for £17 million. The new owners soon disposed of the cumbersome subsidiaries Switzer's, Aynsley, and the Smith Group for a combined price of £32.7 million.[111]

The detrimental impact on Avenue of the sale of Waterford for well below its value was exacerbated by failures in some of its other flagship acquisitions. In 1982 Avenue and Waterford sold their shareholdings in Memory Computer (a company established by Owen Dalton, son of Joseph McGrath's close associate Charles Dalton), for £1.45 million and £865,670 respectively. Not long afterwards Memory floated on the stock market and was valued at £16.5 million.[112] Ferrier Pollock, a clothing distributor that owned the Powerscourt Townhouse shopping centre, had been acquired in 1972 and went into receivership in 1980. Waltham Holdings also went into receivership, Avair collapsed, and Irish Glass Bottle was underperforming.[113] A banner headline in the magazine *Irish Business* summed up what had happened at Avenue. The front cover reads: 'THE MCGRATH FORTUNE: FIFTY YEARS TO BUILD IT AND FIVE YEARS TO BLOW IT!' Between 1973 and 1984 it estimated that £18 million had been lost as a result of bad timing, bad investments, bad luck, and Patrick McGrath's misplaced patriotism that insisted upon investing in solely Irish companies.[114]

During the early 1980s the McGrath family also began to sell off much of its property in south county Dublin, leading to a landmark case in Irish taxation law. In order to avoid paying a hefty capital gains bill on profits of over £2.4 million, the three McGrath brothers (Patrick, Séamus, and Joseph Jnr) engaged in a complicated tax avoidance scheme whereby share-dealings in tax havens such as Jersey and the Isle of Man created artificial losses of £1 million. Both the High and Supreme Courts found in favour of the McGraths against the Revenue Commissioners on the grounds that a loophole in Irish tax law allowed them to conduct these transactions. Their victory resulted in specific legislative changes to ensure such loopholes could not be exploited again.[115]

The rapidly declining fortunes of the sweepstake led to suggestions of replacing it with a national lottery. As early as 1968 students at the Historical Society in Trinity College carried a motion in support of a national lottery.[116] At the height of the recognition dispute between Hospitals Trust and the WUI, Denis Larkin proposed the replacement of the hospitals sweepstake with a 'National Sweepstake'.[117] The various proposals from Hospitals Trust itself to transform the sweepstake into a weekly competition were the surest sign that the existing format did not have a long-term future.

Legislators began to give serious thought to the idea of a national lottery in the early 1980s. Initially it was intended that it would be used primarily to finance sports facilities. In 1983 proposals for the establishment of a national lottery were submitted to the government by Cospóir, the National Sports Council. Definite plans to set it up were included in the Fine Gael–Labour coalition's plan for government, *Building on Reality*, published in October 1984 and management consultants were engaged to draw up a plan for it.[118]

A decision was taken to advertise the franchise to run the lottery and then enact legislation to govern it. By mid-1985 a number of contenders for the lottery franchise had emerged: Hospitals Trust; An Post; a consortium led by Frank Flannery comprising the Mater Hospital (Dublin), Central Remedial Clinic, and the Rehabilitation Institute, all three of which already had well-established and lucrative lotteries; a joint venture between Independent Newspapers and Vernon's Football Pools; and an international bidder, United National Charities Ltd. However, it was felt that only the Flannery group and An Post had a serious chance of success. These two bids appeared to enjoy most support within the government: Labour TDs Dick Spring and Michael D. Higgins and Minister for Finance, Alan Dukes, were believed to favour the An Post application, while Frank Flannery had the support of some members of Fine Gael, a party with which he was personally closely associated.[119]

In October 1985 it was announced officially that An Post had won the franchise. The existence of an extensive network of post offices throughout the country in which lottery tickets could be sold was an important factor in the company's favour, as was the fact that it had an established and trusted reputation. The status of An Post as a semi-state company was also in its favour; independent consultants Touche Ross supported it for this reason.[120] A subsidiary company, An Post National Lottery Company was formed to run the lottery, which was officially launched on 12 March 1987, with the introduction of a scratch card lottery ticket. Two years later the more popular lotto game was introduced, and this has subsequently become the most popular form of the Irish national lottery.

THE CLOSURE OF THE SWEEPSTAKE

The inevitable result of the setting up of the national lottery was the closure of the sweepstake, although no formal machinery was put in place by the government to shut it down. Patrick McGrath had 'several meetings' with the government during 1985 to discuss the future of the sweepstake after the lottery was established.[121] The principal concern was no longer for hospitals, given that the sweepstake was producing so little revenue for the Hospitals Trust Fund, but for the future of the approximately 200 remaining staff; at one point Hospitals Trust suggested nationalising the sweepstakes to protect their employment.[122] If the sweepstake could have been kept as a going concern for even five or six more years, that would have been sufficient to take most of the staff to retirement age.[123]

In 1986 Hospitals Trust submitted a proposal to the government that would allow them to continue to promote fortnightly sweepstakes, but this scheme was rejected by Alan Dukes (who had moved from Finance to Justice) because 'the operation of more than one lottery of the magnitude of the national lottery and the sweepstake they had proposed could result in wasteful duplication'. Dukes subsequently agreed in principle to a further proposal for occasional sweepstakes with tickets costing £10 or £20, but this never came to fruition.[124] Following the last hospitals sweepstake on the Sweeps Hurdle in January 1986, the workforce at Hospitals Trust was laid off and subsequently made redundant when the company officially went into liquidation on 16 March 1987.[125] The national lottery had previously announced that it did not intend to offer employment to them.[126]

THE FATE OF HOSPITALS TRUST'S EMPLOYEES

The unemployed sweepstake workers were entitled to statutory redundancy only. Initially, Hospitals Trust intended to pay an enhanced redundancy that would be financed by the sale of the remaining fourteen years of the lease of the Ballsbridge site back to the Hospitals Trust Board for £1.4 million, but this plan was scuppered by the Revenue Commissioners who claimed £700,000 of that transaction in capital gains tax.[127] Another option was to divert a proportion of the sale of the Ballsbridge site to compensating the redundant workers, but this was rejected by Fianna Fáil Health Minister, Rory O'Hanlon.[128] The eleven-acre site, 'probably the most valuable single piece of real estate left in Dublin', was put up for sale in 1987 but taken off the market a year later when no suitable bids were received, in spite of reported interest from a number of hotel chains. The controversial delay in disposing of it led to the resignation of three members of the Hospitals Trust Board. It was eventually sold at auction in July 1988 for £6.6 million, 'the highest price yet paid at auction for a property in the Republic.' It is now a mixed development of offices, retail units, and an apartment complex named 'The Sweepstakes'.[129]

After the failure of efforts to enhance the redundancy payments, the Hospitals Trust House Association took its case to the Labour Court in May 1987. They argued that the government had a responsibility to them because the loss of their jobs stemmed directly from the decision to establish the national lottery and the refusal to permit sweepstakes to continue to operate alongside it. It was also argued that the government could afford compensation because it had benefited to the tune of £1.2 million from the closure of the sweepstake; £700,000 in capital gains tax from the lease sale-back and a £500,000 insurance payment for damage done to the building during Hurricane Charlie in July 1986. Other potential sources of finance included the proceeds of the pending liquidation sale, unclaimed prize money, and the government rebate on the statutory redundancy entitlement, estimated at '60% of the total paid out Redundancy'.[130] The Labour Court subsequently recommended that the liquidators, Craig Gardner, pay an additional two weeks' wages per year of service, but the liquidator stated that he did not have the power to comply; nor did he have control over the dispersal of unclaimed prize money.[131]

The failure to have the Labour Court recommendation acted upon left many redundant workers in severe financial difficulty. Some of those who had the longest service received only £3,000, whereas this could have risen to £10,000 had the recommendation been implemented. Many of them had difficulty finding alternative employment, because of their age and the unfavourable economic climate, and others were unable to continue paying rent on their accommodation.[132] The strict regulations governing social welfare entitlements also made life difficult. In 1991 the *Irish Times* highlighted the case of a 62-year-old who had 'worked all her life' in the sweepstake until it closed. Unable to afford her own accommodation, she lived with her brother and sister-in-law, so that for the purposes of a means test his income was also deemed to be hers, resulting in the withdrawal of a weekly payment of £40.[133]

The redundant sweepstake workers clearly felt that the government bore a responsibility to them, but the government disagreed because Hospitals Trust was a private company. The employees also felt harshly treated by the directors of Hospitals Trust. Many of them had worked for the sweepstake for up to forty years, and most had shunned the efforts of the WUI to unionise them in opposition to management. According to John Slevin, who had been the financial controller of the company until its closure, 'This was the betrayal. They just could not believe that the company that they had worked for so loyally for so long could do this to them.'[134]

They sustained a campaign to highlight their plight and seek some redress. Public events, including the official launch of the national lottery and the auction of the Ballsbridge site, were picketed peacefully.[135] Some restitution was conceded by the government when it decided to distribute the remaining unclaimed sweepstake prize money among them. After the closure of the sweepstake, £480,000 remained from unclaimed prizes and the accrued interest. The Public Hospitals (Amendment) Act (1990) permitted the Minister for Health to distribute this among former Hospitals Trust employees. Should any claims for payment of these prizes emerge subsequently, this would be met by the exchequer, provided the claim was made within four years of the passing of the act. It was thought unlikely that any such claims would be made as most of the unclaimed prize money dated back to the start of the sweepstake.[136]

Confusion existed concerning the categories of former employees that were eligible for the payments. One hundred and forty-seven people had lost their jobs on 16 March 1987, and a small number had left a few days before this date for alternative employment. It was intended to give these a payment of between £500 and £4,000 each, depending on length of service. A further 200, who had availed of voluntary redundancy between 1978 and 1980 and who had lost an *ex gratia* portion of their pensions when the company folded in 1987, were to receive approximately £1,000 each. Although such payments were technically liable for taxation, none would reach the threshold of £6,000 in order to incur it.[137]

While the passage of this legislation, which received all-party support in the Oireachtas, was an admission by the government of the hardship suffered by the redundant workers, the state was still reluctant to concede any liability. Rory O'Hanlon again rejected the idea of allocating a portion of the £6.6 million raised form the sale of the Ballsbridge site; by 1990 'virtually all the proceeds of that sale [had] now been used up, the bulk of it supporting the public health capital programme'. The government remained wedded to the principle that it had no responsibility to meet the obligations of a private company to its erstwhile workforce.[138]

The second category of former employees compensated, those who had taken voluntary redundancy in the 1970s, continued to pursue their claims for the *ex gratia* portion of their pension with the liquidators. On retirement these women had been given a standard pension payment, that was topped up with an additional *ex gratia* payment, but when the company was wound up they were informed that this latter portion would no longer be paid to them. They claimed that they had never been made aware that there was a difference between both types of payment, and as a result the company was obliged to pay them the full pension for life, a claim supported by Hospitals Trust's former financial controller, John Slevin, who stated that 'nowhere in the company's books had he come across an *ex gratia* account to deal with the funding of pensions for 25 women workers who took early retirement in 1980'.[139] In 1993 the High Court upheld these claims to a full pension. While Hospitals Trust had informed the employees of the situation in a memorandum, Mr Justice Geoghegan held that they could not be expected to understand the implications of it and he had 'no hesitation in concluding that they never understood that any part of the pension was *ex gratia*. The term *ex gratia* was not used in the memo and even if it had been, they would have needed a personal explanation' of its import.[140]

The 147 who were made redundant in March 1986 still remained without the additional redundancy recommended by the Labour Court and only received relatively small payments under the 1990 Act. Led by John Slevin, this group kept up pressure on politicians throughout the 1990s. Eventually, in 2000, the Fianna Fáil–Progressive Democrat coalition government reversed the policy of their predecessors since 1987 and legislation was passed in July of that year awarding those still living, and the next-of-kin of those who had died in the meantime, a lump sum of £20,000 each. The credit for the government's change of heart rests with the then Minister for Enterprise and Employment, Mary Harney, who was extremely sympathetic to the plight of the sweepstake workers.[141] In the Dáil Harney also pointed to the perseverance of the workers themselves, and especially John Slevin, in ensuring a successful conclusion to their campaign: 'If it was not for his determination and for the fact that he was so resolute and such a good campaigner for the former workers, I doubt we would have legislation of this kind before us today. Those former workers, in particular, owe him a great deal of gratitude.'[142]

Harney conceded that the government had some obligation because of the statutory nature of the sweepstake. However, she was anxious to establish that this move did not 'involve setting a precedent for former employees in other organisations, either public or private'.[143] Nevertheless, it could be argued that the government was in fact following a precedent already established in two high-profile redundancies, in the Talbot motor assembly plant and Irish Shipping. When the privately owned Talbot plant in Dublin closed in 1981, Taoiseach Charles Haughey, in whose constituency it had been based, used exchequer funds to tide the workers over for a period.[144] A more appropriate comparison with the sweepstake workers was the case of Irish Shipping

Limited; in 1994 compensation was paid to former workers of the company, which had folded ten years previously, although there was a significant difference in that Irish Shipping was a state-owned company.[145]

The belated award of compensation to the sweepstake workers made redundant in 1987 was the final act in the eventful and contentious history of the Irish hospitals sweepstake, and of its complicated and often fractious relationship with the Irish state, which must have been relieved to be rid of the problematic child to which it have given birth seventy years previously.

EIGHT

THE SWEEPSTAKE AND HOSPITAL DEVELOPMENT, 1939–87

—

HOSPITAL DEVELOPMENT DURING THE EMERGENCY

Between 1939 and 1941 hospital construction was affected adversely by the war and the consequent shortage of building materials. Nevertheless, projects which had been in train were brought to completion, including the provision of a significant number of additional beds for the Mater and Sir Patrick Dun's, an extension to Cappagh Orthopaedic Hospital, new outpatient and X-ray departments for the Richmond, a new outpatient department for Jervis St, and a new X-ray department for Cork city's North Infirmary.[1] With regards to the plan for rationalising general hospital provision on the south side of Dublin city, the amalgamation of Mercer's, Sir Patrick Dun's and the Royal City of Dublin was ready to proceed after the alteration of existing arrangements between Dun's and Trinity College's School of Physics had been approved. The refusal of the Meath to join forced a delay as the scheme had to be adjusted. Plans were also said to be under way for the construction of the new St Vincent's.[2]

Very little additional progress on hospital development took place for the duration of the war. The Hospitals Commission's sixth report, dealing with the period from 1942 to 1944, explained how:

> The severe limitations imposed by the World War on the importation of building materials, and the inadequacy of internal supplies to meet the demands of large scale schemes, continued to militate against hospital development during the years 1942, 1943 and 1944.[3]

A disagreement between the government and the Sisters of Charity, who were supported by the Archbishop of Dublin, delayed progress on the new St Vincent's, 'until an agreement was signed that there would be no interference in the control and management of the Hospital'.[4] Such an agreement appears to have been reached in 1942, though by late 1946 progress was still said to be 'slow', with only the architectural competition completed.[5]

The only real progress had been the passing of the St Laurence's Hospital
Act in 1943 to allow for the construction of the new incarnation of the
Richmond Hospital in Cabra, north of Dublin city.[6] The saga of St Laurence's
encapsulates many of the difficulties encountered in rationalising voluntary
hospital provision in Dublin city. The initial plan had been for the re-building
of a 5–600 bed hospital on the existing site of the Richmond Hospital in
North Brunswick Street, and by 1938 the architect Michael Scott had almost
completed the relevant plans. However, when it was discovered that Dublin
Corporation intended to redevelop the hospital's hinterland, these plans were
shelved temporarily. In March 1939 the board of the Richmond agreed to
move to a larger green-field site in the 'more salubrious' environs of Cabra, in
spite of opposition from the medical staff who feared that being so far
removed from the city centre medical schools would jeopardise its future as a
teaching hospital.

It took four years for the St Laurence's Hospital Act, which provided for
the replacement of the old House of Industry hospitals – the Richmond,
Hardwicke and Whitworth – with the new St Laurence's General Hospital,
to pass through the Oireachtas. In addition to moving from their city centre
location, another contention between the hospital governors and the government was the decision to rename the institution, which the governors claimed
they only became aware of from a newspaper report. Echoing the long-
running dispute over increased state control of voluntary hospitals, objections
were also raised to the greater level of control that the Minister for Local
Government and Public Health would have over the management of the new
hospital, including the appointment and replacement of members of the
hospital's board and the right to 'alter the constitution of the Board in such
manner as he thinks fit'. According to one supporter of the voluntary hospitals,
the act made the Richmond Hospital into 'a Department of State'. In 1944 a
suitable site was finally identified and the following year a compulsory
acquisition order was made and an architect and consulting engineer
appointed. No more progress would be made until the 1950s.[7]

The St Laurence's Hospital Act was not the first occasion on which
legislation was used to dilute voluntary control of hospitals. Under the Dublin
Fever Hospital Act, passed in 1936, the board of Cork Street Fever Hospital
was dissolved and replaced by a commission, bringing the hospital 'absolutely
under Departmental control'. A third instance of such ministerial heavy-
handedness, as the voluntary hospitals saw it, was the enactment of the
Tuberculosis Act in 1945, that provided for the use of money in the Hospitals
Trust Fund to build sanatoria; having already seen the Hospitals Trust Fund
applied to local authority hospitals, the voluntaries bristled at this further
deviation from the original purpose of funding their institutions.[8] The extended

use of legislation in this way to increase state control of certain hospitals, to the detriment of the voluntary tradition, heightened further the tensions between voluntary hospitals and the state during the 1940s.

The upward trend in the deficits of the voluntary hospitals continued during the 1940s. Following a substantial rise in the 1941 deficit, which, at £37,702, was more than twice that for 1940 (£16,426), the Minister for Local Government and Public Health lamented 'that no effective steps have so far been taken to improve the financial position' of the hospitals. Noting that 'a contributing factor to the growing deficits is the practice of treating large numbers of patients free, or at a rate much below the actual cost of mainten-ance', it was recommended that hospital governors investigate the extent to which patients were not paying enough for their treatment and possi-bly requiring patients unable to pay to seek treatment through their local authority.[9] This stern warning appears to have had some salutary effect, as the deficit increase for 1942 was only £90 and 1943 saw a decrease in the deficit by over £21,000. However, the upward trajectory returned in 1944, with a jump of £33,144.[10]

Table 8.1: Total annual deficits of voluntary hospitals, 1940–4 (£)

Year	Total deficits	Increase /decrease over previous year	Increase since 1933
1940	173,401	+ 16,426	118,533
1941	211,103	+ 37,702	156,235
1942	211,193	+ 90	156,325
1943	189,322	– 21,871	134,454
1944	222,466	+ 33,144	167,598
1945	240,020	+ 17,554	185,152

Hospitals Commission, *Seventh general report*, p. 4

The only explanation that the Hospitals Commission was able to offer for these fluctuations was that 'in the year 1943 a determined effort was made by the hospital authorities to control expenditure, but for that year only, as in the year 1944 expenditure again increased at an abnormal rate'. A divergence among the hospitals in the total cost per occupied bed led the commission to reject the catch-all excuse of rising prices being largely responsible for the increased expenditure. In particular there was a noticeable difference in cost per occupied bed between lay and religious-controlled hospitals, leading to the conclusion that 'some reorganisation of administrative methods was necessary in the case of the lay-controlled General Hospitals'.[11] This assessment appeared to ignore the fact that staffing costs were higher in the lay hospitals, which were unable to draw upon the nursing services of nuns, as in the cases of hospitals run by religious communities.

The drastic reduction in income derived from sweepstakes forced the commission to consider alternative sources of income for the voluntary hospitals, if the entire sweepstake surplus was not to be used to meet deficits. Possible sources included an increase in the fees paid by local authorities for the treatment of patients within their jurisdictions, the introduction of a contributory scheme (previously mooted by the commission), and increasing the proportion of beds made available to paying patients.[12]

THE DUBLIN HOSPITALS BUREAU (BED BUREAU)

The establishment of the Dublin Hospitals Bureau, or bed bureau as it was more popularly known, in 1941, was interpreted by the voluntary hospitals as further evidence of the dilution of their autonomy by the state. In February 1941 Professor Henry Moore warned an audience of the Trinity College Historical Society that if officials were to gain control over hospital admissions, the hospitals would have no freedom left. His address also made it clear that the voluntaries were becoming very disillusioned with the direction the sweepstake had taken:

> . . . they soon came to be considered as an industry of national importance; not only were many private fortunes built up through their agency, but they provided a vast amount of employment; incidentally, they gave this country an advertisement abroad which might be considered by some to be of dubious value. As a consequence of State supervision, Government departments soon began to control the distribution of money to the hospitals, and consequently worked themselves into a position whereby they could attempt to dictate hospital policy . . . [13]

The bureau commenced operation on 3 June 1941, initially offering a nighttime service from 11 p.m. until 7 a.m., and from 1 July it operated on a 24-hour basis. Participating hospitals were required to provide the bureau with a daily list of vacant beds available for urgent cases seeking admission. Medical practitioners referring a patient made an application to the bureau which then attempted to find accommodation for the patient either by a direct approach to a hospital or giving the patient details of the accommodation available. As far as practicable the bureau sought to accommodate patients in the hospitals of their choice.[14] In ceding such control to the bureau 'a cherished privilege of the voluntary system was lost – the right to refuse admission'.[15]

The voluntary hospitals' resentment at being obliged by law to state how many vacant beds they had, which could then be filled by an external agency, led to them often not making complete returns. The Hospitals Commission complained of instances 'which seemed to suggest that the Bureau was not receiving full cooperation from the participating hospitals'.[16] The scarcity of beds created by the tradition of scaling back admissions during the summer months was also a problem that the bureau and the Hospitals Commission sought to rectify. An impression also seems to have been created that the existence of the bureau 'relieved the hospitals of the responsibility . . . of putting down a stretcher for an emergency case in default of alternative accommodation'.[17]

In its first six and a half years of operation the bureau satisfied 62 per cent of its applications immediately and 75 per cent in total.[18] The bureau was satisfied with this success rate and reported that its activities were 'regarded by general medical practitioners, unattached to hospitals, as providing an invaluable service for securing speedy admission to hospital of patients who otherwise might have been delayed indefinitely, with consequent deterioration of their condition'. The hospitals themselves were also said to have used the bureau to accommodate patients they did not have room for in other participating hospitals.[19]

The existence and activities of the bureau highlighted the fact that there was still a serious shortage of beds in the Dublin general hospitals to meet the growing demand for hospital treatment. In 1942 it reported that 'its capacity for meeting the public demand must be limited by the number of beds placed at its disposal'.[20] By 1944 the main obstacle it faced was still the shortage of beds:

> The Bureau must . . . continue to work under difficulties until the position is eased either by a diminution in demand for hospital beds or by a considerable expansion in hospital bed complements. Now that a wider public has experienced the benefit and convenience of hospital treatment, it is unlikely that there will be any relief from the former source.[21]

The participation of the municipal St Kevin's Hospital, and the introduction of a rota for admitting patients in 1947, eased the problems created by the scarcity of beds to a degree.[22] Nevertheless, the fact that as late as 1947 there was still a serious shortage of hospital beds in Dublin for the treatment of acute medical and emergency cases highlighted the slow progress that had been made in the implementation of the plans for general hospital provision in the capital, first drawn up by the Hospitals Commission more than ten years previously.

THE PROBLEM OF HOSPITAL FINANCE

The lack of progress in implementing the recommendations of the Hospitals Commission led Senator Sir John Keane to table a motion in the Seanad in March 1943 calling on the government

> to set up a commission to inquire into and make recommendations upon the matter of hospital finance generally; and, more particularly, upon the relations between the voluntary hospitals and the State, with a view to the establishment of the organisation best suited to the efficient operation of the whole hospital system.[23]

The debate that ensued brought to the fore the long running issue of increasing state control of the hospital sector, which the voluntary hospitals had been attempting to withstand since the introduction of the sweepstake.

Unlike practitioners within the voluntary system, Keane was not completely opposed to state control, realising that 'the unseemly scramble that took place among certain hospitals in the beginning of the Sweepstakes to get funds and spend them as they thought fit' necessitated some measure of it to 'control the distribution of these considerable sums of money that had, somewhat unexpectedly, and rather surprisingly, come in'.[24] He shared many of the frustrations that voluntary hospital staff felt with the activities of the Hospitals Commission, criticising its failure to produce any report since 1938. Furthermore, the reports it had produced were laden down with a surfeit of statistics, the usefulness of which was often unclear to him, leading to the opinion that the commission had become 'merely a statistics-collecting body'. He also criticised the lack of progress made on plans for hospital amalgamation and construction, highlighting the particular example of the problems encountered in finding a new site on which to rebuild Cork Street Fever Hospital, and the level of duplication between the functions of the Hospitals Commission and the Department of Local Government and Public Health.[25] Clearly of the opinion that the commission was not up to carrying out its current functions, he posed the question 'what is going to happen, and what view have the Government about what is going to be done, if the Sweepstakes are not revived, or if they are just revived on a more modest scale?' In such an eventuality he saw no option other than state intervention: 'I feel that the need is so great, and the demands for better hospital services so pressing, that the money should be found by the State.'[26]

Appalled at a remedy that called for even greater state control, Dr Robert Rowlette rejected Keane's motion, arguing that the solution to the difficulties of hospital finance was for state control 'to be steadily diminished and disappear altogether'.[27] Echoing opinions expressed on a number of occasions by other defenders of the voluntary sector, most notably Henry Moore, he complained of the state's usurpation of the sweepstake, which had been intended originally for voluntary hospitals, to fund local authority hospitals and provide additional government revenue in the form of stamp duty: 'very large sums of money were diverted from the sweepstakes receipts for the purpose of relieving taxes on the one hand and of relieving rates on the other hand.'[28]

Other senators who spoke to Keane's motion were prepared to accept a system that would accommodate the retention of voluntary hospitals, but also include some element of state control. Trade unionist Thomas Foran complained that this was necessary because the outdated voluntary hospitals had 'become a law unto themselves'.[29] Joseph Brennan conceded 'that some measure of State control is inevitable', but was wary of it becoming as pervasive as in Britain: 'I am not in favour of . . . anything in the nature of the Beveridge plan.'[30] Replying on behalf of the government, Dr Con Ward favoured the forging of a closer relationship between the voluntary hospitals and the state and proposed the best solution to the financial crisis created by growing hospital deficits and reduced sweepstake income was through increased treatment fees: 'if everybody receiving treatment in the voluntary hospitals contributed two guineas per week, or had two guineas contributed in respect of them, it would make a very material difference in the finances of these hospitals.'[31]

The debate on Keane's motion raised legitimate criticisms of the Hospitals Commission, especially its obsession with compiling statistics and the incredibly slow progress that had been made in its plans for hospital rationalisation and development within the first decade of its operation. The debate it generated showed that the representatives of the voluntary hospitals were still in denial about the nature of their relationship with the state; there would never be a return to Dr Rowlette's pre-sweepstake Utopia in which the voluntaries were solely responsible for their own affairs. The majority opinion, including that of the government, appeared to have coalesced around a binary system that would retain the voluntary hospitals but recognise the need for a state role in overseeing hospital finance, while staying well clear of any suggestions of nationalising the health service along the lines being suggested in the United Kingdom.

HEALTH AND HOSPITALS IN THE POST-WAR YEARS

After the war successive ministers for health were determined to pursue ambitious plans to introduce a comprehensive modern general hospital system in Ireland, none more so than the young controversial and crusading Clann na Poblachta minister, Dr Noël Browne, in his three years at the

Custom House from 1948 to 1951. The immediate post-war years saw health policy take a more prominent role in government, due to the impact on the thinking of civil servants and ministers of Sir William Beveridge's 1942 report on *Social Insurance and Allied Services*, that contributed to the establishment of the welfare state in the United Kingdom; the creation of a separate Department of Health in 1947; and the determination to tackle the scourge of high mortality from tuberculosis.

The popular belief in Ireland is that Noël Browne was the architect of the most important post-war health initiatives such as the campaign against TB, the mother-and-child scheme, and the hospital building programme, a perception that owes much to Browne's self-serving, inaccurate and misleading memoir, *Against the Tide*, published in 1986. It is now clear that many of these schemes were being planned from the mid-1940s, before Browne even entered politics.[32] However, Browne is still credited largely with piloting the post-war hospital building programme, in particular taking the decision to tap into the capital resources of the Hospitals Trust Fund to free up the necessary funding for construction.[33] His own account of this is as follows:

> I enjoyed the added advantage that all my predecessors had followed the same miserly spending on hospital building work. They spent only the income from the interest on the accumulated capital invested from successive sweeps. This amounted to a mere £100,000, but I needed millions. The £100,000 annually could not possibly build badly-needed hospitals all over Ireland. We decided to alter that policy radically, and proceeded to liquidate all the available assets in the Sweeps funds invested.[34]

This statement is poorly expressed, giving the impression that only £100,000 was spent on hospital building before 1948. What Browne is referring to is the sum given each year to voluntary hospitals for capital expenditure. From the setting up of the Hospitals Trust Fund in 1933 until the end of 1947, this figure amounted to £1,189,224. In addition, £2,367,179 was paid to local authorities to fund the extensive county hospital building scheme during the same period. Browne's calculations also fail to include the figures of £2,762,501 and £1,159,184 paid to the voluntary hospitals and the Minister for Local Government and Public Health respectively from the sweepstakes organised before the establishment of the Hospitals Trust Fund. Therefore, the total amount spent on hospital construction, not counting that spent on relieving hospital deficits or the expenditure on sanatoria after 1945, in the seventeen years from the start of the sweepstake until the end of 1947 was £7,478,088, more than £3.5 million of which had been spent since the establishment of the Hospitals Trust Fund in 1933.[35]

A closer examination of Department of Health files from the war years reveals that from at least 1944 Dr Con Ward was planning to prioritise hospital construction in the post-war period and to make greater use of the capital in the Hospitals Trust Fund for this purpose. In November 1944 a delegation from the Associated Hospitals Sweepstake Committee, representing the interests of the voluntary hospitals, accompanied by Joseph McGrath, called on Ward 'to see if they could do anything to get the hospital works going or get any information on the subject'. The parliamentary secretary signalled clearly his intentions regarding the Hospitals Trust Fund:

> as he saw things at that moment, assuming that building materials became avail-
> able, they must eat into the Hospitals Trust Funds to meet capital expenditure on
> new buildings and equipment, and that it did not seem possible to keep four, five
> or six millions locked up for the purposes of paying deficits.[36]

To continue paying deficits at an annual level of £200,000 would require the investment of £6.25 million of the approximately £8 million available in the Hospitals Trust Fund, which 'would postpone indefinitely the provision of new hospitals including the hospitals proposed for the City of Dublin'.[37] Such funding was needed especially for what Ward saw as the two most pressing issues in public health: tuberculosis and infectious diseases. A tense meeting concluded with Ward warning the voluntary hospitals that they 'were living in the past' and would need to adapt to the new realities of the post-war world, in part by introducing more charges for their services, echoing the view he expressed in the Seanad the previous year during the debate on Sir John Keane's motion on hospital finance.[38]

THE HOSPITALS TRUST FUND AND TUBERCULOSIS

Ward's intention to widen access to the capital resources of the Hospitals Trust Fund was put into practice with the enactment of the Tuberculosis (Establishment of Sanatoria) Act in March 1945. During the 1930s and 1940s approximately 4,000 people died every year from tuberculosis.[39] The provision of specialist sanatoria was then considered the best option for treating the disease. There were a number of such institutions in the state dating from the late nineteenth and early twentieth centuries.[40]

Ward now proposed to build three additional sanatoria in Dublin, Cork, and Galway that would provide the majority of the additional 4,300 beds that were believed to be needed to treat the extent of the disease.[41] Patients were to be treated free of charge with no income-based means test.[42] The estimated

£1.5 million required to construct these new institutions would be taken from the Hospitals Trust Fund. On completion, control of the sanatoria would be transferred to the relevant local authority and a provision was made for the repayment of up to one-third of the cost of building the sanatoria by the local authority to the Hospitals Trust Fund.[43] The wording of the act gave the minister wide powers to compel the Hospitals Trust Board to release funds to cover any expenses involved in the building of these sanatoria:

> The Minister may direct the Hospitals Trust Board to make payments out of the Hospitals Trust Fund for the purpose of defraying the expenses of the establishment under this Act of a sanatorium and the Hospitals Trust Board shall comply with such direction.[44]

The Tuberculosis Act was a milestone in the use of sweepstake funds to build hospitals, as it signalled a new policy of dipping deeply into the capital of the fund to build local authority institutions. As such it foreshadowed the hospital building programme of the 1950s.

Not surprisingly, the voluntary hospitals and their supporters, who had never come to terms with the usurpation of sweepstake funds for local authority hospitals, were outraged at the principle behind the bill, although in light of its purpose had to tread carefully when criticising it. As usual Fine Gael TDs were the most prominent defenders of the voluntary hospitals; former party leader W. T. Cosgrave, while conceding that 'It is certainly desirable that sufficient money should be made available to deal with TB', warned that the principle of 'encroaching on that [Hospitals Trust] fund' ran the risk of returning the voluntary hospitals to 'the position in which they were prior to the advent of the sweepstakes'. He also prophesied that 'If we spend limitlessly, the Hospitals Trust Fund will soon be exhausted'.[45]

Dr Ward made it clear that he would 'build and equip the institutions that are necessary so long as there is money in that fund', and reiterated his belief that it was time for the Dublin voluntary hospitals to seek financial aid from their local authorities: 'it is not unreasonable to ask the Dublin local authorities to pay voluntary hospitals for the maintenance of their patients.'[46] Rural TDs, such as Clann na Talmhan's Michael Donnellan, who had seen the vast bulk of sweepstake funds used to maintain Dublin voluntary hospitals while their constituents had to pay rates for local authority hospitals, approved wholeheartedly of the new principle governing the expenditure of Hospitals Trust Fund capital.[47]

THE POST-WAR HOSPITAL BUILDING PROGRAMME

The determination of health administrators to extend public health services on an unprecedented scale in post-war Ireland can be seen in the 1945 *Report of the Departmental Committee on the Health Services*, described by Ruth Barrington as 'probably the most radical document ever produced on the Irish health services', and effectively quashed by the Department of Finance which balked at the financial implications, estimated at £7 million, of the proposed extension of public health services.[48] Regarding hospital provision, the report favoured implementing the regionalisation plan proposed by the Hospitals Commission ten years previously.[49] It also favoured the centralisation of services provided by both voluntary hospitals and public health authorities in Dublin city and Dr Ward's view that local authorities needed to undertake more of the financial burden of financing the treatment of Dublin voluntary hospital patients.[50]

In spite of the report's suppression, its recommendations on hospital provision were largely pursued by successive governments during the late 1940s and 1950s. In 1947, when a separate Department of Health was established, a dedicated hospital construction section was formed in it.[51] By 1948 the wartime shortage of building materials had eased somewhat to allow for the re-commencement of hospital construction. The first inter-party government's short-term hospital building programme was announced by Dr Browne in the Dáil in July 1948. On assuming his portfolio some months previously, Browne found requests for 135 hospital building projects, costing an estimated £27 million, on his desk. As there was neither sufficient finance nor building materials to satisfy these claims, he was compelled to choose the most essential ones, and announced a programme that would see £15 million spent over the next seven years to 1955, in the following manner:[52]

General Medical and Surgical Hospitals	£5,900,000
Maternity and Children's Hospitals	£1,600,000
Tuberculosis Hospitals	£3,800,000
Clinics and Dispensaries	£500,000
Mental Hospitals	£1,500,000
Fever Hospitals	£1,250,000

The most controversial aspect of Browne's programme was the announcement that it was to be financed from the capital resources of the Hospitals Trust Fund.[53] Browne's party leader, Seán MacBride, claimed credit for including the deal in the negotiations on the formation of the inter-party government and also for gaining the approval of Joseph McGrath, although

McGrath had no personal control over how the Hospitals Trust Fund was spent.[54] However, as illustrated above, this was not the novel idea it has been subsequently presented as. Dr Ward was clearly eyeing up the fund's capital reserves from 1944 and had established the precedent of using them for construction in the 1945 Tuberculosis Act. In the same way that Browne should be credited less with initiating the mother-and-child scheme and the tuberculosis eradication campaign, than with carrying them to a level not previously envisaged, so too with hospital building his plans for the utilisation of the Hospitals Trust Fund's capital were probably more grandiose than Ward had contemplated. The assessment of Browne's biographer that 'it is hard to imagine that any Fianna Fáil administration would have agreed to the utilisation of the capital in the way that it was utilised by Browne' is probably correct.[55]

Nevertheless, Browne's Fianna Fáil predecessors in Health, Seán MacEntee and Dr James Ryan, criticised him initially for 'not spending enough money' on hospital building.[56] A year later the opposition's criticism had switched to scrutinising Browne's financial calculations. When announcing his programme in 1948, Browne conceded that 'it will no longer be possible to pay annual deficits of unlimited magnitude'.[57] The Dublin Fianna Fáil TD, John McCann, wanted to know how he could continue to finance both buildings and deficits, pointing out that the construction of more hospitals would lead to higher operating costs. Browne's response was that while the capital sum would finance construction, current sweepstake income would allay deficits: 'When the fund is exhausted, we can hope that the sweeps money will continue to flow in and in that way finance any deficits and new building', a policy that relied on the sweepstake recovering its pre-war profitability, something that was yet to be proven in 1949.[58]

Alarm bells went off in the Department of Finance immediately after Browne's announcement of his intention to raid the Hospitals Trust Fund capital. Most of the fund was invested in a range of Irish government, Irish and British local authority, and commonwealth stocks.[59] To realise the capital necessary to fund the hospital construction programme, much of this stock would have to be liquidated. An angry J. J. McElligott, the fiscally conservative Secretary General of Finance, complained that there was 'no intimation of Government approval for a programme of the magnitude contemplated', and warned that the plan to liquidate substantial holdings of Dublin Corporation and Irish government bonds was a 'serious matter' that would 'be a source of great embarrassment to us and to the Corporation if these stocks were thrown on the market even in limited amounts over a long period'. The Hospitals Trust Board was asked to retain its Irish holdings for the present.[60]

A war of words ensued between Finance and Health during 1949, with the secretary of Health informing Finance that Browne 'could not for one

moment agree that he should be precluded from using for hospitals construction outlay that part of the Hospitals Trust Fund invested in Irish
Government Securities and Dublin Corporation Stocks', and Finance
continuing to warn of the damage this would do to the state's financial
holdings: 'It will, if persisted in, entail not only a writing down of the credit of
borrowers whose securities are being pressed for sale (like the Dublin and
Cork Corporations and ourselves), but also a heavy loss to the Hospitals'
Trust Board, thus still further reducing the amount of its income available for
meeting hospitals' deficits.'[61] During the next three years, from 1949 to 1951
inclusive, over £4 million of these investments were liquidated.[62]

McElligott's consternation at Browne's plan was occasioned by the fact
that the Minister for Health was refusing to show the traditional deference
expected by Finance from other government ministers, the upward revision of
the estimate for completing the hospital building programme, and the belief
that Browne's hidden motive was to pass the liability for paying the maintenance deficits of the voluntary hospitals over to the state: 'the conclusion
seems to be inescapable that you have the Exchequer ultimately in mind as
the source of meeting hospital deficits, and my Minister wishes to make it
clear now that any such course of action is completely out of the question.'[63]

By the end of 1949 the estimated cost of the seven-year programme had
risen by over £11 million to £26.6 million, and Browne's civil servants, under
pressure from their colleagues in Finance, were urging the minister to 'prune'
his programme. Reluctant 'to delete any item from the programme which he
had already settled and upon which he had embarked', an optimistic Browne
reassured his officials that they 'need not have qualms about the necessary
funds becoming available'. Quite simply, half-built hospitals would not be
abandoned for lack of resources in the Hospitals Trust Fund:

> no government would or could refuse to make the necessary moneys available if
> the Hospitals Trust Fund petered out, say, about the fourth year of the programme
> or at a later stage. The country must have the hospitals it needed and it was just not
> to be contemplated that the funds would not be provided when they were required.

McElligott's fear that Browne intended hospitals to become a charge on the
exchequer was well founded. Browne conceded that the programme required
some modification and agreed to stretch it out over ten years, allowing for the
use of three more years' worth of sweepstake income.[64]

As the projects went to tender and construction commenced the estimated
overall cost continued to rise, climbing to £35.5 million in 1952. This was due to
a combination of factors including monetary devaluation, the inflationary
effects and shortage of necessary materials occasioned by the Korean War, the

increase in wages for construction workers, the availability of more accurate estimates as the projects reached more advanced stages of planning, and the addition of some new projects, in particular the need to provide more accommodation for the mentally handicapped and wider provision for dispensaries.[65]

The cost of the short-term hospital building programme had more than doubled in the space of four years, from £15 million in 1948 to £35.5 million in 1952. As a consequence, the capital resources and current income of the Hospitals Trust Fund were no longer sufficient to fund both this construction and continue alleviating the operating deficits of the voluntary hospitals. In 1951, for the first time since the establishment of the sweepstake, the new Minister for Health, Dr James Ryan,[66] was forced to seek a grant-in-aid to the Hospitals Trust Fund from the exchequer. Browne's prediction that no government would be prepared to abandon hospitals in the middle of construction proved correct; Ryan's request was acceded to, but he failed to have the stamp duty charged on the Hospitals Trust Fund repealed.[67] Between 1953 and 1957, the Hospitals Trust Fund was topped up by £6,780,000; Ryan had initially anticipated that £11 million would be required for these years, but the unexpected success of the sweepstake resulted in a smaller demand being made upon the exchequer.[68]

By early 1952 the government had little option other than to supplement the Hospitals Trust Fund because the hospital building programme was beginning to have practical effects. Approximately £300,000 a month was being spent from the capital of the fund, leading to fears that it would soon be exhausted.[69] Between 1951 and 1953 £7 million was spent on construction. Most progress was made on the TB sanatoria; Ballyowen in Dublin was finished in 1953 and the Galway Regional Sanatorium was on course for completion by mid-1954.[70] The safety blanket provided by the exchequer ensured that projects in progress could continue, and some of the programme's most important projects were realised by 1956, including the regional hospitals in Galway and Limerick, the regional sanatoria for Dublin and Cork, St Mary's Orthopaedic Hospital in Cork, and Our Lady's Hospital for Sick Children in the Dublin suburb of Crumlin.[71]

Buoyed by the success of the programme, officials in the Department of Health began to prepare a supplementary hospital building programme that would include projects Browne had been forced to exclude in 1948 and some new ones, the need for which had become apparent in the meantime.[72] Aside from this, the department was asked to focus attention on some smaller projects that could be completed relatively quickly, as part of a government decision in 1953 to seek to relieve unemployment by providing construction jobs in capital projects financed by the state. Early in 1954 plans were formulated for a variety of works costing up to £500,000.[73]

After this brief diversion plans for the supplementary programme resumed. Costing up to £10.25 million, approximately three-quarters of which would come from the Hospitals Trust Fund, the principal aim of the new programme was to provide adequate hospital accommodation for psychiatric and mentally handicapped patients, sectors where overcrowding was particularly acute.[74] These ambitious plans were soon shelved as the domestic economic situation deteriorated during 1954. At the end of the year the new second inter-party government decided 'that the whole capital expenditure programme should be reviewed', resulting in the indefinite postponement of the supplementary programme.[75] The urgency of some of the projects contemplated resulted in approval for a shortlist to be drawn up based on the supplementary programme that would cost approximately £1.5 million.[76]

The state's finances deteriorated further during 1955; by November the balance of trade deficit was £25 million, and there was a projected balance of payments deficit of £30 million. The Fine Gael Finance Minister, Gerard Sweetman, warned that hospitals would have to bear a significant share of the overall reduction in capital expenditure.[77] The Minister for Health, T. F. O'Higgins, agreed to forego £500,000 of the grant-in-aid from the exchequer to the Hospitals Trust Fund for 1956–7 and the full grant for the following two years, representing a shortfall of almost £3 million.[78] The combined effect of the rapid expenditure of the Hospitals Trust Fund's capital in the early 1950s, the continuing drain on the current income of the fund to pay operating deficits, and O'Higgins's self-denying ordinance was that the balance remaining in the fund on 31 December 1955 was just over £400,000. Were it not for the continued success of the sweepstake throughout the 1950s there would have been a serious crisis in the construction and financing of Irish hospitals.[79]

Table 8.2: Fungible assets (cash, investments, and premises) of the Hospitals Trust Fund at year ended 31 December (£)

1947	1948	1949	1950	1951	1952
9,704,767	10,131,898	7,427,639	7,635,946	4,933,674	1,227,989

1953	1954	1955	1956	1957	1958
396,906	851,807	436,833	164,062	606,000	1,626,000

Source: Annual reports of the Department of Health from 1951–2 to 1956–7 and the *Statistical Abstract of Ireland.*[80]

The priorities for hospital building at the end of the 1950s were the two new Dublin general hospitals, St Laurence's on the north side and the transfer of St Vincent's to Elm Park, the replacement of the Coombe maternity hospital, and the provision of a new regional hospital for Cork, most of which had their origins in the first report of the Hospitals Commission in 1936. The restrictions imposed by Finance resulted in only £2.5 million being designated for hospital construction, resulting in the abandonment for the foreseeable future of the Cork and St Laurence's projects. In order to allow for the replenishment of the Hospitals Trust Fund, work on St Vincent's and the Coombe would not commence until 1959.[81] Hopes that some work could proceed on local authority hospitals were also dashed when Finance effectively barred use of the Local Loans Fund for that purpose.[82]

When Fianna Fáil resumed office in March 1957, the incoming Health Minister, Seán MacEntee, was appalled by the depleted state of the Hospitals Trust Fund, finding 'that the resources of the Fund, apart from current income, were exhausted'. He was highly critical of his predecessor's decision to forsake the handout from the exchequer. The fund was largely dependent on its current income from sweepstakes of about £2 million per year, almost half of which had to be diverted to maintaining the voluntary hospitals, leaving only £1 million available each year for building. In fact, the situation was so bad that to ensure the solvency of the fund in early 1957 Joseph McGrath made available an advance of £700,000 from the projected surplus of the 1957 Grand National sweepstake.[83]

The precarious situation in the Hospitals Trust Fund resulted in work on the two most urgent projects, St Vincent's and the Coombe, which had not been due to start until 1959, being postponed further into the 1960s. In the meantime only some minor improvements to district hospitals and county homes would be carried out.[84] The shelving of major hospital construction projects was also in tune with the policy of the new Fianna Fáil government concerning public expenditure; in a departure from its previous term of office when it sought to stimulate employment through state-financed construction, it now favoured conserving resources by focusing on the adaptation, repair and maintenance of public buildings, such as hospitals and schools, rather than spending considerable capital constructing new ones.[85]

MacEntee decided the best way to secure the future of the Hospitals Trust Fund and allow for the eventual resumption of hospital building in the 1960s was to replenish the capital of the fund through the creation of a reserve fund. A contingency fund was also established to provide a cushion against unforeseen expenses, such as wage increases, which had wreaked particular havoc on the costs of the original short-term programme. Greater prudence would be exercised regarding the disbursement of Hospitals Trust Fund monies in future: no commitments would be entered into that could not be kept safely within the limits of available funds; the starting dates of major construction projects would be staggered; no commitments would be undertaken until proper estimates, based on tenders, were received; and projects which had not actually commenced would be delayed if finances again became tight.[86]

The salutary effects of these measures soon became clear; the balance of the fund rose to over £5 million in 1961, remaining at that level until the end of the decade.[87] Hopes that the fund's recovery would allow for a resumption of hospital building were dashed, however, because it coincided with a sustained decline in sweepstake income after 1961. Although the Hospitals Trust Fund still received about £2 million a year from the sweepstakes, an increasingly larger proportion of this was being diverted to covering deficits, so that by November 1962 there was still no surplus available in the Hospitals Trust Fund that could be used for building and long awaited projects like St Laurence's and Cork Regional Hospital had little prospect of being realised in the immediate future.[88] The diversion of an increasingly large portion of the Hospitals Trust Fund to cover deficits effectively postponed any serious discussion of further hospital building until the end of the 1960s.

VOLUNTARY HOSPITAL DEFICITS

In 1944, when Dr Ward signalled his intention to begin utilising the capital of the Hospitals Trust Fund for hospital construction, he intended that voluntary hospital deficits would in future account for a lesser portion of the fund. On a number of occasions he made it clear that these expenses should be covered in large part by rates. Throughout the war years approximately 54 voluntary hospitals participating in the sweepstake continued to return a combined deficit in excess of £200,000. This rose sharply to £340,000 in 1947. At this stage it was still unclear that the sweepstake would return to its pre-war success, and the risk of diminished income led the secretary of the Hospitals Commission to warn in 1945 that 'unless the authorities of the Voluntary Hospitals themselves . . . can succeed in introducing prompt remedial measures, the Voluntary Hospitals will in the near future be faced with a more acute financial crisis than at any period prior to the Sweepstakes'.[89]

Browne's ambitious plans for the Hospitals Trust Fund necessitated further measures to reduce the draw of the voluntary hospitals on the fund to cover their operating losses. To produce an annual income of £340,000, £10 million of the Hospitals Trust Fund would need to be set aside as an endowment, money that Browne intended for building hospitals and sanatoria. In October 1948 he asked the Hospitals Commission to consider new methods for paying deficits, based around a fixed sum.[90] This resulted in his announcement in July 1950 that a ceiling of £400,000 would be put on payments for the years 1950 to 1952 inclusive. This figure was calculated on the basis of the deficit figure for 1948.[91] As Barrington has pointed out, this did little to endear him to a medical profession already suspicious of the greater encroachment of the state into medicine during his tenure as minister.[92]

Browne's plan to curtail deficit payments was widely criticised by supporters of the voluntaries who howled loudly at any attempts to interfere with their activities. In the first place it appeared incompatible with his hospital building programme. A plan to increase the number of hospital beds in the country could only have the effect of raising hospital expenditure. Hospitals that succeeded in making savings during 1948 complained that they were penalised by having the deficit fixed to their 1948 figure. The new policy was only introduced in mid-1950 although it was to apply to all of that year. There was no elasticity to allow for increases in salaries and wages, which were largely responsible for the increased deficits as they were for the re-valuation of the cost of the hospital building programme.

A vicious circle emerged when a hospital's deficit exceeded the permitted limit and its bank overdraft was extended, resulting in higher interest charges and a further rise in its operating deficit. This made many lay governors fear they would be held personally liable for debts.[93] Lord Wicklow warned that this problem threatened the future of the National Children's Hospital: 'I have been directed to inform the Hospitals Commission that unless some satisfactory arrangements are made at once, regarding the unsecured deficit of this Hospital, my board will be reluctantly compelled to take drastic steps and close the Hospital in the very near future.'[94]

A serious situation also developed at Sir Patrick Dun's. In 1951 the two governors appointed by Dublin Corporation resigned and the Corporation refused to appoint replacements until it received guarantees that it would have no liability for the hospital's debts. Dun's operating deficit of approximately £10,000 was attributed to a sizeable increase in its bed complement from 117 to 168 between 1947 and 1949, which was not accounted for by pegging the deficit payment to 1948 levels.[95] Eventually, special private legislation had to be enacted by the Oireachtas to limit the liability of Dun's Board of Governors.[96]

In practice Browne's fixed deficit policy was unenforceable. Initially he agreed to withdraw the £400,000 limit for 1950 and base the payment for that year on an average of the deficit for the preceding three years.[97] In 1952 applications from the Mater, Temple Street, the Coombe, and the Harold's Cross Hospice to have the outstanding balance of their 1950 deficits reimbursed was acceded to.[98] The ceiling for 1951 was raised by 25 per cent to take account of increased bed occupancy and higher commodities' prices.[99] The fixed deficit level was abandoned for 1953 and raised to £600,000 in 1954 and £700,000 in 1956. Also in 1956 a special exchequer subvention of £250,000 was used to clear the remaining uncovered deficits up to 1953.[100] In effect, the threat to the financial viability of the voluntary hospitals proved greater than the desire to force the hospitals to curtail their expenditure.

During the 1930s the Hospitals Commission held that the deficits were due largely to profligacy on the part of the hospitals, a view that had changed by the 1950s. In 1951 the commission declared itself 'satisfied that the hospital authorities and their staffs did in general make genuine efforts to keep their deficits within the prescribed limits and it is to their credit that some did succeed in doing so'. Significant increases in salaries and commodities and the long-term effect of sweepstake funding in the form of larger hospitals with increased bed complements appear largely to account for the indebtedness of the voluntary hospitals in the post-war years.[101]

The fixed payments policy failed to have any impact on reducing voluntary hospital deficits. The incomplete nature of the Hospitals Commission's archives has made it difficult to calculate the exact figures. The tables below, which show the deficit figure returned by the commission between 1946 and 1953 and the sum paid from the Hospitals Trust Fund to cover shortfalls from 1954 to 1958, give the most accurate publicly available figures:

Table 8.3: Annual figure for hospital deficits, 1946–53 (£)

1946	1947	1948	1949	1950	1951	1952	1953
237,624	340,448	399,523	473,761	543,783	628,644	612,131	668,824

Source: Hospitals Commission final reports on yearly hospital deficits, NAI, DH A104/5 (vol. v), A104/6 (vol. vi), A104/7 (vol. vii), A104/9 (vol. viii), A104/10 (vol. x), A104/14.

Table 8.4: Amount paid from Hospitals Trust Fund to cover deficits to the year ended 31 March, 1954–8 (£)

1954	1955	1957	1958
656,434	683,107	699,950	1,249,980

Source: Report of the Department of Health, 1953–4, p. 72; *1954–5*, p. 80; *1956–7*, p. 71; *1957–8*, p. 73; no figure was provided in the report for 1955–6.

An examination of hospital expenditure and income carried out by the Department of Health showed that salaries and wages continued to be the largest charge on the hospitals, followed by provisions and the physical maintenance of the institutions:

Table 8.5: Expenditure of voluntary hospitals, 1947–55 (£000s)

Year	1947	1948	1949	1950	1951	1952	1953	1954	1955
Provisions	333	360	384	422	466	514	566	588	620
Surgery & dispensary	143	176	204	242	263	338	365	391	402
Salaries & wages	310	357	418	467	542	598	675	766	829
Maintenance	340	390	423	475	528	542	567	567	640
Administration	60	69	73	80	154	104	111	118	129
Finance	26	33	35	34	41	46	51	53	68

Table 8.6: Income of voluntary hospitals, 1947–55 (£000s)

Year	1947	1948	1949	1950	1951	1952	1953	1954	1955
Patient contributions	249	277	288	310	372	500	540	548	542
Health authorities	458	546	606	682	746	800	947	975	1043

Source: 'Grants towards deficits', *c.*Oct. 1956, NAI, DH, H34/8A (vol. IV).

Table 8.6 indicates that the hospitals sought to implement Dr Ward's solution of making local authorities take greater responsibility for the maintenance of their patients. Following an approach to Dublin Corporation from the city's voluntary hospitals, the corporation began in 1946 to contribute towards the maintenance of poor patients from the Dublin County Borough area, but this additional funding was largely swallowed up by increases in salaries and the cost of drugs and other provisions.[102] The reform of national insurance and social welfare during the 1940s and 1950s led to increased contributions for insured patients.[103] The planned extension of access to hospital services to the majority of the population under the 1953 Health Act, due to be phased in after 1956, would increase both the demand for hospital services and the dependence of hospitals on income from public authorities.[104] The recovery of the sweepstake during the 1950s, and the greater availability of public funding, kept the voluntary hospitals afloat.

Other efforts were undertaken to effect a decrease in debts, including the employment of professional consultants to examine the problem.[105] However, the deficit figure, and the proportion of sweepstake income required to cover it, both continued to rise dramatically towards the end of the decade. In 1958 34.4 per cent of sweepstake income was set aside for deficits; by 1961 this had risen to 65 per cent. Indications that income from the sweepstake was starting to decline from 1962 onwards raised serious questions about future financing. The future of the Hospitals Trust Fund was now in doubt; insufficient funds had caused the indefinite postponement of major hospital construction projects and deficits were increasing at a higher rate than income from the sweepstake.[106]

THE ADELAIDE AND VICTORIA HOSPITALS AND THE SWEEPSTAKE

Throughout the 1930s and 1940s one of the leading Protestant-managed hospitals in Dublin, the Adelaide, had remained steadfast in its opposition to the sweepstake. The Victoria Hospital in Cork, which had close links with the Adelaide, also refused to accept the proceeds of gambling. However, by the early 1950s these institutions were having difficulty surviving on their traditional sources of charitable income. In 1951 the *Church of Ireland Gazette* prodded the conscience of Dublin's Protestants: 'The writing is on the wall and, unless attention is paid to it, there will soon be in Dublin no hospital which Protestants may call their own.' The Hospital Sunday Fund had brought in a total of £2,111 for the Adelaide in 1950, not nearly enough to cover its debt of £18,000. The choice was stark; if the Adelaide was not to have to go cap in hand to the sweepstake, its supporters would have to dig deeper into their pockets: 'It is not enough to hold up holy hands of horror in condemnation of sweeps. If we, who are not actively engaged in running the hospital, are still convinced that it should have nothing to do with the accursed thing our convictions should take the form of increased subscriptions.'[107]

The situation had not improved much by 1953, when the hospital's governors sought state funding in order to avert closure. The payment made by Dublin Corporation to the Dublin voluntary hospitals for the treatment of its patients was of little use to the Adelaide, which treated mostly Protestants, and as such this was a small grant. Dr James Ryan believed that as some of the Hospitals Trust Fund was now coming directly from the exchequer, in the form of the grant-in-aid, the Adelaide could avoid accusations of taking the sweepstake's shilling, as they could argue that the money was coming directly to them from state funds, logic that was not shared by the hospital's representatives who felt 'that as long as the money was associated with the Hospitals Trust Fund some of their members would object'. Instead they preferred to receive a grant while avoiding 'the appearance of the money being a portion of the Hospitals Trust Fund'. The Minister for Health was not prepared to enter into such a unique agreement with one hospital; if the Adelaide wanted state funding it would have to apply for it from the Hospitals Trust Fund like all other hospitals in the state.[108]

The fear of alienating its traditional supporters by consorting with the Hospitals Trust Fund kept the Adelaide out for the remainder of the 1950s.

Eventually, the decision was taken in 1960 to apply for grants from the fund, leading the smaller Victoria Hospital to lament that 'Today we stand alone'. By tomorrow the Victoria had followed suit, receiving grants totalling £41,026 in the first three years after joining the sweepstake in 1961.[109]

THE SUCCESSES AND FAILURES OF THE 1950S

The uncertain future of both hospital construction and the financial future of the voluntary hospitals, due to the perilous state of the Hospitals Trust Fund in the early 1960s, necessitate an assessment of the decision to liquidate its capital. It has already been shown that this idea did not originate with Noël Browne. However, it is probably the case that no other minister would have forged ahead with it on such a grand scale, especially as it became clear during the 1950s that growing voluntary hospital deficits would continue to be a significant charge on the Hospitals Trust Fund into the future.

The successes of Browne's hospital building plans are clearly visible even today in Ireland, in institutions such as the new St Vincent's Hospital (eventually opened in November 1970), the flagship St James's General Hospital in Dublin (previously St Kevin's), St Luke's Cancer Hospital in Dublin, and the University College Hospital in Galway (formerly the Regional Hospital). Writing in 1960, Dr Joseph Robins, an official in the Department of Health, boasted that 'Every city and practically every major town in the country has some visible token of its achievement either in the form of a new or renovated hospital, a new clinic or a modern dispensary premises'.[110] James Deeny was proud to have taken part in 'one of the greatest achievements of this state since its foundation . . . the building of hospitals'.[111]

However, a strong case can also be made that the liquidation of so much of the capital of the Hospitals Trust Fund was short-sighted and that Browne's profligacy was ultimately damaging to the Irish hospital system. The principal argument for the prosecution in this case is that the Hospitals Trust Fund was almost bankrupt by the late 1950s and serious hospital building was effectively postponed for over a decade, without some of the most important schemes such as the new Coombe, St Laurence's and Cork Regional Hospital being completed, projects that dated back thirty years to the first report of the Hospitals Commission.

Some commentators at the time and subsequently have questioned the wisdom of expending large sums of money on certain projects. James Deeny opposed building both St Luke's and the new Dublin Fever Hospital at Cherry Orchard, on the grounds that the city's existing cancer and fever hospitals were adequate.[112] A crucial aspect of the programme was the construction of sanatoria to treat TB, a public health scourge that had been practically eradicated by the end of the 1950s, due largely to the development of effective drugs such as streptomycin. At least the maintenance costs of these institutions were low and by the 1960s when no longer required for their original purpose were converted to other hospital uses, as in the case of the Dublin Regional Sanatorium (now the James Connolly Memorial Hospital).

In defence of Browne, he was only Minister for Health for three years. The spiralling costs of the hospital building programme and of voluntary hospital deficits continued under his successors. O'Higgins can be criticised for submitting easily to the will of Finance in forsaking lucrative grants-in-aid. The hospital building programme was also a victim of the vicissitudes of Irish governments in the post-war years. Four different governments between 1948 and 1957 resulted in changes, often contradictory, in the direction of the hospital building programme. Initially Fianna Fáil encouraged public expenditure on capital projects to relieve unemployment, but subsequently preferred to conserve resources and maintain existing public buildings in preference to building new ones, an indication that hospital building policy was also at the mercy of wider economic considerations. Nor can Noël Browne be blamed for the poor economic condition of Ireland in the latter half of the 1950s or unforeseen events like the Korean War, which had an adverse effect on building by driving up costs and resulting in a shortage of building materials.

Any assessment of the wisdom of Browne's raiding of the Hospitals Trust Fund must examine what the intentions behind it were. If he hoped to implement successfully the programme he announced in 1948 within seven years, at the cost to the fund of £15 million, then he was a failure. James Deeny considered Browne to be 'ruthless and much more calculating than people thought', and another contemporary, J. J. McElligott, believed that Browne was aiming to make the exchequer responsible for funding hospitals. Browne's declaration to his officials in 1949 that governments would not refuse to subsidise hospitals even if the Hospitals Trust Fund was exhausted indicates that his intention was to build the hospitals regardless of whether the fund was adequate for the purpose. If his intention was effectively to nationalise the hospitals, from the point of view of funding if not administration, by making them a charge on the exchequer, his liquidation of the Hospitals Trust Fund was a success; by the early 1960s the state was effectively financing Irish hospitals. Sweepstake proceeds continued to cover voluntary hospital deficits, but all of the indications were that this would no longer be sufficient even for that purpose. The success of the sweepstake had indemnified successive Irish governments against having to undertake full responsibility for funding hospitals. As the gradual demise of the sweepstake began during the 1960s the state was finally forced to face that responsibility.

HOSPITAL PLANNING AND CONSTRUCTION IN THE 1960s
AND 1970s

After the hiatus of the late 1950s and early 1960s caused by the financial limitations of the Hospitals Trust Fund, planning for the health services, and especially the hospital sector, resumed in the mid-1960s. A white paper on *The health services and their further development*, published in January 1966, outlined the improvements that were needed in the health service. In relation to hospitals it recommended further regionalisation, administrative changes in the running of local authority hospitals by transferring their control to regional health boards, greater liaison between county hospitals and larger regional and teaching hospitals, and reiterated the need to revive plans for the new St Laurence's and Cork Regional Hospitals and a long-term replacement for the Federated Dublin Voluntary Hospitals.[113] This latter statutory body was established in 1961, comprising the Adelaide, Meath, National Children's, Baggot Street, Sir Patrick Dun's, Mercer's and Dr Steevens' hospitals, initially to improve the quality of medical education in Dublin, and eventually to amalgamate the hospitals in some form. An initial effort to merge most of them on the site of Sir Patrick Dun's was abandoned in 1965 when plans to run a new road through the site were discovered.[114]

In November 1967 a Consultative Council on the General Hospital Services was established to produce more concrete proposals for hospital development based on the ideas of the previous year's white paper. The subsequent report, known as the FitzGerald Report after the council's chair, Professor Patrick FitzGerald of UCD and St Vincent's, was a detailed, radical, and inevitably controversial blueprint for the future of hospital provision in Ireland. Echoing many of the themes of its predecessor thirty years before, the first report of the Hospitals Commission, FitzGerald argued that there were still too many hospitals (169) in the state and recommended 'a considerable reduction in the number of centres providing acute treatment'. With 27 different local authorities responsible for public hospitals there was a 'lack of coordination . . . and the absence of a planned organisation of services'. Quite simply, Irish hospitals were 'too many, too small and too independent of each other'.[115]

The answer to this problem was, as it had been for the Hospitals Commission in 1936, regionalisation. The hospital system should be reorganised into three regions based in Dublin, Cork, and Galway, each of which would have a regional hospital (Dublin would have two, one each on the north and south side) and a number of large general hospitals. The existing district and county hospitals were to be downgraded to district nursing homes and community health centres respectively.[116] Administrative changes, including centralising the appointment of consultants and establishing regional health boards and hospital management committees, were also recommended.[117]

Specifically in regards to hospital provision for Dublin city, FitzGerald suggested that the two regional hospitals consist of an amalgamation of Jervis Street and St Laurence's into a new institution to be built on a site adjacent to the Mater, while on the south side land adjoining St Vincent's in Elm Park would accommodate a new regional hospital formed from the amalgamation of the Federated Hospitals. These would be complemented by two large general hospitals, St Kevin's on the south side and the converted Dublin Regional Sanatorium, now the James Connolly Memorial Hospital, on the north side.[118]

Civil servants in Health immediately recognised that 'some of the proposals have far reaching implications and will require close examination as to their practicability'.[119] One of the leading sources of opposition was local interest groups who campaigned actively against the downgrading of their local district and county hospitals; one of the most vociferous regions in this regard was Mallow in County Cork.[120] Neither the Catholic St Vincent's nor the pre-dominantly Protestant Federated Hospitals showed any enthusiasm for the suggestion that they be located close by one another and share facilities.[121] Alarmed that Education Minister Donogh O'Malley's recently announced plans to merge Dublin's two universities might curtail the Protestant input into medical education, supporters of the Feds undoubtedly feared a further erosion of Protestant identity if forced into some form of alliance with St Vincent's, on the basis of a plan largely drawn up by a professor at UCD and St Vincent's.

Although FitzGerald recommended that there be no change to voluntary hospital management, the Catholic religious orders involved in running hospitals feared that the new administrative changes 'would unduly limit their freedom of action as hospital proprietors', and in order to placate them an agreement had to be drawn up by the Department of Health reassuring them of 'the basic measure of control which voluntary hospitals should have over the hospitals' affairs' and rejecting 'any idea of reducing or diluting this to such an extent that ownership ceases to be significant'.[122]

This opposition from so many vested interests resulted in a consider-able delay in implementing many of the recommendations. Most of the administrative reforms were enacted in the 1970 Health Act, including the establishment of regional health boards to take over the management of public hospitals from local authorities and the establishment of Comhairle na nOispidéal to govern the appointment of specialists and consultants.[123] It fell to a new Health Minister, Brendan Corish, leader of the Labour Party and Tánaiste in the Fine Gael–Labour coalition (1973–7), to tackle the thornier issue of regionalisation. Eventually, he settled on implementing a modified version of the FitzGerald proposals, produced by Comhairle na nOispidéal, based on more extensive general hospital provision. Under the new scheme Dublin was to have three general hospitals on the north side of the city – the existing Mater and James Connolly as well as an entirely new one at

Beaumont – and three on the south side, St Vincent's, St James's (as St Kevin's had been redesignated in 1971) and a new one to be built on a site at Newlands Cross, which would become Tallaght hospital.[124]

AMALGAMATION, CLOSURE AND CONSOLIDATION
IN THE 1980s

By the 1980s the insignificant sums accruing to the Hospitals Trust Fund from the sweepstake made a negligible contribution to offsetting the deficits of the voluntary hospitals, and the fund was largely dependent on grants-in-aid from the exchequer. For example, in 1980 the fund received just over £1.5 million from the sweepstake compared to £34.5 million from the exchequer.[125] The Irish hospital system was now effectively state funded. Nevertheless the process of reforming the Irish hospital service continued. The new St Vincent's at Elm Park finally opened in 1970 and the contract for Cork Regional Hospital was signed in 1972.[126] Both projects had been initiated by the Hospitals Commission in 1936.

Many of the other recommendations of the Hospitals Commission and its successors, particularly relating to the rationalisation of Dublin general hospitals, were implemented in a short space of time during the late 1980s, in what the then chairman of St James's described as 'probably the largest and swiftest closure and transfer of acute hospital services in the history of the voluntary hospital movement'.[127] In 1983 Mercer's was closed and its functions transferred to St James's, with Sir Patrick Dun's, Dr Steevens', and Baggot Street following between August 1986 and January 1988.[128] The new Dublin general hospital at Beaumont, approved by Brendan Corish in 1974, was officially opened in November 1987, incorporating Jervis Street and the abortive St Laurence's–Richmond.[129] Also in the 1980s the small infant hospital, St Ultan's, one of the participants in the first sweepstake, joined forces with the nearby National Children's Hospital.[130]

The suddenness of the closures and the loss of so many well-established Protestant hospitals made Dublin Protestant leaders wary of the plan to rush the Adelaide into a merger with the Meath and National Children's hospitals in the proposed new Tallaght Hospital. During the late 1980s and early 1990s a campaign to ensure the maintenance of the Adelaide's unique Protestant and voluntary ethos was carried forth by lay Protestants, medical professionals, and clergy who feared that successive governments and the Department of Health were trying to abolish the Adelaide in a manner similar to that of the smaller hospitals like Dr Steevens'. This effort was ultimately successful when a charter was agreed that gave identical status to the three hospitals comprising the new entity, and the Adelaide, Meath and National Children's hospitals finally closed in 1998 on the transfer of their functions to the new purpose-built general hospital in Tallaght.[131] Sixty-two years after the publication of the first general report of the Hospitals Commission, and eleven after the closure of the hospitals sweepstake, the process of reforming and rationalising the Irish hospital service, set in train by the opportunity created by the availability of vast sweepstake funding, had eventually been realised.

NINE

CONCLUSION

—

During the Dáil debate on the bill to compensate the redundant Hospitals Trust employees in 2000 it was noted that in the 57 years of its existence, the Irish state benefited to the tune of £170 million from the sweepstake – £135 million for hospitals and £35 million in stamp duty.[1] The sweepstake was introduced for a specific purpose – to save Dublin's voluntary hospitals from financial ruin and closure. Within a short space of time it had succeeded so well in achieving this aim that its remit was extended to providing an entirely new public hospital infrastructure for the country. By the end of the 1930s the voluntary hospitals' future had been secured and most counties could boast a brand new hospital. On this basis alone should the sweepstake not be judged as one of the greatest successes of the infant Irish state? In addition there were the ancillary benefits of the large sums of foreign currency brought in the country; the employment of thousands, directly in Hospitals Trust and in companies which supplied it, like the printers of tickets; and revenue accruing to the state in postage, radio advertising, and the 25 per cent stamp duty levied on the hospitals' portion of the sweepstake surplus.

Yet the sweepstake represents one of the greatest missed opportunities in the history of independent Ireland. A plan for a comprehensive reform of the country's hospital provision (the first report of the Hospitals Commission), and the wherewithal to achieve it, existed during the 1930s, but it would take until 1987 to implement the final parts of the Hospitals Commission's ambitious blueprint. Undoubtedly, the voluntary hospitals must shoulder much of the blame for this failure. They wanted to enjoy the full benefit of the sweepstake without any accountability to the state which had provided this new source of unprecedented funding. In the early years of the sweepstake they showed themselves incapable of applying the funds in an efficient and constructive manner, a failure that forced the government to intervene and establish a structure for dispensing grants. An abiding resentment at the state's usurpation of sweepstake revenue to build public hospitals, and the inability and unwillingness to keep expenditure within reasonable limits, can also be identified as failings on the part of the voluntary hospitals. The fractious relationship that resulted between the voluntary hospitals and the

Hospitals Commission militated further against the successful implementation of the reform agenda, as did the bureaucratic quagmire into which the statistics-laden Hospitals Commission had descended by the late 1940s.

However, successive Irish governments must share the blame for failing to capitalise to the fullest extent on the unique opportunity created by the availability of such massive funds. In this regard the unwillingness of any government to undertake financial responsibility for its hospitals must be highlighted. In 1930 the only alternative to either the sweepstake or the closure of hospitals was some form of state funding, a step that neither the Cumann na nGaedheal administration nor its Fianna Fáil successor was prepared to take. As a result, citizens of Great Britain, the USA and Canada provided the bulk of the money to build and equip Irish hospitals. Ten years after independence, Ireland was still reliant on its old colonial master for such vital revenue, a point not lost on the sweepstake's most vociferous opponent, Thomas Johnson. It was not until the 1950s, when sweepstake income was no longer adequate, that the Irish state finally accepted this responsibility to provide for the health of its citizens, largely because Dr Noël Browne had presented it with a *fait accompli*; he had committed the state to building hospitals in the knowledge that such a promise could not be reneged upon. Browne and many of his supporters are guilty of overstating his achievements as Minister for Health, especially concerning TB and the liquidation of the Hospitals Trust Fund's capital; unfortunately, in doing so, real achievements such as this are lost sight of.

Any assessment of the success of the sweepstake must take into account the price paid for its achievements. For over 50 years successive Irish governments turned a blind eye to the various illegal methods adopted by Hospitals Trust and its agents to sell millions of tickets abroad in countries where their sale was not lawful. The wording of the Public Hospitals Act allowed Irish governments to distance themselves from direct involvement in such activities, but nonetheless they colluded willingly in them, earning the enmity of governments in Britain, America and elsewhere.

The role of Hospitals Trust Ltd as a buffer between the state and the source of its hospital funding did not permit sufficient oversight of how sweepstake revenue was spent. This is most blatantly obvious in the case of the large personal fortunes compiled by the three promoters, Joseph McGrath, Richard Duggan and Spencer Freeman. In the immediate post-war years as the sweepstake began to revive, Irish government ministers and civil servants had begun to realise how problematic this was. Aware of the significance of the sweepstake to the Irish economy, Hospitals Trust dealt in a very arrogant manner with government departments, demanding that many arms of the state, including foreign embassies, the postal service and telecommunications, serve its interests ahead of those of the state itself. In later years, when the sweepstake was no longer even a useful source of hospital funding for the state, it had become a serious embarrassment, and the only reason it was allowed to continue for so long after it outlived its usefulness was that no government wished to make redundant hundreds of vulnerable workers who were unlikely to gain employment elsewhere. The Irish government had learned its lesson by 1987 and did not award the national lottery franchise to a private corporation.

Files in the National Archives indicate that the unsavoury nature of Hospitals Trust's operation was well known to the government, but the perceived charitable nature of its activities prevented any questions about its propriety being raised until the 1970s. Questions were asked, particularly by journalists in Canada and the USA, but this never filtered back to Ireland. When Irish journalists and politicians began to ask the questions that governments did not want to hear, they were branded as unpatriotic or forced to pursue their careers elsewhere, as in the case of Joe MacAnthony. The recent revelations of various judicial tribunals investigating political and corporate corruption in Ireland reveal the sort of society in which an organisation like the sweepstake was allowed to flourish. If the sweepstake still existed there would probably be a tribunal sitting in Dublin Castle to examine it.

The money generated by the Irish hospitals sweepstake allowed the infant Irish state to provide an extensive and modern hospital system that was of great benefit to its citizens. Given the huge sums of money available, an even better infrastructure could have been built, and stricter legislative oversight would have ensured that the reputation and legacy of the sweepstake was less tainted.

Appendix Accounts of Sweepstake Draws

Sweepstake	Gross proceeds	Prize fund	Hospitals fund	Stamp duty	Expenses (excl. promoters' fee)	Promoters' fee
1930 Manchester November Handicap	666,710	409,233	131,671		71,367	46,085
1931 Grand National	1,761,963	1,182,415	438,990		94,380	42,119
1931 Derby	2,827,696	1,902,500	697,424		134,259	58,266
1931 Manchester November Handicap	2,979,851	2,206,388	735,154		206,711	65,837
1932 Grand National	3,409,744	2,247,719	841,436		209,483	74,314
1932 Derby	4,184,485	2,804,552	774,091	258,030	205,789	89,569
1932 Cesarewitch	3,670,302	2,384,373	679,556	226,518	255,664	79,486
1933 Grand National	3,139,321	1,987,730	581,497	193,832	270,239	69,026
1933 Derby	3,010,694	1,943,430	557,380	185,793	220,318	66,453
1933 Cambridgeshire	2,726,558	1,707,857	504,854	168,284	251,541	60,851
1934 Grand National	3,000,086	1,871,198	735,284	183,821	269,692	65,822
1934 Derby	2,835,152	1,802,442	519,103	173,034	212,307	62,371
1934 Cambridgeshire	3,234,126	2,002,535	590,774	196,914	291,419	70,012
1935 Grand National	2,825,520	1,681,963	520,485	173,495	338,275	62,518
1935 Derby	1,935,695	1,161,363	354,847	118,282	213,176	44,850
1935 Cambridgeshire	2,267,665	1,322,758	414,584	138,194	285,355	51,222
1936 Grand National	2,491,392	1,454,770	458,670	152,890	324,631	55,924
1936 Derby	2,063,841	1,254,078	378,026	126,008	211,247	47,322
1936 Cambridgeshire	2,706,474	1,610,878	497,038	165,679	318,234	60,017
1937 Grand National	2,785,490	1,662,382	512,004	170,668	324,829	61,613
1937 Derby	2,682,812	1,662,975	491,402	163,800	243,217	59,416
1937 Cesarewitch	2,695,411	1,583,034	493,366	164,455	331,547	59,625
1938 Grand National	2,747,656	1,613,189	503,485	167,828	340,937	60,705

Sweepstake	Gross proceeds	Prize fund	Hospitals fund	Stamp duty	Expenses (excl. promoters' fee)	Promoters' fee
1938 Derby	2,384,495	1,460,075	437,511	145,837	236,898	53,667
1938 Cesarewitch	2,446,282	1,409,837	448,177	149,392	328,836	54,805
1939 Grand National	2,433,981	1,346,328	447,474	149,158	388,838	54,730
1939 Derby	1,670,839	956,713	306,194	102,064	228,851	39,660
1939 Cesarewitch	1,353,719	616,085	248,900	82,966	346,722	33,549
1940 Irish Red Cross Steeplechase	333,624	164,775	*	20,467	80,852	
1940 Grand National	554,631	224,762	102,718	34,239	225,978	
1940 Phoenix Plate	93,225	45,561	13,664	4,554	28,317	- 988
1940 Irish Cesarewitch	69,046	33,589	10,075	3,358	22,035	- 1,885
1940 Irish Red Cross Chase	78,439	38,806	*	3,879	20,519	2,760
1941 Irish Lincolnshire	53,103	26,111	7,832	2,610	13,637	2,026
1941 Irish Red Cross Chase	53,989	26,588	*	2,658	14,052	1,898
1941 Galway Plate	49,641	24,437	*	2,443	13,807	855
1941 Irish Cesarewitch	57,741	28,410	8,521	2,840	15,237	1,805
1942 Irish Red Cross Chase	65,185	32,202	*	3,219	18,342	976
1942 Irish Lincolnshire	70,751	34,900	10,468	3,489	17,169	3,768
1942 Irish Derby	69,630	34,355	10,305	3,435	14,555	6,055
1942 Baldoyle Red Cross Chase	72,536	35,928	*	3,592	16,348	5,205
1942 Naas Chase	93,590	45,992	13,795	4,598	20,524	7,066
1943 Hospital Chase	107,839	53,157	15,944	5,314	22,009	9,880
1943 Irish Lincolnshire	128,702	62,907	*	6,289	22,875	14,862
1943 Baldoyle Derby	133,338	65,585	19,672	6,557	24,596	14,747
1943 Phoenix Nursery Handicap	137,659	67,733	*	6,771	26,578	14,052
1943 Leopardstown Chase	176,051	86,285	25,879	8,626	30,426	21,333
1944 Baldoyle Chase	213,064	104,680	31,397	10,465	37,960	24,833
1944 Phoenix Handicap	200,541	98,515	29,547	9,849	44,785	14,309

Race						
1944 Golden Jubilee Handicap	146,733	71,924	*	7,191	39,409	3,737
1944 Phoenix Nursery Handicap	201,864	99,375	29,805	9,935	49,132	10,479
1945 Baldoyle Chase	271,086	133,299	39,979	13,326	58,144	31,813
1945 Phoenix Park Handicap	333,295	162,762	*	16,272	56,244	41,392
1945 Leopardstown Handicap Hurdle	373,906	182,900	54,857	18,285	64,865	44,849
1945 Curragh Nursery Handicap (10)	586,080	144,240	86,544	28,848	67,355	76,884
1946 Leopardstown Chase	802,740	502,850	117,921	39,307	103,507	22,722
1946 Derby	1,313,544	772,144	239,427	79,809	153,311	32,538
1946 Cambridgeshire	1,851,622	1,059,345	336,784	112,261	245,431	42,923
1947 Grand National	2,146,477	1,174,290	392,028	130,676	345,642	48,816
1947 Derby	1,999,651	1,155,635	368,897	122,965	273,953	46,349
1947 Cambridgeshire	2,074,204	1,067,920	381,589	127,196	411,278	47,702
1948 Grand National	1,790,225	843,400	328,887	109,629	430,612	42,081
1948 Derby	1,010,180	444,200	184,249	61,416	266,344	26,653
1948 Cambridgeshire	1,162,071	568,088	170,351	56,783	320,470	20,233
1949 Grand National	1,467,657	717,616	215,192	71,731	394,699	35,686
1949 Derby	1,436,666	723,633	261,995	87,332	289,649	34,946
1949 Cambridgeshire	1,543,637	794,900	225,695	75,232	372,118	37,093
1950 Grand National	1,703,574	835,000	312,937	104,312	378,619	38,630
1950 Derby	1,582,745	842,131	292,407	97,469	289,308	38,190
1950 Cambridgeshire	1,847,568	906,856	339,163	113,054	407,129	43,177
1951 Grand National	2,269,368	1,154,066	417,406	139,136	464,531	51,523
1951 Derby	1,725,644	935,144	318,781	106,260	299,260	41,003
1951 Cambridgeshire	2,323,278	1,215,613	425,039	141,680	432,841	52,338
1952 Grand National	2,308,643	1,216,013	432,871	144,290	463,337	53,173
1952 Derby	1,974,299	1,119,910	485,565	121,391	291,478	45,845
1952 Cambridgeshire	2,510,666	1,329,090	458,870	152,957	451,717	55,946

* Red Cross sweepstakes.

Sweepstake	Gross proceeds	Prize fund	Hospitals fund	Stamp duty	Expenses (excl. promoters' fee)	Promoters' fee
1953 Grand National	2,808,430	1,501,338	515,781	171,927	501,341	62,017
1953 Derby	2,712,952	1,597,155	500,781	166,927	346,486	60,417
1953 Cambridgeshire	3,098,251	1,689,983	567,167	189,056	512,639	67,498
1954 Grand National	3,203,189	1,740,390	589,678	196,559	549,965	69,899
1954 Derby	2,988,325	1,760,357	552,646	184,215	384,823	65,949
1954 Cambridgeshire	3,448,183	1,883,900	632,135	210,711	571,330	74,428
1955 Grand National	3,556,506	1,946,900	653,645	217,882	592,135	76,722
1955 Derby	3,095,186	1,805,815	571,460	190,487	412,685	67,956
1955 Cambridgeshire	3,683,990	2,011,277	673,468	224,490	605,006	78,836
1956 Grand National	3,977,623	2,186,910	731,224	243,742	655,490	84,997
1956 Derby	3,624,191	2,105,530	668,571	222,857	492,042	78,314
1956 Cambridgeshire	4,315,973	2,394,100	791,717	263,906	684,196	91,450
1957 Grand National	4,430,377	2,445,877	813,446	271,148	716,692	93,768
1957 Derby	3,810,233	2,220,200	704,698	234,900	517,955	82,168
1957 Cambridgeshire	4,551,769	2,561,050	832,667	277,555	678,196	95,818
1958 Grand National	4,752,036	2,693,300	891,007	297,002	773,600	102,041
1958 Derby	4,158,812	2,462,100	779,777	259,926	569,113	90,176
1958 Cambridgeshire	5,110,081	2,891,015	936,000	312,000	748,804	106,840
1959 Grand National	5,345,426	3,137,450	1,002,267	334,089	759,226	113,909
1959 Derby	5,246,139	3,074,500	969,776	323,259	695,207	110,443
1959 Cambridgeshire	5,752,241	3,276,800	1,051,613	350,537	812,486	119,172
1960 Grand National	6,008,230	3,486,400	1,126,543	375,514	896,585	127,165
1960 Derby	5,260,555	3,108,100	972,854	324,285	674,740	110,771
1960 Cambridgeshire	6,027,428	3,402,050	1,102,213	367,404	887,967	124,569
1961 Grand National	6,167,056	3,418,780	1,127,186	375,728	966,652	127,233
1961 Derby	5,488,924	3,260,080	1,029,173	343,058	741,784	116,779

1961 Cambridgeshire	6,161,956	3,400,980	1,123,342	374,447	973,378	126,823
1962 Grand National	5,857,808	3,251,500	1,098,339	366,113	1,022,339	124,156
1962 Irish Sweeps Derby	5,545,804	3,171,500	1,039,838	346,613	871,975	117,916
1962 Cambridgeshire	4,488,884	2,361,850	841,666	280,555	910,321	96,778
1963 Grand National	5,130,824	2,655,400	962,030	320,676	1,085,061	109,6161
1963 Irish Sweeps Derby	5,026,574	2,809,850	942,482	341,161	853,611	107,531
1963 Cambridgeshire	4,953,084	2,720,450	928,703	309,568	889,606	106,062
1964 Grand National	5,311,500	2,729,600	971,775	323,925	1,049,056	110,656
1964 Irish Sweeps Derby	5,311,296	2,926,600	980,793	326,931	887,177	111,618
1964 Cambridgeshire	4,898,660	2,558,900	892,905	297,635	912,852	102,243
1965 Grand National	5,151,480	2,715,300	965,903	321,967	1,045,946	110,030
1965 Irish Sweeps Derby	4,972,080	2,813,350	932,265	310,755	812,732	106,441
1965 Cambridgeshire	5,020,000	2,720,800	916,088	305,362	844,619	104,716
1966 Lincoln	5,072,200	2,599,850	929,775	309,925	1,020,116	106,176
1966 Irish Sweeps Derby	4,636,640	2,495,500	853,058	284,352	827,742	97,993
1966 Cambridgeshire	4,551,000	2,402,050	828,938	276,312	831,243	95,420
1967 Lincoln	5,118,000	2,600,750	941,906	313,969	1,083,045	107,470
1967 Irish Sweeps Derby	4,730,390	2,572,650	869,820	289,940	816,917	99,781
1967 Cambridgeshire	4,310,752	2,198,200	788,354	262,784	876,747	91,091
1968 Lincoln	4,645,740	2,214,400	855,720	285,240	1,120,700	98,277
1968 Irish Sweeps Derby	4,479,010	2,337,600	826,455	275,485	888,675	95,155
1968 Cambridgeshire	4,168,174	2,041,250	763,842	254,614	939,752	88,477
1969 Lincoln	4,455,744	2,080,050	820,152	273,384	1,118,782	94,483
1969 Irish Sweeps Derby	4,392,544	2,268,500	811,452	270,484	897,404	93,555
1969 Cambridgeshire	4,055,392	1,941,200	741,186	247,062	947,997	86,060
1969 Sweeps Hurdle	3,720,048	1,818,350	685,697	228,565	855,893	80,141
1970 Lincoln	4,086,204	2,017,500	752,663	250,663	916,495	87,284
1970 Irish Sweeps Derby	4,240,922	2,109,830	784,176	261,392	945,029	90,645
1970 Cambridgeshire	3,795,808	1,778,930	697,014	232,338	958,560	81,348

Sweepstake	Gross proceeds	Prize fund	Hospitals fund	Stamp duty	Expenses (excl. promoters' fee)	Promoters' fee
1970 Sweeps Hurdle	4,128,000	2,032,420	762,000	254,000	940,381	88,280
1971 Lincoln	3,876,516	1,829,600	713,787	237,929	979,009	83,137
11971 Irish Sweeps Derby	4,554,560	2,218,320	839,730	279,910	1,061,651	96,571
1971 Cambridgeshire	4,234,464	2,002,500	776,337	258,779	1,029,003	89,809
1971 Sweeps Hurdle	4,156,622	1,855,950	766,551	255,517	1,132,830	88,765
1972 Lincoln	4,296,672	2,011,450	793,626	264,542	1,079,588	91,653
1972 Irish Sweeps Derby	4,425,988	2,091,700	816,748	272,249	1,095,279	94,120
1972 Cambridgeshire	3,993,136	1,894,700	734,313	244,771	965,976	85,326
1972 Sweeps Hurdle	4,080,800	1,901,050	749,831	249,944	1,027,280	86,982
1973 Lincoln	4,076,820	1,928,050	749,610	249,870	1,002,596	86,958
1973 Irish Sweeps Derby	4,077,828	1,853,050	752,874	250,958	1,086,359	87,307
1973 Cambridgeshire	3,757,726	1,654,600	675,399	225,133	984,475	79,042
1973 Sweeps Hurdle	3,630,248	1,687,300	653,297	217,765	870,251	76,685
1974 Lincoln	3,607,100	1,584,350	650,306	216,769	953,460	76,366
1974 Irish Sweeps Derby	3,745,060	1,642,550	672,799	224,266	1,055,320	−21,158†
1974 Cambridgeshire***	3,357,644	1,470,550	603,871	201,290	unavailable	unavailable
1974 Sweeps Hurdle	3,187,510	1,395,600	576,949	192,316	921,965	−68,451†
1975 Lincoln	3,030,108	1,321,950	545,664	181,888	937,113	−65,204†
1975 Irish Sweeps Derby	3,034,770	1,332,600	550,672	183,558	982,172	−65,738†
1975 Cambridgeshire	3,382,930	1,331,950	741,877	247,292	925,623	−65,021†
1975 Sweeps Hurdle	2,758,538	1,087,150	607,307	202,435	869,620	−54,735†
1976 Lincoln	2,814,980	1,106,500	618,926	206,308	799,104	−55,639†
1976 Irish Sweeps Derby	2,708,526	854,500	598,979	199,659	968,980	54,087
1976 Cambridgeshire	2,554,404	760,900	565,381	188,460	953,648	42,680‡
1976 Sweeps Hurdle	2,459,960	732,200	544,356	181,452	927,796	−49,839†
1977 Irish Sweeps Derby	2,523,484	748,000	557,276	185,759	944,911	−50,844†
1977 Cambridgeshire	2,476,821	730,600	545,225	181,741	997,579	−49,906†

1977 Sweeps Hurdle	2,409,350	710,350	530,517	176,839	999,083	-48,762†
1978 Lincoln	2,498,760	737,650	550,802	183,601	1,010,528	-50,340†
1978 Irish Sweeps Derby	2,169,450	640,700	477,957	159,318	854,674	-44,674†
1978 National Stakes	1,790,116	524,250	391,368	130,456	669,450	-37,940†
1978 Irish Sweeps Autumn Handicap	1,704,180	501,540	374,238	124,746	636,657	-36,607†
1979 Philips Rockingham Stakes	1,805,886	536,350	397,370	132,456	1,458,539	-38,407†
1980 Grand National	1,555,554	465,050	342,484	114,162	799,874	-34,138†
1980 Irish Sweeps Derby	1,963,340	580,650	428,521	142,841	970,955	-40,829†
1980 Irish Sweeps Autumn Handicap	1,923,478	571,050	421,810	140,604	1,003,920	-40,308†
1980 Irish Sweeps Hurdle	1,472,804	437,750	323,664	107,888	556,292	-32,674†
1981 Terry Rogers Hurdle **	506,132	153,300	110,505	36,835	121,535	9,823
1981 Grand National	1,831,956	543,150	400,614	133,538	733,984	38,659
1981 Irish 2,000 Guineas **	397,967	120,800	88,046	29,349	123,585	7,826
1981 Irish Sweeps Derby	1,799,632	602,900	395,063	131,687	619,319	38,227
1981 Philips Electrical Stakes **	385,167	116,850	84,885	28,295	130,465	7,545
1981 Cambridgeshire	1,739,672	515,600	383,866	127,956	675,417	-37,356†
1981 RTV Hurdle **	424,856	130,750	93,973	31,324	141,010	8,353
1982 Irish Sweeps Hurdle	1,959,344	580,700	429,782	143,261	741,017	35,812‡
1982 Rogers Fairview Hurdle **	369,817	111,650	81,240	27,080	119,414	7,221
1982 Grand National	1,924,566	569,150	421,688	140,562	727,160	15,185‡
1982 Irish 2,000 Guineas **	324,574	99,450	72,280	24,094	122,075	369‡
1982 Irish Sweeps Derby	1,954,512	585,000	429,944	143,315	719,697	40,940
1982 Philips Electrical Stakes **	355,620	108,000	78,361	26,120	132,343	6,278‡
1982 Cambridgeshire	1,855,636	548,400	406,043	135,348	682,773	6,316‡
1982 RTV Rentals Hurdle **	347,341	103,700	76,306	25,436	128,873	4,873‡
1983 Irish Sweeps Hurdle	2,012,356	595,550	442,149	147,383	773,124	-41,889†

** Shamrock sweeps.
*** Audited accounts unavailable. Figures are from *Ir. Times*, 3 Oct. 1974 and do not provide amount paid in expenses.
† Fee abated in full as expenses exceeded permitted level.
‡ Fee abated in part as expenses exceeded permitted level.

Sweepstake	Gross proceeds	Prize fund	Hospitals fund	Stamp duty	Expenses (excl. promoters' fee)	Promoters' fee
1983 Toyota Sweeps Hurdle **	346,322	103,900	75,920	25,307	124,100	6,748
1983 Lincoln	1,687,412	501,200	372,378	124,126	749,594	- 36,463†
1983 Nijinsky Stakes **	275,998	82,900	61,340	20,447	111,188	- 5,425†
1983 Irish Sweeps Derby	1,968,248	584,000	433,068	144,356	728,716	21,603‡
1983 Kildare Handicap **	380,726	114,050	84,066	28,022	139,007	unavailable
1983 Tote Cesarewitch	1,970,592	586,400	436,678	145,560	878,356	- 41,464†
1983 RTV Hurdle **	269,757	82,100	59,919	19,973	112,781	- 5,326†
1984 Irish Sweeps Hurdle	2,029,200	601,200	446,951	148,984	761,841	- 42,263†
1984 Oberstown Hurdle **	339,770	101,450	74,862	24,954	122,576	6,654
1984 Grand National	1,950,688	579,350	431,074	143,692	757,046	- 41,028†
1984 [Irish ?] 2,000 Guineas **	319,973	96,300	71,252	23,750	113,809	6,333
1984 Irish Sweeps Derby	2,119,105	629,650	467,417	155,805	793,635	29,146‡
1984 Horgan Livestock Handicap **	305,462	92,200	67,919	22,639	116,526	unavailable
1984 Tote Cesarewitch	1,920,855	572,300	425,532	141,844	720,124	24,444‡
1984 Killeen Hurdle **	270,134	80,600	59,942	19,981	103,259	5,328
1985 Irish Sweeps Hurdle	1,768,313	526,850	391,346	130,448	657,787	9,415‡
1985 National trial **	306,836	92,500	68,239	22,747	117,470	unavailable
1985 Grand National	1,838,303	544,400	405,518	135,173	685,725	3,042‡
1985 Saval Beg Stakes **	280,420	83,700	62,318	20,773	105,249	3,965‡
1985 Joe McGrath Irish Sweeps Derby	1,901,263	567,700	421,124	140,375	758,877	- 40,254†
1985 Philips Electrical Stakes **	324,815	97,550	72,324	24,108	118,317	6,429
1985 Tote Cesarewitch §	1,737,680					
1986 Irish Sweeps Hurdle §	1,411,149					

** Shamrock sweeps.

§ Accounts not in Oireachtas Library and full details not given in newspaper reports.

† Fee abated in full as expenses exceeded permitted level.

‡ Fee abated in part as expenses exceeded permitted level.

Ticket prices:

1930 Manchester November Handicap to 1940 Irish Cesarewitch	10 shillings
1940 Irish Red Cross Chase to 1945 Leopardstown Handicap Hurdle	5 shillings
1945 Curragh Nursery Handicap to 1950 Cambridgeshire	10 Shillings
1951 Grand National to 1974 Sweeps Hurdle	£1
1975 Lincoln to 1985 Sweeps Hurdle	£2
1985 Grand National to 1986 Irish Sweeps Hurdle	£3
Shamrock Sweeps	£1

Notes

—

INTRODUCTION

1   Arthur Webb, *The clean sweep: The story of the Irish hospitals sweepstake* (London, 1968); Joe MacAnthony, 'Where the sweep millions go', *Sunday Independent*, 21 Jan. 1973; *Today Tonight Special: The Sweep*, 22 Jan. 1992; *Hidden history: If you're not in...*, RTÉ 1 television, 2 Dec. 2003.
2   Ruth Barrington, *Health, medicine and politics in Ireland, 1900–1970* (Dublin, 1987); Mary E. Daly, '"An atmosphere of sturdy independence": The state and Dublin hospitals in the 1930s', in Greta Jones and Elizabeth Malcolm (eds), *Medicine, disease and the state in Ireland, 1650–1940* (Cork, 1999), pp. 234–52.
3   John Horgan, *Noël Browne: Passionate outsider* (Dublin, 2000); Greta Jones, *'Captain of all these men to death': The history of tuberculosis in nineteenth and twentieth-century Ireland* (Amsterdam, 2001).

ONE: THE ORIGINS OF THE IRISH HOSPITALS SWEEPSTAKE

1   Roger Munting, *An economic and social history of gambling in Great Britain and the USA* (Manchester, 1996), pp. 13–14 and pp. 55–7; Joan Vance, *An analysis of the costs and benefits of public lotteries: The Canadian experience* (New York/Ottawa, 1989), pp. 35–8; C. L'Estrange Ewen, *Lotteries and sweepstakes* (London, 1932), pp. 332–3 and p. 360.
2   Rowena Dudley, *The Irish Lottery, 1780–1801* (Dublin, 2005), pp. 13–22 and p. 42. This book provides a detailed and comprehensive account of the eighteenth-century Irish state lottery.
3   Arthur Webb, *The clean sweep: The story of the Irish Hospitals Sweepstake* (London, 1968), pp. 24–7; 'Richard Duggan' in Royal Irish Academy, *Dictionary of Irish Biography* (*DIB*) (Cambridge, 2009); *Irish Independent, Irish Press* and *Irish Times*, 5 Nov. 1934.
4   Webb, *The clean sweep*, pp. 39–41.
5   *Ir. Times*, 11 Nov. 1922; extract from *Daily Mail*, 10 Nov. 1922, in National Archives of Ireland (NAI), Department of Justice (DJ) H69/8.
6   *Ir. Times*, 14 Nov. 1922; 'C. Hayes, Inspector of Taxes, v. R. J. Duggan', in *Reports of Irish tax cases, vol. I: 1923–32* (Dublin, 1932), p. 270.
7   Webb, *The clean sweep*, p. 41.
8   J. B. Lyons, *The quality of Mercer's: The story of Mercer's Hospital, 1734–1991* (Sandycove, 1991), p. 135.
9   Marie Coleman, 'The origins of the Irish Hospitals Sweepstake', in *Irish Economic and Social History*, XXIX (2002), p. 43.
10 Secretary, Dept of Home Affairs to Law Officer, Jan. 1923, NAI, DJ H69/20.

11 NAI, DJ H69/20.

12 NAI, DJ H69/22, H69/25, H69/24.

13 NAI, DJ H69/21.

14 *Freeman's Journal (FJ)*, 4 June 1923; Peter Gatenby, *Dublin's Meath Hospital, 1753–1996* (Dublin, 1996), p. 99.

15 Chief State Solicitor to Minister for Home Affairs, 2 May 1923, NAI, DJ H69/45.

16 Warrant from Minister for Home Affairs to Postmaster General, 24 May 1923, NAI, DJ H69/45.

17 Assistant Secretary, General Post Office to Minister for Home Affairs, 31 May 1923, NAI, DJ H69/45.

18 *Cork Examiner*, 4 June 1923; NAI, DJ, H69/55.

19 Gatenby, *Dublin's Meath Hospital*, p. 99.

20 Attorney General to Chief State Solicitor, May 1924, NAI, DJ H240/3.

21 NAI, DJ H240/14; *Irish Independent (Ir. Ind.)*, 28 Nov. 1924.

22 Coleman, 'The origins of the Irish Hospitals Sweepstake', p. 45.

23 'C. Hayes, Inspector of Taxes, v. R. J. Duggan', pp. 269–81.

24 T. A. Finlay to Messrs R. Rice & Son, 3 Mar. 1925, NAI, DJ H240/23(1).

25 The name of the Department of Home Affairs changed officially to the Department of Justice on 2 June 1924.

26 NAI, DJ H240/23(1–2).

27 NAI, Department of An Taoiseach (DT) s3828/a, DJ H240/38.

28 NAI, DJ H240/23(2) and (5).

29 Memo. on illegal lotteries, 24 Nov. 1928, NAI, DJ H240/23(5).

30 Henry O'Friel to Chief State Solicitor, 6 Sept. 1926, NAI, DJ H240/23(2).

31 Adelaide Hospital, *Annual report, 1922*, p. 15.

32 Barrington, *Health, medicine and politics in Ireland*, p. 108; Daly, '"An atmosphere of sturdy independence"', pp. 237–8; Tony Farmar, *Holles Street, 1894–1994: The National Maternity Hospital, a centenary history* (Dublin, 1994), pp. 75–9.

33 Barrington, *Health, medicine and politics in Ireland*, p. 108.

34 Sir Patrick Dun's Hospital, *Annual report, 1927*, p. 6, *1928*, p. 7, *1929*, p. 5.

35 Incorporated Dental Hospital, *Annual report, 1920*, pp. 6–7.

36 Teach Ultain, *Annual report, 1928–9*, p. 7; National Children's Hospital, *Annual report, 1930*, p. 14.

37 Farmar, *Holles Street*, p. 80.

38 Sir Patrick Dun's Hospital, *Annual report, 1922*, p. 6; Adelaide Hospital, *Annual report, 1926*, p. 16.

39 David Mitchell, *A peculiar place: The Adelaide Hospital, 1839–1989* (Dublin, 1989), pp. 161–2; Sir Patrick Dun's Hospital, *Annual report, 1923–4*, pp. 8–9.

40 Sir Patrick Dun's Hospital, *Annual report, 1923–4*, p. 9.

41 Greta Jones, 'The Rockefeller Foundation and medical education in Ireland in the 1920s', in *Irish Historical Studies*, vol. XXX, no. 120 (Nov. 1997), pp. 564–80, quote on p. 579.

42 Sir Patrick Dun's Hospital, *Annual report, 1925*, p. 9.

43 Sir Patrick Dun's Hospital, *Annual report, 1927*, pp. 5–7.

44 Minutes of the Board of Governors of Sir Patrick Dun's Hospital, 24 Mar. 1927–23 Feb. 1928, Royal College of Physicians of Ireland (RCPI), minute books of Sir Patrick Dun's Hospital.

45 NAI, DJ H69/81; *Ir. Times*, 2 Mar. 1923.

46 *Ir. Times*, 2 Mar. 1923.

47 Adelaide Hospital, *Annual report, 1918*, p. 14; Sir Patrick Dun's Hospital, *Annual report, 1927*, p. 5.

48 National Maternity Hospital, *Annual report, 1928*, p. 16.

49 Ibid., p. 17.

50 Farmar, *Holles Street*, pp. 78–80; National Maternity Hospital, *Annual report, 1926*, pp. 17–19.

51 *Dáil Debates (DD)*, vol. 3 (11 May 1923), col. 884.

52 Public Charitable Hospitals (Temporary Provisions) Bill (1923).

53 *DD*, vol. 2 (2 Mar. 1923), cols 1999–2001.

54 Ibid., vol. 2 (2 Mar. 1923), cols 2001–2.

55 'Reasons why any measure introduced for the purpose of legalising sweepstakes should be opposed', NAI, DJ H69/1.

56 *DD*, vol. 2 (2 Mar. 1923), cols 2011–12.

57 Ibid., vol. 2, (2 Mar. 1923), col. 2016.

58 *Ir. Times*, 26 Feb. 1923.

59 *FJ*, 27 Feb. 1923.

60 *Ir. Times*, 5 Mar. 1923.

61 E. W. Young to Secretary, Minister for Home Affairs, 5 Feb. 1923, NAI, DJ H69/37.

62 Rev. David Barry, 'The moral aspect of sweepstakes – from a Catholic and a Protestant viewpoint', in *Irish Ecclesiastical Record*, 5th series, vol. xxxviii (Sept. 1931), pp. 307–9.

63 *Catholic Bulletin*, vol. xxii, no. 2 (Jan. 1932), p. 5.

64 *DD*, vol. 2 (2 Mar. 1923), cols 1991–3 and 2007–9.

65 Ibid., vol. 2 (2 Mar. 1923), cols 1995–9.

66 Ibid., vol. 2 (2 Mar. 1923), col. 2008.

67 Ibid., vol. 3 (11 May 1923), cols 865–8.

68 Ibid., vol. 3 (11 May 1923) cols 873–5.

69 Dáil Éireann, *Report of the special committee on the Public Charitable Hospitals (Temporary Provisions) Bill, 1923*, NAI, DT s3828/A.

70 Barrington, *Health, medicine and politics in Ireland*, p. 109.

71 Letter to W. T. Cosgrave, 4 Nov. 1929, NAI, DT s3828/A.

72 Henry O'Friel to Michael McDunphy, 11 Nov. 1929, NAI, DJ H240/51(1).

73 Barrington, *Health, medicine and politics in Ireland*, p. 109.

74 National Children's Hospital, *Annual report, 1929*, p. 9.

75 Adelaide Hospital, *Annual report, 1929*, p. 18.

76 *DD*, vol. 34 (10 Apr. 1930), col. 901.

77 Public Charitable Hospitals (Temporary Provisions) Act (1930), section 1.

78 *DD*, vol. 33 (20 Feb. 1930), col. 717.

79 Ibid., vol. 33 (20 Feb. 1930), col. 727.

80 Public Charitable Hospitals (Temporary Provisions) Act (1930), section 4.

81 Ibid., section 6.

82 Ibid., section 7.

83 Ibid., section, 9; *Seanad Debates (SD)*, vol. 13 (28 May 1930), col. 1310.

84 Public Charitable Hospitals (Temporary Provisions) Act (1930), section 2.

85 Public Charitable Hospitals (Temporary Provisions) Bill (1929): as amended in special committee; *SD*, vol. 13 (21 May 1930), cols 1214–24.

86 Public Charitable Hospitals (Temporary Provisions) Act (1930), section 5.

87 *SD*, vol. 13 (21 May 1930), cols 1225–31.

88 Public Charitable Hospitals (Temporary Provisions) Act (1930), section 10.

89 St Ultan's Hospital, board minutes, 16 Oct. 1930, RCPI.

90 The biographical information in the following paragraphs is from Marie Coleman, 'Joseph McGrath', in *DIB*.

91 John M. Regan, *The Irish counter-revolution, 1921–1936* (Dublin, 1999), p. 93.

92 Michael McCarthy, 'The Shannon scheme strike', in *Old Limerick Journal*, 5 (Dec. 1980), pp. 21–6.

93 W. T. Cosgrave to Minister for Home Affairs, 31 July 1922, NAI, DJ H69/8.

94 'Spencer Freeman', in *DIB*; Webb, *Clean sweep*, pp. 120–6; *Who was who, VIII: 1981–1990*.

95 Hospitals Trust to Count Gerald O'Kelly de Gallagh, 24 July 1930, NAI, Department of Foreign Affairs (DFA), 34/13.

96 *Ir. Times*, 10 Nov. 1930.

97 Ibid., 15 Nov. 1930.

98 Ibid., 11 Nov. 1930.

99 Ibid., 15 Nov. 1930.

100 Ibid., 18 Nov. 1930.

101 Ibid., 18 Nov. 1930; Webb, *Clean sweep*, pp. 63–41; *Times*, 24 Nov. 1930. This process became quite common during the 1930s. The holders of potential winners often sold a portion of the ticket, usually to a bookmaker, for cash. Therefore, if the horse did not win they would at least have some monetary reward.

102 *Ir. Times*, 18 Nov. 1930.

103 Craig Gardner & Co. to Minister for Justice, 28 Jan. 1931, NAI, DJ H240/51 (Part 1).

104 Audited accounts of the 1930 Manchester November Handicap sweepstake, Oireachtas Éireann Library (OÉL).

TWO: THE SWEEPSTAKE IN IRELAND IN THE 1930s

1 'Sweepstakes under the Public Hospitals Acts', n/d [*c.* Oct. 1945], National Archives of Ireland (NAI), Department of An Taoiseach (DT) s13,774/A.

2 *Ir. Times*, 14 Jan. 1932; Irish hospitals sweepstake, *1937 Derby draw programme*, p. 157.

3 *Ir. Times*, 17 Feb. 1931, 4 Apr. 1931.

4 Ibid., 21 Nov. 1930.

5 Ibid., 25 May 1932.

6 *1937 Cesarewitch draw programme*, p. 60; *Ir. Times*, 1 Feb. 1936.

7 *1939 Grand National draw programme*, p. 11.

8 *Cork Examiner*, 7 Oct. 1939.

9 *1937 Cesarewitch draw programme*, p. 60.

10 *1934 Grand National draw programme*, pp. 40–3.

11 *Ir. Times*, 7 July 1934.

12 Ibid., 22 Sept. 1932.

13 *1938 Grand National draw programme*, p. 11.

14 Irish lottery and sweepstake tickets, collected and arranged by C. L'Estrange Ewen [n/d, *c.*1944], British Library, London.

15 *1937 Cesarewitch draw programme*, p. 60.

16 *1932 Derby draw programme*, p. 27.

17 *1932 Cesarewitch draw programme*, p. 7.

18 *1933 Grand National draw programme*, p. 7, *Ir. Times*, 21 Jan. 1933, 28 Oct. 1935.

19 The detail in the foregoing paragraphs is based on Laurence-Marie Gemma Bradley, 'John Keating, 1889–1977: His life and work', unpublished MA thesis (University College Dublin, 1991), vol. I, pp. 125–31 and p. 302.

20 *Ir. Times*, 10 Sept. 1932, 29 Apr. 1933.

21 Ibid., 16 Apr. 1932, 1 July 1933.

22 *Evening Mail*, 24 Oct. 1935.

23 *1932 Cesarewitch draw programme*, pp. 7–9. A detailed description of the arrangements for the 1938 Derby draw can be found in NAI, Office of the Secretary to the President (PRES) I/P354.

24 *Evening Herald*, 26 Nov. 1936 and 19 Oct. 1935; *Ir. Times*, 7 Nov. 1940.

25 *Irish News* [Tipperary], 15 Sept. 1932.

26 Tony Farmar, *A history of Craig Gardner & Co.: The first hundred years* (Dublin, 1988), pp. 147–59.

27 *Ir. Times*, 22 Oct. 1931.

28 Ibid., 14 Mar. 1931.

29 Ibid., 2 Apr. 1931.

30 Ibid., 14 Oct. 1931.

31 Ibid., 22 Oct. 1931.

32 Ibid., 16 Oct. 1931.

33 Ibid., 17 Oct. 1931.

34 Ibid., 15 Oct. 1931.

35 Ibid., 22 Oct. 1931.

36 Ibid., 28 Oct. 1931.

37 Ibid., 15 and 22 Oct. 1931.

38 Ibid., 27 Oct. 1931.

39 Ibid., 28 Oct. 1931.

40 Ibid.

41 Ibid., 5 Dec. 1931.

42 Ibid.

43 *Ir. Times*, 27 Apr. 1932.

44 Mim Scala, *Diary of a teddy boy* (Dublin, 2000), pp. 10–11.

45 *Evening Telegraph*, 3 Aug. 1932.

46 *Ir. Times*, 11 Mar. 1933.

47 Ibid., 13 July 1933.

48 Ibid., 27 May 1933.

49 *Evening Herald*, 4 Jan. 1936.

50 Joan Vance, *An analysis of the costs and benefits of public lotteries: The Canadian experience* (New York/Ottawa, 1989), p. 3.

51 *Ir. Times*, 24 Nov. 1930.

52 Ibid., 28 Mar. 1931.

53 Ibid., 19 Oct. 1931.

54 *Irish hospitals sweepstakes, draw programmes, 1935–9.*

55 Barry, 'The moral aspect of sweepstakes', p. 310.

56 'Functional chart [provisional] – main lines of responsibility – Hospitals Trust [1940] Ltd.', 28 Mar. 1946, in possession of Mr John Slevin; 'Paddy McGrath', in Ivor Kenny (ed.), *In good company: Conversations with Irish leaders* (Dublin, 1987), p. 82.

57 Coleman, 'Joseph McGrath', in *Dictionary of Irish Biography (DIB)*.

58 S. A. Roche to Lord Powerscourt, 13 Aug. 1932, NAI, Department of Justice (DJ) H240/76.

59 Joseph McGrath to Lord Powerscourt, 15 Aug. 1932, NAI, DJ H240/76.

60 Lord Powerscourt to James Geoghegan, 15 Aug. 1932, NAI, DJ H240/76.

61 S. A. Roche to Lord Powerscourt, 19 Aug. 1932, NAI, DJ H240/76.

62 Public Charitable Hospitals (Temporary Provisions) Act (1930), section 9; Public Hospitals Act, (1933) section 2.

63 *The Sweep*, RTÉ 1, 22 Jan. 1992, RTÉ television archive.

64 *Seanad Debates (SD)*, vol. 16 (5 July 1933), cols 2109–10.

65 *Ir. Times*, 10 Sept. 1932.

66 Ibid., 25 Apr. 1935.

67 Ibid., 5 Oct. 1937.

68 *Dáil Debates (DD)*, vol. 72 (7 July 1938), cols 417–18.

69 Sean Rothery, *Ireland and the new architecture, 1900–1940* (Dublin, 1991), p. 148.

70 Annette Becker, John Olley and Wilfried Wang (eds), *20th century architecture: Ireland* (Munich/New York, 1997), p. 197.

71 'The Irish Sweep offices, an art deco loss', www.geocites.com/Paris/Salon/6941/sweep.htm on 14 Dec. 2000.

72 *1939 Grand National draw programme*, pp. 24–5; Frederick O'Dwyer, *Lost Dublin* (Dublin, 1981), p. 145.

73 *Cork Examiner*, 19 Sept. 1938; *Dundalk Examiner*, 14 Jan. 1939.

74 Interview with Mr John Slevin, Dublin, 7 Aug. 2007.

75 O'Dwyer, *Lost Dublin*, p. 145.

76 Helen V. Smith to James Fitzgerald-Kenney, 27 Sept. 1930, NAI, DJ H240/51(11).

77 *Irish Catholic*, 3 June 1937.

78 Minutes of the executive committee, 30 Oct. 1935, Irish Labour History Museum (ILHM), Irish Women Workers' Union Papers (IWWU) 19/1/9.

79 *Irish Catholic*, 3 June 1937; Minutes of the executive committee, 12 Mar. 1936, ILHM, IWWU 19/1/9.

80 Minutes of the executive committee, 19 Sept. 1935, ILHM, IWWU 19/1/8, 30 Oct. 1935, IWWU 19/1/9.

81 Minutes of the executive committee, 19 Sept. 1935, ILHM, IWWU 19/1/8.

82 *Ir. Times*, 6 Nov. 1935.

83 Ibid.

84 *Watchword*, 31 Jan. 1931.

85 Ibid., 24 Jan. 1931; 7 Feb. 1931.

86 *Report of the Commission of Inquiry into the Civil Service: Final report* (1936), p. 140: Fifth Appendix, 'Return showing non-industrial members of the Civil Service set out according to inclusive pay as on the 1st January, 1934'.

87 Minutes of the executive committee, 21 Jan. 1932, ILHM, IWWU 19/1/7.

88 Minutes of the executive committee, 31 Aug. 1933, ILHM, IWWU 19/1/8.

89 IWWU, *Annual report, 1939*, p. 3, ILHM, IWWU 19/1/10.

90 *DD*, vol. 79 (30 Apr. 1940), col. 2072.

91 Minutes of the executive committee, 17 Aug. 1933, ILHM, IWWU 19/1/8.

92 *DD*, vol. 76 (21 June 1939), col. 1376.

93 Mary E. Daly, *Women and work in Ireland* (Dundalk, 1997), p. 49.

94 *Watchword*, 24 Jan. 1931.

95 Ibid., 7 Feb. 1931.

96 Ibid., 3 Jan. 1931.

97 Ibid., 7 Feb. 1931, 24 Jan. 1931.

98 National Library of Ireland (NLI), Piaras Béaslaí papers (PB), MS 33,963 (6), MS 33,966 (5), MS 33,967 (5); University College Dublin Archives Department (UCDA), Michael Hayes papers, P53/295.

99 *Watchword*, 7 Feb. 1931.

100 *Ir. Times*, 18 Aug. 1932; *DD*, vol. 47 (3 May 1933), col. 494.

101 *DD*, vol. 76 (21 June 1939), col. 1376.

102 *Watchword*, 7 Feb. 1931.

103 *Ir. Press*, 28 Oct. 1935.

104 *Watchword*, 24 Jan. 1931.

105 Minutes of the executive committee, 17 Dec. 1931, ILHM, IWWU 19/1/7.

106 IWWU, *Annual report, 1939*, p. 4, ILHM, IWWU 19/1/10.

107 Maurice Gorham, *Forty years of Irish broadcasting* (Dublin, 1967), pp. 64–5; Alacoque Kealy, 'Irish radio data, 1926–1980', Radio Telefís Éireann Occasional Papers Series, no. 1 (May 1981), p. 33; *Irish Radio News* (*IRN*) (18 Oct. 1930), p. 11.

108 Quoted in Gorham, *Forty years of Irish broadcasting*, p. 55; J. B. Clark, BBC internal circulating memo. on Irish Free State Broadcasting Service, 23 Nov. 1937, BBC Written Archive (BBCWA), Reading.

109 *IRN* (4 Oct. 1930), p. 3.

110 Gorham, *Forty years of Irish broadcasting*, p. 88.

111 *IRN* (10 Jan. 1931), p. 3.

112 Ibid. (22 Nov. 1930), p. 6.

113 Ibid. (12 Sept. 1931), p. 11.

114 *DD*, vol. 38 (23 Apr. 1931), col. 256.

115 Ibid., vol. 66 (22 Apr. 1937), col. 1547.

116 Ibid., vol. 61 (26 Mar. 1936), col. 375.

117 *IRN* (6 May 1933), p. 5; (1 July 1933), p. 3.

118 Ibid. (4 Nov. 1933), p. 4; (18 Nov. 1933), p. 4.

119 Ibid. (25 Nov. 1933), p. 4; (16 Dec. 1933), p. 7.

120 J. B. Clark, BBC internal circulating memo. on Irish Free State Broadcasting Service, 23 Nov. 1937, BBCWA.

121 *IRN* (2 Dec. 1933), p. 6; *DD*, vol. 56 (15 May 1935), col. 1021.

122 'Memorandum submitted by the Minister for Posts and Telegraphs for consideration by the government on the subject of commercial advertising from radio stations in Eire', 21 Oct. 1938, NAI, DT s9520(A).

123 *DD*, vol. 52 (9 May 1934), col. 614.

124 'Advertising (sponsored) programmes – question of future policy in regard to', *c.* Apr. 1934, NAI, DT s9520(A).

125 Kealy, 'Irish radio data', pp. 34–5; *DD*, vol. 41 (22 Apr. 1932), col. 492; vol. 70 (31 Mar. 1938), col. 1255.

126 Gorham, *Forty years of Irish broadcasting*, p. 65.

127 *1935 Grand National draw programme*, p. 79.

128 Richard Pine, *2RN and the origins of Irish radio* (Dublin, 2001), p. 168, n. 147.

129 Gorham, *Forty years of Irish broadcasting*, p. 56, NAI, Department of Transport, Tourism & Communications (DTT&C) 20/57 (vol. 3).

130 Kealy, 'Irish radio data', p. 57, Table 1: Radio licences from 1926 to 1972.

131 Hospitals Trust broadcasting scheme, NAI, DT s7095.

132 Spencer Freeman to P. S. O'Hegarty, 29 May 1934, NAI, DTT&C tw8160 (vol. 1).

133 Dept of Posts and Telegraphs memo., 29 May 1934, NAI, DTT&C tw8160 (vol. 1).

134 Memo. prepared by Mr Shanks, 'Commercial Broadcasting Station', Tomás Ó Fiaich Memorial Library and Archive (ÓFLA), Armagh, Joseph Cardinal MacRory papers, box 1, folder 1.

135 Frank O'Reilly to Cardinal MacRory, 13 June 1934, ÓFLA MacRory papers, box 1, folder 1; Lord French to Private Secretary, Department of the President, 22 Feb. 1934, NAI, DT s2726.

136 Frank O'Reilly to Cardinal MacRory, 13 June 1934, ÓFLA MacRory papers, box 1, folder 1.

137 Fr John Charles McQuaid to Eamon de Valera, 20 Feb. 1934, NAI, DT s2726.

138 'Proposal to erect in Cork a high power broadcasting station for commercial purposes', 3 Mar. 1934, NAI, DT s2726.

139 Seán Ó Muimhneacháin to Private Secretary, Minister for Industry and Commerce, 9 Oct. 1934, NAI, DT s2726.

140 NAI DT s9520/B.

141 NAI, DT s7095.

142 Ibid.

143 Ibid.

144 Ibid.

145 T. Monaghan to Secretary, Dept of Posts and Telegraphs, 25 Apr. 1935; P. S. O'Hegarty to Joseph McGrath, 8 May 1935, NAI, DTT&C 20/57 (vol. 1).

146 Joseph McGrath to P. S. O'Hegarty, 14 Sept. 1935, NAI, DTT&C 20/57 (vol. 1).

147 'Athlone high power station: proposals by the hospitals trust limited for increase of power of station', n/d [*c.* Dec. 1935], NAI, DTT&C 20/57 (vol. 1).

148 Memo. from Mr Codling, 22 Jan. 1936, NAI, DTT&C 20/57 (vol. 1).

149 NAI, DTT&C 20/57 (vol. 1) & (vol. 2).

150 Eamonn Ó Gallchobhair, 'Music – Free State broadcasting II', in *Ireland Today*, (Aug. 1937), p. 64.

151 *1934 Derby draw programme*, p. 47; *Ir. Times*, 13 May 1934; *1935 Grand National draw programme*, p. 70.

152 *Ir. Times*, 7 July 1934.

153 *1935 Grand National draw programme*, pp. 74–6.

154 *1935 Derby draw programme*, p. 63.

155 *Ir. Times*, 11 Apr. 1934.

156 Teddy Fennelly, *Fitz – and the famous flight* (Portlaoise, 1997), p. 307.

157 Ibid., pp. 301–2.

158 Ibid., p. 304.

159 Arthur Swinson, *The great air race: England–Australia, 1934* (London, 1968), p. 95.

160 Fennelly, *Fitz*, p. 309.

161 Ibid., p. 308, p. 306.

162 Ibid., pp. 309–13; *Ir. Times*, 17 Oct. 1934; Swinson, *Great air race*, pp. 95–7.

163 Swinson, *Great air race*, p. 108.

164 *Ir. Times*, 23 Oct. 1934.

165 Swinson, *Great air race*, p. 97.

166 Fennelly, *Fitz*, p. 315.

167 *Ir. Times*, 23, 29 and 31 Oct. 1934.

168 *1937 Grand National draw programme*, p. 115.

169 *Ir. Times*, 13 Aug. 1935; *1937 Grand National draw programme*, pp. 116–17. The dispute between Hospitals Trust and Mollison was settled in 1936, *Evening Herald*, 10 Nov. 1936.

170 Memo. from Mr McMenamin to Secretary, Dept of Posts and Telegraphs, 10 Nov. 1930, NAI, DTT&C 1+F41218/62–1.

171 Joseph McGrath to Controller, GPO, 6 Nov. 1930; Memo. to Secretary, Dept of Posts and Telegraphs, 7 Nov. 1930, NAI, DTT&C G7165/52(2).

172 Mr McMenamin to Secretary, Dept of Posts and Telegraphs, 10 Nov. 1930, NAI, DTT&C 1+F41218/62–1.

173 'Posting and delivery of correspondence in connection with the Hospitals Sweeps', Nov. 1930, NAI, DTT&C 1+F41218/62–1.

174 Memo. to Secretary, Dept of Posts and Telegraphs, 19 Dec. 1932, NAI, DTT&C G7165/52(1).

175 Dept of Posts and Telegraphs memo., 11 Apr. 1933, NAI, DTT&C G7165/52(1).

176 Dept of Posts and Telegraphs memos, 22 Mar. 1933, 7 Apr. 1933, NAI, DTT&C G7165/52(1).

177 Letter from Rita O'Donoghue, 8 Maretimo Villas, Blackrock, Dec. 1936, NAI, DTT&C G7165/52(4).

178 R. J. Cremins to Secretary, Dept of Posts and Telegraphs, 30 Dec. 1936, NAI, DTT&C G7165/52(4).

179 Memo. from Michael McDunphy, 24 Jan. 1935, NAI, DT s7333/A.

180 Memo. from Michael McDunphy, 30 Jan. 1935, NAI, DT s7333/A.

181 Memo. from Michael McDunphy to each member of the executive council, 6 Nov. 1935, NAI, DT s7333/A.

182 Memo. from P. S. Ó Muireadhaigh, 28 Sept. 1937, NAI, DT s7333/A.

183 Particulars of remittances transmitted to Hospitals Trust from 1 Jan. 1936 to 11 Sept. 1937; Memo. from P. S. Ó Muireadhaigh, 23 Sept. 1937, NAI, DT s7333/A.

184 P. S. Ó Muireadhaigh to Secretary, Dept of External Affairs, 6 Jan. 1938, NAI, DT s7333/A.

185 See chapter 5.

186 Maurice Moynihan to Assistant Secretary, Dept of Taoiseach, 1 Apr. 1938; Reply to Maurice Moynihan, 4 Apr. 1938, NAI, DT s7333/A.

187 Memo. from Maurice Moynihan, 3 May 1938, cabinet decision, 17 May 1938, NAI, DT s7333/A.

188 See chapter 5.

189 P. Ó Cinneide to Secretary, Dept of Finance, 4 Aug. 1938, NAI, DT s7333/A.

190 *News Chronicle*, 13 June 1932, *Evening Telegraph*, 29 July 1932, *Ir. Press*, 22 and 23 July 1932.

191 *Ir. Times*, 5 and 8 Nov. 1932; *Cork Examiner*, 12 Nov. 1932.

192 *Ir. Times*, 8 Nov. 1932.

193 *Ir. Ind.*, 5–7 Nov. 1935; *Donegal Vindicator*, 9 Nov. 1935.

194 *Stanhope* v. *Hospitals Trust Ltd.* (no. 2) [S.C., I.F.S.] [1936] Ir. Jur. Rep. 25, http://www.justis.com/j-net; *Evening Herald*, 16–17 June 1936.

195 Memo. of Joseph Andrews, original in the possession of John Horgan, pp. 20–3.

THREE: THE DEVELOPMENT OF IRISH HOSPITALS IN THE 1930s

1 J. K. Feeney, *The Coombe Lying-in Hospital* (Dublin, *c*.1983), p. 132.

2 Davis Coakley, *Baggot Street: A short history of the Royal City of Dublin Hospital* (Dublin, 1995), p. 72.

3 David Mitchell, *A peculiar place: The Adelaide Hospital, 1839–1989* (Dublin, 1989), p. 164.

4 *Ir. Times*, 25 Nov. 1930.

5 Mark Tierney, 'The Irish Hospitals Sweepstake and Barrington's Hospital', in *Old Limerick Journal*, no. 24 (winter 1988), p. 116.

6 J. B. Lyons, *The quality of Mercer's: The story of Mercer's Hospital, 1734–1991* (Sandycove, 1991), pp. 131 and 135–6.

7 O'Donel T. D. Browne, *The Rotunda Hospital, 1745–1945* (Edinburgh, 1947), p. 82.

8 Gearóid Crookes, *Dublin's 'Eye and Ear': The making of a monument* (Dublin, 1993), p. 127; *Ir. Times*, 27 June 1931; Tierney, 'The Irish Hospitals Sweepstake and Barrington's Hospital', p. 116.

9 Mitchell, *A peculiar place*, p. 164.

10 Helen Burke, *The Royal Hospital Donnybrook: A heritage of caring, 1743–1993* (Dublin, 1993), pp. 203–4 and 219.

11 Hospitals Commission, *First general report, 1933–4* (Dublin, 1936), pp. 29 and 33.

12 Diary of Dr Kathleen Lynn, 26 Feb. 1930, Royal College of Physicians of Ireland (RCPI).

13 The Public Charitable Hospitals (Amendment) Act (1931), admitted Our Lady of Lourdes Hospital, Rochestown Ave, Dublin; Peamount Sanatorium; the Royal Victoria Eye and Ear; St Anne's, Dublin; St Mary's Open Air Hospital, Cappagh; and St Joseph's Orthopaedic, Westmeath. The Public Charitable Hospitals (Amendment) Act (1931), admitted the Eye, Ear and Throat Hospital, Cork. The Public Charitable Hospitals (Amendment) Act (1932), admitted Newcastle Sanatorium, Wicklow.

14 *Dáil Debates* (*DD*), vol. 36 (26 Nov. 1930), cols 410–11.

15 Ibid., vol. 37 (20 Feb. 1931), cols 382–93.

16 Memo. from the Hospitals Committee re. scheme for 1931 Grand National Sweepstake, National Archives of Ireland (NAI), Department of Justice (DJ) H240/52 (1).

17 Public Charitable Hospitals (Amendment) Act (1931), section 6.

18 *Ir. Times*, 25 Nov. 1930.

19 National Children's Hospital, *Annual report, 1930*, p. 15; St Ultan's Hospital, *Annual report, 1931*, p. 6.

20 Sir Patrick Dun's Hospital, *Annual report, 1931*, pp. 7 and 9–10.

21 *Ir. Times*, 25 Nov. 1930.

22 Bethel Solomons, *One doctor in his time* (London, 1956), p. 117.

23 Tony Farmar, *Holles Street, 1894–1994: The National Maternity Hospital, a centenary history* (Dublin, 1994), p. 83.

24 J. F. Stokes to Secretary, Associated Hospitals Sweepstake Committee, 13 Jan. 1931; Lord Powerscourt to J. F. Stokes, 16 Jan. 1931; J. F. Stokes to Secretary, Associated Hospitals Sweepstake Committee, 23 Jan. 1931, NAI, DJ H240/56.

25 Feeney, *Coombe Lying-in Hospital*, p. 132.

26 Peter Gatenby, *Dublin's Meath Hospital, 1753–1996* (Dublin, 1996), pp. 105–6.

27 Farmar, *Holles Street*, pp. 84 and 89.

28 *Ir. Times*, 3 Dec. 1930.

29 Ibid., 29 Dec. 1930.

30 St Ultan's Hospital, *Annual report, 1932*, p. 8.

31 Ibid., *1931*, p. 16; *1935*, p. 16.

32 Sir Patrick Dun's Hospital, *Annual reports, 1930*, p. 70; *1931*, p. 57.

33 Tierney, 'The Irish Hospitals Sweepstake and Barrington's Hospital', p. 118.

34 *Ir. Times*, 27 June 1934.

35 National Children's Hospital, *Annual report, 1931*, p. 13.

36 St Ultan's Hospital, *Annual reports, 1933*, p. 11; *1938*, p. 9.

37 Martin Gorsky, John Mohan and Martin Powell, 'The financial health of voluntary hospitals in interwar Britain', *Economic History Review*, LV, 3 (2002), p. 552.

38 Public Charitable Hospitals (Amendment) (no. 2) Act (1931).

39 Public Charitable Hospitals (Amendment) Act (1931), section 3.

40 NAI, DJ H240/57.

41 *Ir. Times*, 29 Apr. 1933.

42 *Report of the Committee of Reference presented to the Minister for Justice: Manchester November Handicap Sweepstake, 1931* (Dublin, 1932), p. 6.

43 Ibid., pp. 6–7.

44 Ibid., pp. 9–10.

45 Ibid., p. 11.

46 Ibid., pp. 13–14.

47 *Report of the Committee of Reference: Grand National, 1932*, pp. 12–13 and p. 7.

48 *Report of the Committee of Reference: Derby, 1932*, p. 7.

49 S. A. Roche to Secretary, Dept of Local Govt and Public Health, 18 Aug. 1932, NAI, DJ H240/60.

50 James Geoghegan to Lord Powerscourt, 15 Aug. 1932, NAI, DJ H240/60.

51 Cappagh Hospital's claim for endowment, 28 May 1932, NAI, DJ H240/74.

52 Sr M. Peter to James Geoghegan, 23 June 1932, NAI, DJ H240/74.

53 Cappagh Hospital's renewed claim for endowment, c.Jan. 1933, NAI, DJ H240/74.

54 *Ir. Times*, 10 Aug. 1932.

55 Lord Powerscourt to Minister for Justice, 17 Feb. 1933, NAI, DJ H240/67.

56 'Memorandum in regard to the Public Charitable Hospitals Acts, 1930 and 1931', 16 Sept. 1932, NAI, Department of Health (DH) H39/48.

57 E. P. McCarron to Secretary, Dept of Finance, 21 Oct. 1932, NAI, DH H39/48.

58 Public Hospitals Act (1933), section 14.

59 Ibid., section 17.

60 Ibid., section 18.

61 Ibid., sections 17 and 23.

62 Ruth Barrington, *Health, medicine and politics in Ireland, 1900–1970* (Dublin, 1987), p. 118.

63 Public Hospitals Act (1933), section 20.

64 Ibid., section 24.

65 Ibid., section 25 (1).

66 Barrington, *Health, medicine and politics in Ireland*, pp. 117–18.

67 'Memorandum in regard to the Public Charitable Hospitals Acts, 1930 and 1931', 16 Sept. 1932, NAI, DH H39/48.

68 Dept of Local Govt and Public Health memorandum, 22 Feb. 1933, NAI, DH H39/48.

69 Barrington, *Health, medicine and politics in Ireland*, p. 116.

70 Public Hospitals Act (1933), section 26.

71 *DD*, vol. 47 (28 Apr. 1933), cols 321–30.

72 Memorandum from León Ó Broin to Mr Redmond, 10 June 1933, NAI, Department of Finance (DF) supply files, s84/40/32(MF).

73 *DD*, vol. 47 (28 Apr. 1933), cols 330–7.

74 Ibid., vol. 47 (3 May 1933), cols 468–72 and 481–2.

75 *Seanad Debates (SD)*, vol. 16 (28 June 1933), cols 2037 and 2043–4; (5 July 1933) col. 2101.

76 Hospitals Commission, *First general report*, p. v.

77 M. O'Callaghan to the editor, *Ir. Times*, 26 Sept. 1933.

78 *DD*, vol. 58 (11 July 1935), col. 304.

79 Hospitals Commission, *First general report*, p. 3.

80 Ibid., p. 4.

81 Ibid., pp. 10–11.

82 Ibid., pp. 12–13.

83 See chapter 1.

84 Minutes of the board of governors of Sir Patrick Dun's Hospital, 3 Sept. 1931, RCPI.

85 Letter from T. G. Moorhead to editor, *Ir. Times*, 9 Feb. 1932.

86 *Ir. Times*, 8 Feb. 1931.

87 Minutes of the board of governors of Sir Patrick Dun's Hospital, 12 Oct. 1931; 14 Jan. 1932; 28 Jan. 1932; 22 Nov. 1933; 11 Apr. 1935, RCPI.

88 Hospitals Commission, *First general report*, pp. 13–15.

89 Ibid., pp. 16–17.

90 Ibid., pp. 17–18.

91 Ibid., p. 20.

92 Ibid., p. 24.

93 Ibid., pp. 9–10.

94 Ibid., pp. 29–32.

95 Ibid., pp. 35–6.

96 Ibid., pp. 36–8.

97 Ibid., pp. 42–53.

98 Hospitals Commission, *Sixth general report, 1942, 1943 and 1944* (Dublin 1946), p. 5.

99 Hospitals Commission, *Fourth general report, 1938* (Dublin 1940), pp. 4–5.

100 Hospitals Commission, *First general report*, p. 80.

101 'Recommendations of the Hospitals Commission in respect of hospital deficits for the year 1935', NAI, DH A104/1 (vol. 1).

102 Secretary Dept of Local Govt and Public Health to Messrs Craig Gardner and Co., 1 Sept. 1936, NAI, DH A104/1 (vol. 1).

103 A. F. Cooney to Secretary, Dept of Local Govt and Public Health, 3 Oct. 1936, NAI, DH A104/1 (vol. 1).

104 Eamonn de Barra to Secretary, Dept of Local Govt and Public Health, 24 Sept. 1936, NAI, DH A104/1 (vol. 1).

105 'Recommendation of the Hospitals Commission in respect of hospital deficits on maintenance for the year 1937', NAI, DH A104/1 (vol. 1).

106 Hospitals Commission, *Third general report, 1937* (Dublin 1938), p. 4.

107 Ibid., p. 3.

108 A. F. Cooney to Secretary, Dept of Local Govt and Public Health, 3 Oct. 1936, NAI, DH A104/1 (vol. 1).

109 Hospitals Commission, *Third general report*, p. 4.

110 Ibid., p. 3; 'Recommendation of the Hospitals Commission in respect of hospital deficits on maintenance for the year 1937', NAI, DH A104/1 (vol. 1).

111 'Recommendation of the Hospitals Commission in respect of hospital deficits on maintenance for the year 1937', NAI, DH A104/1 (vol. 1).

112 'Maintenance deficits of voluntary hospitals', 4 Apr. 1939, NAI, DH A104/1 (vol. 2).

113 Ibid.

114 'Recommendation of the Hospitals Commission in respect of hospital deficits on maintenance for the year 1935', NAI, DH A104/1 (vol. 1).

115 J. Hubbard Clark to Secretary, Dept of Local Government and Public Health, 26 Sept. 1936, NAI, DH A104/1 (vol. 1).

116 Sr M. Brigid to Secretary, Dept of Local Government and Public Health, 8 Nov. 1938, NAI, DH A104/1 (vol. 1).

117 W. R. Burne to Secretary, Dept of Local Government and Public Health, 14 Nov. 1938, NAI, DH A104/1 (vol. 1).

118 *Ir. Times*, 21 Nov. 1938.

119 Ibid.

120 Ibid., 29 Nov. 1938.

121 Ibid., 12 Dec. 1938.

122 Diary of Kathleen Lynn, 29 Nov. 1938, RCPI.

123 'Recommendation in respect of maintenance deficits of voluntary hospitals for the year 1938', NAI, DH A104/1 (vol. 2).

124 Minutes of the board of governors of Sir Patrick Dun's Hospital, 11 Aug. 1938 and 9 Mar. 1939, RCPI.

125 'Recommendation in respect of maintenance deficits of voluntary hospitals for the year 1938', NAI, DH A104/1 (vol. 2).

126 Martin Gorsky and John Mohan, 'London's voluntary hospitals in the interwar period: Growth, transformation and crisis', in *Nonprofit and Voluntary Sector Quarterly*, vol. 30, no. 2 (June 2001), pp. 251–6.

127 Ibid., p. 263.

128 Gorsky, Mohan and Powell, 'The financial health of the voluntary hospitals in interwar Britain', pp. 545–6.

129 Ibid., p. 543.

130 'Maintenance deficits of voluntary hospitals', 4 Apr. 1939, NAI, DH A104/1 (vol. 2).

131 'Report and recommendations of the Hospitals Commission in respect of maintenance deficits of voluntary hospitals for the year 1939', NAI, DH A104/1 (vol. 2).

132 Ibid.

133 Timothy B. Smith, 'The social transformation of hospitals and the rise of medical insurance in France, 1914–1943', in *Historical Journal*, vol. 41, no. 4 (1998), pp. 1,055–87.

134 'Report and recommendations of the Hospitals Commission in respect of maintenance deficits of voluntary hospitals for the year 1939', NAI, DH A104/1 (vol. 2); Mel Cousins, *The birth of social welfare in Ireland, 1922–1952* (Dublin, 2003), pp. 81–3.

135 Circular letter from Dept of Local Govt and Public Health to secretaries of each voluntary hospital, Sept. 1939, NAI, DH A104/1 (vol. 2).

136 A. F. Cooney to Secretary, Dept of Local Govt and Public Health, 14 Dec. 1939, NAI, DH A104/1 (vol. 2).

137 E. de Barra to J. Hurson, 31 Aug. 1940, NAI, DH A104/1 (vol. 2).

138 Hospitals Commission, *Second general report, 1935–6* (Dublin, 1937), p. 1.

139 Ibid., pp. 5–7.

140 Ibid., pp. 7–9.

141 Margaret Ó hÓgartaigh, *Kathleen Lynn: Irishwoman, patriot, doctor* (Dublin, 2006), pp. 94–105.

142 Hospitals Commission, *Second general report*, p. 35.

143 Ibid., pp. 35–8.

144 Ibid., pp. 41–2.

145 *Ir. Times*, 28 Apr. 1936.

146 Hospitals Commission, *Third general report*, pp. 8–9.

147 'Report on conditions in Ireland, May 26th to June 11th 1942', by George E. Allen and Dr Daniel P. O'Brien, folder 2, box 1, series 403, RG 1.1, Rockefeller Foundation Archives (RFA), Rockefeller Archive Center (RAC).

148 Hospitals Commission, *Third general report*, p. 9 and pp. 5–7.

149 Hospitals Commission, *Fourth general report*, pp. 6–7 and 9–10.

150 Hospitals Commission, *Second general report*, p. 40.

151 'Proposal to establish a hospitals bureau', 13 Mar. 1936, NAI, DH A117/2 (vol. 1).

152 A. F. Cooney to Secretary, Dept of Local Govt and Public Health, 25 Apr. 1936, NAI, DH A117/2 (vol. 1).

153 Edward T. Freeman to Secretary, Dept of Local Govt and Public Health, 6 Nov. 1936, NAI, DH A117/2 (vol. 1).

154 A. F. Cooney to Secretary, Dept of Local Govt and Public Health, 17 Dec. 1936, NAI, DH A117/2 (vol. 1).

155 Mary E. Daly, '"An atmosphere of sturdy independence": The state and Dublin hospitals in the 1930s', in Greta Jones and Elizabeth Malcolm (eds), *Medicine, disease and the state in Ireland, 1650–1940* (Cork, 1999), p. 246.

156 Henry Moore, 'Future hospital policy in Dublin', in *Irish Journal of Medical Science* (June 1936), pp. 242–6.

157 William Doolin, 'Future hospital policy in Dublin', in ibid., pp. 252–5.

158 T. G. Moorhead, 'Future hospital policy in Dublin', in ibid., p. 259.

159 *Ir. Times*, 15 Nov. 1937.

160 Ibid., 7 Feb. 1938.

161 Ibid., 19 Feb. 1938; Daly, '"An atmosphere of sturdy independence"', p. 246.

162 K. Mangan to Attorney General, 4 Mar. 1940; Dept of Local Govt and Public Health to Secretary Dept of Finance, 8 Mar. 1940, NAI, DH A117/2.

163 Public Hospitals (Amendment) Act (1940), section 2 (1).

164 Ibid., section 4.

165 *Ir. Times*, 29 Feb. 1936.

166 Hospitals Commission, *First general report*, pp. 72–3.

167 *Ir. Times*, 29 Feb. 1936.

168 Henry Moore to Alan Gregg, 28 July 1925, folder 5, box 1, series 403, RG 1.1, RFA, RAC.

169 Royal Academy of Medicine in Ireland, 'Draft scheme for the endowment of medical research in Saorstát Éireann', 9 Apr. 1932, NAI, DJ H240/72.

170 S. A. Roche to General Secretary, RAMI, 14 Apr. 1932, NAI, DJ H240/72.

171 Private Secretary to the Minister for Justice, to Maurice Moynihan, 4 May 1932, NAI, DJ H240/72.

172 Maurice Moynihan to Henry Moore, 19 May 1932, NAI, DJ H240/72.

173 John F. Fleetwood, *The history of medicine in Ireland* (Dublin, 1983), p. 274.

174 Medical Research Council of Ireland (MRCI), *Annual report, 1939*, pp. 2–3.

175 MRCI, *Annual report, 1941*, p. 2.

176 Hospitals Commission, *Fourth general report*, p. 10.

177 MRCI, *Annual report, 1945*, p. 3; *1944*, p. 6.

178 *Ir. Times*, 27 Dec. 1940.

179 MRCI, *Annual reports, 1937, 1938* and *1939*.

180 Patrick N. Meenan to Gerard R. Pomerat, 5 Mar. 1956, folder 387, box 59, series 403, RG 2.1956, RFA, RAC.

181 Nancy Mary Panella, 'The patients' library movement: an overview of early efforts in the United States to establish organized libraries for hospital patients', in *Bulletin of the Medical Library Association*, vol. 84, no. 1 (Jan. 1996), pp. 52–61; Stephen J. Brown, 'Librarians at Cambridge, 22–27 Sept. 1930', in *Studies* (Dec. 1930), p. 675.

182 Brown, 'Librarians at Cambridge', pp. 671–6.

183 *Hospital Library Council of Ireland, 1937–58* [Pamphlet in NLI], p. 1.

184 Ibid., pp. 1–2; Public Hospitals Act (1933), section 26.

185 Christina Keogh to Minister for Local Govt and Public Health, 2 Jan. 1934, 'Library services for hospitals in Saorstát Éireann: draft scheme', NAI, DH AF101/1 (vol. 1).

186 Christina Keogh, to Minister for Local Govt and Public Health, 27 Oct. 1933, NAI, DH AF101/1 (vol. 1).

187 'Suggested amendment to draft scheme of library service for hospitals', 15 May 1935, NAI, DH AF101/1 (vol. 1).

188 Hospitals Commission to Secretary, Library Association of Ireland (LAI), 11 Jan. 1936, NAI, DH AF101/1 (vol. 1).

189 J. Hurson to Secretary, Associated Hospitals Sweepstakes Committee, 27 Nov. 1936, NAI, DH AF101/1 (vol. 1).

190 *Hospital Library Council of Ireland (HLCI), 1937–58*, pp. 3–5.

191 'Deputation from Hospital Library Council, Thursday, 15 Feb. 1940', NAI, DH AFIOI/1 (vol. 1).

192 Secretary, Dept of Local Govt and Public Health to Secretary, Hospital Library Council, 16 Apr. 1940, NAI, DH AFIOI/1 (vol. 1).

193 Christina Keogh to Minister for Local Govt and Public Health, 31 May 1940; J. Hurson to Christina Keogh, 23 July 1940, NAI, DH AFIOI/1 (vol. 1).

194 Christina Keogh to P. J. Ruttledge, 11 July 1941, DH AFIOI/1 (vol. 1).

195 Hospital Library Council, Chief Executive Officer's report for year ending 31 Dec. 1938, NAI, DH AFIOI/4 (part 1).

196 *Sixth annual report of the Hospital Library Council, 1942*, p. 7, NAI, DH AFIOI/4 (part 1).

197 *Ninth annual report of the Hospital Library Council, 1945*, pp. 5–6, NAI, DH AFIOI/4 (part 1).

198 *Annual reports of the Hospital Library Council*, NAI, DH AFIOI/4 (part 1).

199 Hospital Library Council, Chief Executive Officer's report for year ending 31 Dec. 1938, NAI, DH AFIOI/4 (part 1).

200 *Third annual report of the Hospital Library Council, 1939*, p. 18, NAI, DH AFIOI/4 (part 1).

201 *Fifth annual report of the Hospital Library Council, 1941*, p. 7, NAI, DH AFIOI/4 (part 1).

202 Marie Coleman, 'The development of the Irish hospital library service', unpublished paper delivered to the Irish Economic and Social History Society Conference, 18 Nov. 2006.

FOUR: THE SWEEPSTAKE IN GREAT BRITAIN IN THE 1930s

1 *Royal Commission on Lotteries and Betting (RCLB), 1932–3: Final report* (1933), p. 17.

2 *Hansard, series 5 (Commons)*, vol. 164 (7 June 1923), 2352.

3 Ibid., vol. 179 (18 Dec. 1924), 1188; vol. 181 (19 Mar. 1925), 2447; vol. 182 (2 Apr. 1925), 1502; vol. 227 (9 May 1929), 2304.

4 Roger Munting, *An economic and social history of gambling in Great Britain and the USA* (Manchester, 1996), pp. 32–3.

5 Note on the Betting and Lotteries Act for the Chancellor, The National Archives (TNA), Home Office (HO), HO45/16318.

6 B. E. Astbury, 'The Betting and Lotteries Act, 1934', in *Social Science Review* (Jan. 1935), p. 5, TNA, HO45/18783.

7 Note on the Betting and Lotteries Act for the Chancellor, TNA, HO45/16318.

8 Attorney General to Home Secretary, 1 Oct. 1929, TNA, HO45/14237.

9 Sir John Anderson to Commissioner, Metropolitan Police, 6 Mar. 1930, TNA, HO45/14238.

10 Home Office to Attorney General, Sept. 1929, TNA, HO45/14237.

11 Ibid.

12 *Hansard, series 5 (Commons)*, vol. 241 (17 July 1930), 1448.

13 Extract from *Daily Express*, 31 July 1930, National Archives of Ireland (NAI), Department of Tourism, Transport and Communications (DTT&C) 1+F41218/62(1).

14 Enda Delaney, *Demography, state and society: Irish migration to Britain, 1921–1971* (Liverpool, 2000), p. 84, Table 2.11 and p. 45; Table 2.3.

15 TNA, Metropolitan Police Office MEPO2/2279.

16 Memo. by T. J. Kiernan, *n/d*, NAI, Department of Justice (DJ) H240/51(11).

17 Letter to Sir Ernley Blackwell, 18 Nov. 1930, TNA, MEPO2/2279.

18 F. Warner, Inspector, Metropolitan Police to Chief Inspector, 5 Dec. 1930, TNA, MEPO2/2279.

19 Lieutenant Colonel Charles Howard-Bury, DSO (1883–1963), of Belvedere House, County Westmeath, Conservative MP for Chelmsford, 1926–31; *Hansard, series 5 (Commons)*, vol. 251 (16 Apr. 1931), 343.

20 *Hansard, series 5 (Commons)*, vol. 253 (10 June 1931), 1014.

21 *Ir. Times*, 2 Oct. 1933.

22 Secretary, Irish Free State High Commission, London, to Secretary, Dept of External Affairs, 6 Sept. 1930, NAI, Department of Foreign Affairs (DFA) 34/13.

23 J. D'Arcy to J. V. Fahy, 1 Oct. 1930, NAI, DFA 34/13.

24 Secretary Irish Free State High Commission, London to Secretary, Dept of External Affairs, 6 Sept. 1930, NAI, DFA 34/13.

25 T. J. Kiernan to Secretary, Dept of External Affairs, 26 Jan. 1931, NAI, DFA 34/13.

26 TNA, HO45/25958.

27 *Hansard, series 5 (Commons)*, vol. 245 (19 Nov. 1930), 433.

28 Extract from *Evening News*, 9 Dec. 1930, TNA, DO35/446/6.

29 'Minutes of evidence taken before the Royal Commission on Lotteries and Betting', evidence of Sir Ernley Blackwell, 30 June 1932, pp. 18–19, TNA, HO45/15218.

30 'Statement submitted by the Deputy Commissioner of the Police of the Metropolis' to the Royal Commission on Lotteries and Betting, TNA, MEPO2/5555.

31 *Hansard, series 5 (Commons)*, vol. 266 (8 June 1932), 1926; vol. 279 (15 June 1933), 309–10.

32 Spencer Freeman, quoted in *Ir. Times*, 20 Sept. 1933.

33 W. Peters, UK Trade Commissioner, Dublin, to Cabinet Irish Situation Committee, 22 Mar. 1933, TNA, DO35/446/6.

34 Ibid.

35 Deirdre McMahon, *Republicans and imperialists: Anglo-Irish relations in the 1930s* (London and New Haven, 1984), pp. 36–8, 41 and 31.

36 *Ir. Times*, 24 Nov. 1930.

37 A. J. Cunningham to J. W. Dulanty, 24 Nov. 1931, NAI, DFA 34/13; *Ir. Times*, 30 Nov. 1930.

38 D. S. London, to J. W. Dulanty, 11 Apr. 1934, NAI DFA 34/13(c).

39 F. E. Dalton to J. W. Dulanty, 30 Oct. 1935, NAI, DFA 34/13 (c).

40 Dept of Local Govt and Public Health to J. J. Walshe, 10 May 1934, NAI, DFA 34/13(c).

41 *Ir. Times*, 29 Nov. 1930.

42 Ibid., 6 Apr. 1932.

43 J. Hutchinson-Cockburn, *The Christian outlook on lotteries, betting and gambling* (London, 1932), p. 1.

44 *Daily Mail*, 20 Nov. 1930, NAI, Department of Finance (DF) Supply Files s84/2/30.

45 *Ir. Times*, 12 Aug. 1932.

46 T. J. Kiernan to Secretary, Dept of External Affairs, 15 Aug. 1932, NAI, DFA 34/13.

47 Spencer Freeman to Minister for Justice, 15 Aug. 1932, NAI, DJ H240/60.

48 Count O'Kelly de Gallagh to Secretary, Dept of External Affairs, 20 Aug. 1932, NAI, DFA 34/13.

49 *Ir. Times*, 1 Sept. 1932.

50 Home Secretary to Cabinet, 9 Dec. 1930, TNA, DO35/446/6.

51 Minute by Mr Bushe, 9 Dec. 1930, TNA, DO35/446/6.

52 Minute of meeting with Home Office, Scottish Office and customs officials, 8 Dec. 1930, TNA, DO35/446/6.

53 Home Secretary to Cabinet, 9 Dec. 1930, TNA, DO35/446/6.

54 'Banks acting as agents for sale or distribution of lottery tickets', 4 Dec. 1934, TNA, HO45/18079.

55 Home Secretary to Cabinet, 24 Feb. 1932, TNA, DO35/446/6.

56 'Statement submitted by the Deputy Commissioner of the Police of the Metropolis', TNA, MEPO2/5555.

57 'Memo. submitted to Royal Commission on Lotteries and Betting by the Scottish Office and Lord Advocate's Department', July 1932, TNA, HO45/18033.

58 *Times*, 16 May 1931, TNA, MEPO2/2279.

59 *Ir. Times*, 13 Jan. 1933.

60 Ibid., 8 July 1931; *Hansard, series 5 (Commons)*, vol. 250 (30 Mar. 1931), 751.

61 Home Secretary to Cabinet, 24 Feb. 1932, TNA, DO35/446/6.

62 *Hansard, series 5 (Commons)*, vol. 264 (7 Apr. 1932), 290; vol. 266 (26 May 1932), 527.

63 Ibid., vol. 264 (7 Apr. 1932), 290.

64 'Suggestions as to amending the law regarding Betting, Gaming and Lotteries', TNA, MEPO2/5555.

65 *RCLB, 1932–3: Final report* (1933), pp. 129–38, TNA, HO45/15218.

66 Ibid., pp. 138–9.

67 Ibid., pp. 139–46.

68 Home Secretary to Cabinet [c.July 1933], TNA, HO45/16661.

69 Memo. on drafting of Betting and Lotteries Act, Mar. 1934, TNA, CO323/1248/17.

70 *Hansard, series 5 (Lords)*, vol. 91 (27 Mar. 1934), 425.

71 Ibid., (26 Apr. 1934), 782.

72 *Hansard, series 5 (Commons)*, vol. 291 (27 June 1934), 1137–8.

73 Ibid., 1235.

74 Ibid., vol. 293 (6 Nov. 1934), 967–98.

75 *Daily Telegraph*, 15 Nov. 1934, TNA, HO45/18783; *Hansard, series 5 (Commons)*, vol. 291 (27 June 1934), 1139–40.

76 *Hansard, series 5 (Commons)*, vol. 291 (27 June 1934), 1148; Circular letter to police on Betting and Lotteries Act, TNA, HO45/18783.

77 TNA, HO45/19481.

78 Ibid.

79 A. Skelton to Secretary, Home Office, 2 Apr. 1935, TNA, HO45/19481.

80 Ibid., HO45/19481.

81 *Daily Mail*, 1 Apr. 1935, TNA, HO45/19481.

82 William Peters to Comptroller-General, Department of Overseas Trade, 27 May 1935, TNA, DO35/446/6.

83 Report of meeting between Dulanty and civil servants from Home Office and Dominions Office, 2 Aug. 1935, TNA, DO35/446/6.

84 Joseph McGrath to P. S. O'Hegarty, 14 Sept. 1935, NAI, DTT&C 20/57 (vol. 1).

85 TNA, DO35/446/6.

86 *Hansard, series 5 (Commons)*, vol. 303 (27 June 1935), 1284.

87 *Ir. Times*, 6 May 1937.

88 Ibid., 20 Mar. 1936.

89 Ibid., 22 Jan. 1938; 1 June 1938.

90 Ibid., 8 Sept. 1937; 17 Aug. 1938.

91 Ibid., 20 Nov. 1937; 5 June 1936.

92 Ibid., 5 Oct. 1937; 20 Oct. 1937, TNA, DO34/898/6.

93 TNA, DO35/446/6.

94 J. W. Dulanty to Secretary, Dept of External Affairs, 6 Feb. 1935, NAI, DFA 34/13(E).

95 Circular issued by Mrs Chapman, NAI, DFA 34/13(E).

96 Minute by J. P. Walshe, 19 Feb. 1935, NAI, DFA 34/13(E).

97 Joseph McGrath to J. P. Walshe, 4 Mar. 1935, NAI, DFA 34/13(E).

98 J. W. Dulanty to Secretary, Dept of External Affairs, 3 Aug. 1935, NAI, DFA 34/13(E).

99 F. A. Newsam to J. E. Stephenson, 21 June 1935, TNA, DO35/446/6.

100 Dominions Office memo., 21 June 1935, TNA, DO35/446/6.

101 F. A. Newsam to J. E. Stephenson, 21 June 1935, TNA, DO35/446/6.

102 Dominions Office memo., 21 June 1935, TNA, DO35/446/6.

103 Dominions Office memo., 31 July 1935, TNA, DO35/446/6.

104 S. A. Roche to Seán Murphy, 19 Aug. 1935, NAI, DFA 34/13(E).

105 F. A. Newsam to J. E. Stephenson, 20 Dec. 1937, 'Sales in this country of tickets in the sweepstake promoted in the Irish Free State by the Irish Hospitals Trust Limited' [c.1938], TNA, DO35/446/6.

106 *Daily Express*, 20 Nov. 1930, TNA, MEPO2/2279.

107 *Ir. Times*, 15 Jan. 1931.

108 Ibid., 10 Mar. 1931; *Hansard, series 5 (Commons)*, vol. 251 (20 Apr. 1931), 612.

109 *Hansard, series 5 (Commons)*, vol. 252 (19 May 1931), 1781–5.

110 Ibid., 1785–8.

111 Ibid., 1790.

112 Ibid., vol. 263 (22 Mar. 1933), 877–86.

113 *Ir. Times*, 10 Oct. 1932; *Times*, 10 Oct. 1932.

114 *Ir. Times*, 12 Oct. 1932.

115 *Times*, 10 Oct. 1932; H. M. Palmer and S. E. Wynn-Jones, 'Sir Arthur Stanley (1869–1947)', in *Oxford Dictionary of National Biography*, www.oxforddnb.com/view/article/36242?docPos=1.

116 *Ir. Times*, 21 Sept. 1933.

117 *Times*, 25 June 1935; see also *Times*, 4 July 1934; 5 Nov. 1936; 21 Apr. 1937; 8 May 1937 and 5 Oct. 1939.

118 *Ir. Times*, 19 Sept. 1933.

119 Ibid., 20 Sept. 1933; 28 Sept. 1933.

120 *New York Times*, 21 June 1933.

121 Opinion of Mr Eustace Fulton on the Duke of Atholl's fund, 24 Oct. 1933, TNA, Treasury Solicitor, TS27/1167.

122 *Ir. Times*, 22 July 1933.

123 Ibid., 30 Sept. 1933; 21 Oct. 1933.

124 Ibid., 15 Nov. 1933; 25 Nov. 1933.

125 Ibid., 27 Feb. 1934.

126 Ibid., 25 Nov. 1933.

127 'Conservative and Unionist Party's hints for speakers on Betting and Lotteries Bill', 10 May 1934, p. 22, TNA, HO45/16316.

FIVE: THE SWEEPSTAKE IN NORTH AMERICA IN THE 1930S

1 Roger Munting, *An economic and social history of gambling in Great Britain and the USA* (Manchester, 1996), pp. 28–36.

2 Joan Vance, *An analysis of the costs and benefits of public lotteries: The Canadian experience* (New York/Ottawa, 1989), pp. 51–2; National Archives of Canada (NAC), RG 25, External Affairs, vol. 1739, file 1935–218; Leon Trepannier, *Sweepstakes: Why they must be legalized for us* (Montréal, 1936), p. 51.

3 Munting, *An economic and social history of gambling in Great Britain and the USA*, pp. 36–9.

4 *NY Times*, 2 July 1932.

5 R. D. McLellan, 'Now it's gambling' in *Readers' Digest* [US edition], vol. 24, no. 142 (Feb. 1934), pp. 25–7.

6 F. A. Sterling, US Legation Dublin to Secretary of State, 25 Apr. 1931, National Archives and Records Administration (NARA), State Decimal Files (State DF) 1930–9, Record Group (RG)59 841D.513/4.

7 *NY Times*, 25 Sept. 1932.

8 James Grafton Rogers to Michael MacWhite, 23 Oct. 1931, NARA, State DF, 1930–9, RG59 841D.513/9.

9 Post Office Department, fraud order case file no. 6079, NARA, RG28.

10 Report by Henry H. Balch, American Consul General, Dublin on 'An estimate of Irish sweepstakes tickets sales in the United States', 29 Mar. 1932, NARA, State DF, 1930–9, RG59 841D.513/18.

11 *NY Times*, 6 June 1934.

12 *Ir. Times*, 24 Nov. 1922; *Freeman's Journal (FJ)*, 22 Mar. 1923; *Cork Examiner*, 4 June 1923.

13 National Archives of Ireland (NAI), Department of Justice (DJ), H69/41 and H69/112.

14 *Ir. Times*, 18 Nov. 1930.

15 Ibid., 25 Nov. 1930.

16 Travers Sweatman to W. W. Kennedy, 5 Oct. 1932, NAC, RG13, Justice, vol. 376, file 1932–778.

17 Hugh Guthrie, Minister for Justice, to Hugh Phillips, KC, Winnipeg, 5 July 1934, NAC, RG13, Justice, vol. 397, file 1934–178 (1).

18 Suzanne Morton, *At odds: Gambling and Canadians, 1919–1969* (Toronto, 2003), p. 54.

19 *1935 Grand National draw programme*, p. 32.

20 Morton, *At odds*, p. 15.

21 G. H. Daniel, Vancouver, to Hugh Guthrie, 28 May 1931, NAC, RG13, Justice, A–2, vol. 356, file 1931–937.

22 P. N. Lambert, Toronto, to R. B. Bennett, 10 Apr. 1932, NAC, RG13, Justice, vol. 397, file 1934–178(1).

23 Morton, *At odds*, p. 54.

24 *Debates of the Senate of the Dominion of Canada*, session 1931 (8 May 1931), pp. 84–5, (17 June 1931), pp. 274–8, (17–18 June 1931), pp. 281–92; session 1932–3 (8 Mar. 1933), pp. 319–20; NAC, RG13, Justice, A–2, vol. 356, file 1931–937; Morton, *At odds*, p. 9.

25 Assistant Secretary of the Treasury to Secretary of State, 29 Mar. 1932, NARA, State DF, 1930–9, RG59 841D.513/16.

26 Fred B. Smith to Henry L. Stimson, 6 Jan. 1931, NARA, State DF, 1930–9, RG59 841D.513/1.

27 Post Office Department, fraud order case files, files 5307, 5332, 5333, NARA, RG28.

28 Office of Postmaster General to Secretary of State, 14 Jan. 1931, NARA, State DF, 1930–9, RG59 841D.513/2.

29 Joseph McGrath to J. V. Fahy, 8 Sept. 1930, NAI, Department of Foreign Affairs (DFA) 34/13.

30 Memo. of Joseph Andrews, original in the possession of John Horgan, p. 19.

31 'Report of Mr Joseph G. Andrews re. workings of Irish Sweepstakes Organization, especially in the United States', enclosed with letter of John K. Davis, American Consul, Dublin to Secretary of State, 12 Feb. 1940, NARA, State DF, 1940–4, RG59 841D.513/83.

32 Andrews memorandum, p. 13.

33 'Report of Mr Joseph G. Andrews'.

34 Andrews memorandum, p. 42.

35 'Report of Mr Joseph G. Andrews'.

36 Andrews memorandum, p. 11.

37 Lot 559, Mealys' independence sale, 15 Apr. 2008, now in the NLI. I am grateful to Mr George Mealy for allowing me see this document prior to the auction.

38 Interview with Professor J. Kevin Kealy, son of William Kealy, Dundrum, Dublin 5, Feb. 2007.

39 'Report of Mr Joseph G. Andrews'.

40 Questionnaire completed by Joseph Andrews for Commissioner of Internal Revenue, July 1940, NARA, State DF, 1940–4, RG59 841D.513/97; Andrews memorandum, p. 39.

41 Post Office Department, fraud order case file 7084, NARA, RG28.

42 Circular letter from A. A. Cooper, Ajax Trading Coy, O'Connell St, Dublin, NARA, State DF, 1930–9, 841D.513/25.

43 Andrews memorandum, pp. 38–9; Eric Boden's *curriculum vitae*, folder 1194, box 163, series 403, RG2.1938, Rockefeller Foundation Archives (RFA), Rockefeller Archive Center (RAC).

44 'Report of Mr Joseph G. Andrews'; Andrews memorandum, pp. 12–15.

45 Andrews memorandum, pp. 27–31.

46 Military Archives (MA), Cathal Brugha Barracks, G2/3216.

47 Andrews memorandum, p. 20 and 33.

48 Ibid., p. 53.

49 Joseph Andrews, 'Information regarding the possible evasion of income tax payments by agents selling Irish sweepstake tickets', enclosed with letter of John K. Davis, American Consul General, Dublin, to the Secretary of State, 12 Feb. 1940, NARA, State DF 1940–4, RG59 841D.513/83.

50 John K. Davis, American Consul General, Dublin, to the Secretary of State, 12 Feb. 1940, NARA, State DF 1940–4, RG59 841D.513/83.

51 John K. Davis to the Secretary of State, 12 Feb. 1940, NARA, State DF 1940–4, RG59 841D.513/83.

52 Ibid., 19 Mar. 1940, NARA, State DF 1940–4, RG59 841D.513/88.

53 K. P. Aldrich, Chief Inspector, Post Office Department, Washington to Chief, Division of European Affairs, Department of State, 22 Apr. 1940, NARA, State DF 1940–4, RG59 841D.513/89.

54 Telegram from John K. Davis to Secretary of State, 1 May 1940, NARA, State DF 1940–4, RG59 92.

55 Francis H. Styles to Secretary of State, 23 July 1940, NARA, State DF 1940–4, RG59 841D.513/97.

56 Ibid., 28 Nov. 1940, NARA, State DF 1940–4, RG59 841D.513/102.

57 Francis H. Styles to Secretary of State, 6 May 1941, NARA, State DF 1940–4, RG59 841D.513/104.

58 Samuel Klaus to Mr Lyon, 2 Jan. 1943, NARA, State DF, 1940–4, RG59 841D.513/111.

59 Francis H. Styles to Secretary of State, 24 June 1941, NARA, State DF 1940–4, RG59 841D.513/107.

60 Elmer L. Irey, Office of Commissioner of Internal Revenue to Thomas Fitch, Department of State, 21 June 1941, NARA, State DF 1940–4, RG59 841D.513/108.

61 Francis H. Styles to Secretary of State, 10 Dec. 1941, NARA, State DF 1940–4, RG59 841D.513/109.

62 Mark Hull, *Irish secrets: German espionage in wartime Ireland, 1939–1945* (Dublin, 2003), pp. 196–7; MA, G2/X/1091.

63 Hull, *Irish secrets*, pp. 197–8; MA, G2/3261.

64 'Activities of German agent in Éire', The National Archives (TNA), DO121/86, 1943.

65 MA, G2/3261.

66 Ibid.

67 'Activities of German agent in Éire', TNA, DO121/86, 1943.

68 MA, G2/3261.

69 Elmer L. Irey to Thomas Fitch, 30 Nov. 1940, NARA, State DF 1940–4, RG59 841D.513/101.

70 Photocopies of correspondence between Joseph Andrews and the Revenue Commissioners, Dublin Castle, Feb.–Apr., 1973, Andrews memorandum, pp. 59–62.

71 'Activities of German agent in Éire', TNA, DO121/86, 1943.

72 Joseph Andrews to An Taoiseach, 3 Oct. 1939; James Andrews [father of Joseph Andrews] to Seán MacEntee, 3 Nov. 1939, NAI, Department of An Taoiseach (DT) S11537.

73 Seán MacEntee to An Taoiseach, 6 Nov. 1939, NAI, DT S11537.

74 Handwritten notes by P. O'Donoghue, NAI, DT S11537.

75 Seán MacEntee to An Taoiseach, 6 Nov. 1939; P. P. O'Donoghue, Department of the Attorney General to P. Kennedy, 26 June 1941, NAI, DT S11537.

76 Handwritten notes by P. O'Donoghue, NAI, DT S11537.

77 Department of Posts and Telegraphs, memo. re. international postal regulations and Hospitals Trust, 1 Dec. 1939, NAI, DT S11537.

78 D. Ó Duinn, Office of the Revenue Commissioners to Private Secretary to the Minister for Finance, 4 June 1940, NAI, DT S11537.

79 Marie V. Tarpey, 'Joseph McGarrity, fighter for Irish freedom', in *Studia Hibernica*, no. 11 (1971), pp. 164–80; D. J. Hickey and J. E. O'Doherty, *A new dictionary of Irish history from 1800* (Dublin, 2003), p. 296; 'Irish activities in the United States', 4 Oct. 1939, FBI file no. 61–7606: 'Irish Republican Army', section 1 (I am grateful to Mr Ed Morrison, Philadelphia for providing me with a copy of this document).

80 Connie Neenan to Moss Twomey, 21 Mar. 1933, University College Dublin Archives (UCDA), Moss Twomey papers P69/185(50).

81 M. H. Enright to Joseph McGarrity, 27 Nov. 1933, NLI, Joseph McGarrity papers, Ms 17,450; Tarpey, 'Joseph McGarrity', p. 178.

82 *Ir. Times*, 26 July 1979; *Cork Examiner*, 26 July 1979.

83 Brian Hanley, *The IRA, 1926–1936* (Dublin, 2002), p. 163.

84 *Ir. Times*, 26 July 1979.

85 J. Edgar Hoover to Arthur M. Thurston, 7 Oct. 1943, FBI file no. 61–7606: 'Irish Republican Army', section 14; FBI report, Philadelphia, 5 Apr. 1943, ibid., section 9; Seán Cronin, *Washington's Irish policy, 1916–1986: Independence, partition, neutrality* (Dublin, 1997), p. 102; Russell: NAI, DJ J8/802 (I am grateful to Caoimhe Nic Daibhéid for this reference).

86 Moss Twomey to Connie Neenan, 28 Mar. 1933, UCDA, Moss Twomey papers P69/185(25).

87 Tom O'Hanlon, 'Drew Pearson – the Sweep's US link man', in *Profile* (July 1973), p. 21. This is contained in the original July 1973 issue of *Profile*, which was removed from sale and replaced with an issue that did not contain this story, a direct result of pressure from Hospitals Trust Ltd.

88 Andrews memorandum, p. 16; *Ir. Press*, 8 Nov. 1937.

89 Andrews memorandum, p. 13.

90 Ibid., p. 16; 'Report of Mr Joseph G. Andrews'.

91 'Joseph McGarrity leaves $20,000', unidentified newspaper report, Villanova University (VU), McGarrity papers, group II, box 6, folder 5.

92 Andrews memorandum, p. 14.

93 Ibid., pp. 38–40.

94 *Ir. Ind.*, 16 Mar. 1940.

95 Andrews memorandum, p. 26.

96 Ibid., pp. 34 and 17.

97 'Report of Mr Joseph G. Andrews'.

98 Andrews memorandum, p. 35.

99 Hull, *Irish secrets*, pp. 43 and 61.

100 J. E. Stephenson to John Maffey, 18 Apr. 1940, TNA, DO130/8.

101 Hull, *Irish secrets*, p. 61.

102 Joseph McGarrity's diary entries for 17 Apr. and 14 June 1939, VU, McGarrity papers, group II, box 2, folder 6.

103 Report of George H. Barringer on 'Irish Sweeps tickets sold in the United States', 29 May 1933, NARA, State DF, 1930–9, RG59 841D.513/31.

104 Criminal Cases, Southern District of New York, c104–68, NARA, North East Regional Archives, New York City.

105 Ibid.; E. E. Conroy to J. Edgar Hoover, 17 May 1943, FBI, file no. 61–7606: 'Irish Republican Army', section 10.

106 FBI file no. 61–555: 'Irish activities in the United States', Apr.–Sept. 1939. I am grateful to Dr Brian Hanley for a copy of this document.

107 Diary entry for 19 Apr. 1939, VU, McGarrity papers, group II, box 2, folder 6. McGarrity had daughters named Ann and Deirdre.

108 Andrew Russell (Drew) Pearson (1897–1969).

109 Ann T. Keene, 'Drew Pearson', in *American National Biography*, vol. 17 (New York/Oxford, 1999), pp. 208–9.

110 Oliver Pilat, *Drew Pearson: An unauthorized biography* (New York, 1973), pp. 93–4.

111 W. J. B. Maculey to Michael MacWhite, 1 Sept. 1931, UCDA, MacWhite papers, P194/319; 'Washington merry-go-round', *Daily Mail*, 2 Mar. 1938, ibid., P194/498.

112 Pilat, *Drew Pearson*, pp. 95–8.

113 Keene, 'Drew Pearson', p. 209.

114 *Ir. Ind.*, 1 Aug. 1930.

115 *NY Times*, 23 Jan. 1931.

116 Ibid., 22 June 1931.

117 Memo. by James Grafton Rogers, Assistant Secretary, Department of State, 22 Sept. 1931, NARA, State DF, 1930–9, RG59 841D.513/6.

118 Cable from Department of External Affairs to Washington Consulate, 6 Sept. 1933, NAI, DFA, Washington Embassy files 1008.

119 John Cudahy to Secretary of State, 5 Oct. 1937, NARA, State DF, 1930–9, RG59 841D.513/33.

120 *Boston Traveller*, 28 July 1939.

121 *NY Times*, 11 Nov. 1941.

122 *New York Post, New York Journal & American, NY Times*, 17 Jan. 1939.

123 Andrews memorandum, p. 25–6.

124 Ibid., pp. 40–1.

125 Hospitals Trust Ltd to Henry J. MacFarland, 26 Feb. 1932, NARA, State DF, 1930–9, RG59 841D.513/47.

126 Andrews memorandum, p. 41.

127 *Stubbs' Weekly Gazette (Irish Free State and Northern Ireland)*, 28 Jan. 1931, 25 Feb. 1931, 8 Apr. 1931, 24 June 1931; *Iris Oifigiúil*, 22 Jan. 1932, p. 48.

128 Documents enclosed with letter of Francis H. Styles to Secretary of State, 24 June 1941. NARA, State DF 1940–4, RG59 841D.513/107.

129 Andrews memorandum, pp. 36–7; *South Bend (Ind.) News-Times*, 31 July 1935; *New York Mirror*, 19 May 1939; *Time*, 12 Nov. 1934.

130 *NY Times*, 6 June 1934.

131 Ibid., 16 Mar. 1937.

132 Fred McDonald and Bob Considine, 'Not a clean sweep: The inside workings of the Irish lottery', in *Collier's* (4 June 1938), p. 57.

133 *Washington Post*, 25 Mar. 1939.

134 *Hidden history: If you're not in. . .*, RTÉ 1 television, 2 Dec. 2003.

135 Michael MacWhite to Joseph P. Walshe, 31 Oct. 1930, UCDA, MacWhite papers P194/228.

136 *NY Times*, 21 June 1931.

137 Ibid., 30 June 1931.

138 J. R. Clark to Minister for External Affairs, 27 Aug. 1931, NAI, DFA, Washington Embassy files 1008.

139 Printed circular letter from Hospitals Trust, 1 Aug. 1931, NARA, State DF, 1930–9, RG59 841D.513/9.

140 Office of Postmaster General to Secretary of State, 10 May 1932, NARA, State DF, 1930–39, RG59 841D.513/19.

141 *NY Times*, 24 Feb. 1932.

142 Ibid., 12 Oct. 1931, NARA, State DF 1930–9, RG59 841D.513/9.

143 J. R. Clark to Minister for External Affairs, 27 Aug. 1931, NAI, DFA, Washington Embassy files 1008.

144 Henry H. Balch to Secretary of State, 10 Mar. 1932, NARA, State DF, 1930–39, RG59 841D.513/15.

145 F. H. Boland to Minister Plenipotentiary, Washington DC, 11 Sept. 1940, NAI, DFA, Washington Embassy files 1008.

146 Henry H. Balch to Secretary of State, 31 Mar. 1932, NARA, State DF, 1930–9, RG59 841D.513/17.

147 James Farley to Secretary of State, 22 Sept. 1938, NARA, State DF, 1930–9, RG59 841D.513/72.

148 D. McC. Watson, Craig Gardner & Co., to William D. Moreland Jr, American Consul, Dublin, 6 Oct. 1947, NARA, State DF, RG59 841D.513/10–1547.

149 J. M. Donaldson to Secretary of State, 19 Apr. 1948, NARA, State DF, RG59 841D.513/1–1948.

150 Edward D. McLaughlin, American Legation, Dublin to Secretary of State, 12 Aug. 1948, NARA, State DF, RG59 841D.513/8–1248.

151 Office of Postmaster General to Secretary of State, 12 Oct. 1931, NARA, State DF 1930–9, RG59 841D.513/9.

152 Circular letter from Joseph McGrath re. return of remittances for 1931, Manchester November Handicap sweep, NARA, State DF 1930–9, RG59 841D.513/9.

153 *NY Times*, 17 Mar. 1934.

154 Andrews memorandum, p. 43.

155 Report from Washington Embassy to Department of External Affairs, 2 Mar. 1937, NAI, DFA, Washington Embassy files 108.

156 *NY Times*, 26 Mar. 1937.

157 Ibid., 27 Mar. 1937.

158 Washington Embassy report to Secretary, Department of External Affairs, 2 Mar. 1937, NAI, DFA, Washington Embassy files 108.

159 Ibid., 1 June 1937, NAI, DFA, Washington Embassy files 108.

160 *Ir. Times*, 13 Apr. 1931.

161 McDonald and Considine, 'Not a clean sweep', p. 57.

162 *NY Times*, 5 Aug. 1938; NARA, State DF, 1930–9, RG59 841D.513/79.

163 *NY Times*, 25 Apr. 1935.

164 Ibid., 25 Apr. 1935, 15 and 28 Aug. 1936; Criminal Cases, Southern District of New York, C97–5, NARA, North East Regional Archives, New York City.

165 *NY Times*, 7 and 11 Aug. 1936.

166 *New York News*, 31 Mar. 1939 and 2 Apr. 1939; *New York World Telegram*, 1 Apr. 1939; *Los Angeles Evening News*, 5 Apr. 1939; *Los Angeles News*, 31 Mar. 1939 and 6 Apr. 1939.

167 Office of Postmaster General to Secretary of State, 10 May 1932, NARA, State DF, 1930–9, RG59 841D.513/19.

168 Department of State, Division of Western European Affairs, memo., 16 June 1932, NARA, State DF, 1930–9, RG59 841D.513/16.

169 Ibid., on 'Conversation between Mr R. E. Eggleton, Post Office Inspector and Mr Reber', 6 Aug. 1936, NARA, State DF, 1930–39, RG59 841D.513/46.

170 Deirdre McMahon, *Republicans and imperialists: Anglo-Irish relations in the 1930s* (London and New Haven, 1984), p. 221.

171 John Cudahy, 'Prevention of violations of United States statutes by the Hospitals Trust, Limited', 27 Oct. 1937, NARA, State DF, 1930–9, RG59 841D.513/52.

172 A. P. Aldrich to Secretary of State, 22 Jan. 1938. NARA, State DF 1930–9, RG59 841D.513/57.

173 Sumner Welles to John Cudahy, 4 Feb. 1938, *Foreign Relations of the United States (FRUS)*, 1938, vol. II, p. 196.

174 John Cuday to Secretary of State, 9 Apr. 1938, *FRUS*, 1938, vol. II, pp. 197–9.

175 Ibid., 23 Apr. 1938, pp. 200–1.

176 Copy of letter from P. J. Fleming to US agents, 5 May 1939, NARA, State DF, 1940–4, RG59 841D.513/83.

177 Department of State memo, 7 June 1938, NARA, State DF, 1930–9, RG59 841D.513/68.

178 *NY Times*, 28 Mar. 1936; McDonald and Considine, 'Not a clean sweep', p. 57.

179 Telegram, Dept of State to American Consul, Dublin, 20 Aug. 1938, NARA, State DF, 1930–9, RG59 841D.513/67A; Henry H. Balch to Secretary of State, 24 Aug. 1938, NARA, State DF, 1930–9, RG59 841D.513/70; Henry H. Balch to Secretary of State, 7 Sept. 1938, NARA, State DF, 1930–9, RG59 841D.513/71.

180 Leo T. McCauley to Secretary, Dept of External Affairs, 30 Aug. 1939, NAI, DFA 234/24.

181 *NY Times Magazine*, 3 June 1934, p. 8.

182 *NY Times*, 21 Mar. 1937.

183 'Elaine', 'An "Irish Sweepstakes" party for St Patrick's Day', in *Good Housekeeping* (Mar. 1934), p. 94.

184 *Washington Post*, 11 Mar. 1934; *Washington Herald*, 11 Oct. 1935; *Bloomington Telephone*, 23 Mar. 1938.

185 *Washington Post*, 17 July 1952.

186 *Gloversville Herald*, 22 Oct. 1935; *Chicago Daily Tribune*, 22 Oct. 1935.

187 *Bridgeport Post*, 18 Sept. 1939.

188 *Boston Herald*, 23 May 1938.

189 *NY Times*, 10 Dec. 1939, 13 Feb. 1940 and 16 Apr. 1941.

190 *Baltimore Sun*, 25 Mar. 1931; *NY Times*, 11 Nov. 1932; *Washington Herald*, 6 and 8 Jan. 1936.

191 *San Diego Tribune*, 4 Mar. 1938.

192 John J. McCarthy, 'The Irish Sweeps', in *Harper's Monthly Magazine*, vol. 169 (June 1934), pp. 49–59.

193 Ibid., p. 55–6.

194 Ibid., p. 52.

195 Shane Speer, 'Westbrook Pegler', in *American National Biography (ANB)*, vol. 17, pp. 246–7.

196 Westbrook Pegler, 'Fair enough', *Washington Post*, 31 Mar. 1936.

197 Ibid., 21 Apr. 1936.

198 Ibid., 30 Mar. 1937.

199 The details which follow are from McDonald and Considine, 'Not a clean sweep', pp. 16–17 and 55–7.

200 *Washington Post*, 10 July 1938.

201 Marion R. Casey, 'Ireland, New York and the Irish image in American popular culture, 1890–1960', PhD., New York University (1998), p. 58.

202 Kevin Rockett (ed.), *The Irish filmography: Fiction films, 1896–1996* (Dublin, 1996), p. 349.

203 Ibid., pp. 370–1.

204 Library of Congress Motion Picture Collection, VBM 0204: *Captain and the kids: The winning ticket* (1938), FAC 0301: *Popeye: Olive's sweepstake ticket* (1941), VBF 5523: *The Flintstones: The sweepstake ticket* (1960).

205 *NY Times*, 11 June 1933.

206 John Samuel Ezell, *Fortune's merry wheel: The lottery in America* (Cambridge, Mass., 1960), p. 277.

207 *Chicago Daily Tribune*, 29 June 1934 and 6 Apr. 1938.

208 *Congressional Record*, 73rd Congress, 1st session (10 June 1933), p. 5,630; 2nd session (30 Jan. 1934), p. 1,638; 2nd session (10 May 1934), p. 8,512.

209 Michael MacWhite to Secretary, Dept of External Affairs, 17 Apr. 1934, NAI, DFA 34/292.

210 *Congressional Record*, 73rd Congress, 2nd session (10 May 1934), p. 8,514.

211 Michael MacWhite to Secretary, Dept of External Affairs, 17 Apr. 1934, NAI, DFA 34/292.

212 Ibid.

213 *Congressional Record*, 74th Congress, 1st session (8 July 1935), p. 10,765.

214 *Boston Herald*, 17 Dec. 1935.

SIX: SURVIVAL AND RECOVERY, 1939–61

1 *Ir. Times*, 2 Apr. 1940; *New York Journal American*, 1 Apr. 1940.

2 *Montreal Gazette*, 25 Mar. 1940, *Johannesburg Forum*, 19 Apr. 1941.

3 *South Wales Echo & Evening Press, South Wales Argus, Midland Daily Telegraph*, 8 Jan. 1940.

4 *St John's (Newfoundland) Evening Telegram*, 10 Jan. 1940; *Bronx Sentinel*, 8 Mar. 1940; *Argus (Melbourne)*, 8 Jan. 1940.

5 *New York Herald Tribune*, 1 Dec. 1939.

6 *Irish Independent (Ir. Ind.)*, 6 Feb. 1940; *Irish Press (Ir. Press)*, 6 Feb. 1940.

7 *Ir. Press*, 2 Apr. 1940.

8 Ibid., 5 July 1940.

9 *Dáil Debates (DD)*, vol. 79 (30 Apr. 1940), col. 2073.

10 *Ir. Press*, 21 Dec. 1940.

11 *Ir. Times*, 5 Apr. 1940.

12 File no. 9974: Hospitals Trust (1940) Ltd., Companies Registration Office, Dublin.

13 *Who Was Who*, vol. VIII, 1981–1990; Spencer Freeman, *You can get to the top* (Dublin, 1972), pp. 19–20; *Times*, 11 June 1942.

14 *Ir. Ind.*, 2 Apr. 1940.

15 *DD*, vol. 76 (21 June 1939), col. 1375.

16 Public Hospitals (Amendment) Act (1939), section 5.

17 'Amendment of the Public Hospitals Act, 1933', 6 May 1939, National Archives of Ireland (NAI), Department of An Taoiseach (DT) S11248.

18 *DD*, vol. 76 (21 June 1939), col. 1376.

19 Ibid., col. 1377.

20 'Grand National Sweepstake', 28 Mar. 1940, NAI, DT S11763.

21 'Holding of future sweepstakes', 16 Apr. 1940, NAI, DT S11763.

22 *Seanad Debates (SD)*, vol. 24 (15 May 1940), cols 1413–14; *DD*, vol. 79 (30 Apr. 1940), cols 2096 and 2073.

23 Donal Ó Drisceoil, *Censorship in Ireland, 1939–1945* (Cork, 1996), pp. 73 and 85; 'Report of Mr Joseph G. Andrews', National Archives and Records Administration (NARA), State Decimal Files (DF) 1940–4, RG59 841D.513/83.

24 Fergus D'Arcy, *Horses, lords and racing men* (Kildare, 1991), p. 305.

25 John Welcome, *Irish horse-racing: An illustrated history* (Dublin, 1982), p. 161.

26 D'Arcy, *Horses, lords and racing men*, pp. 307–8.

27 Welcome, *Irish horse-racing*, pp. 161–2; Brian Smith, *The horse in Ireland* (Dublin, 1991), p. 237; Tony Sweeney, Annie Sweeney and Francis Hyland, *The Sweeney guide to the Irish turf from 1501 to 2001* (Dublin, 2002), Table: 'Ireland's top racehorse owners from 1751 to the present day [2001]', pp. 193–4.

28 Executive Committee minutes, 17 Dec. 1943, Irish Red Cross Archives (IRCA).

29 Public Hospitals (Amendment) (no. 2) Act (1939).

30 Information leaflet on Irish Red Cross Steeplechase, Jan. 1940, National Archives of Ireland (NAI), Secretary to the President (PRES) 1/P1392.

31 Executive Committee minutes, 16 Feb. 1940, IRCA.

32 *Ir. Press*, 1 Feb. 1940.

33 Ibid., 27 Feb. 1940.

34 *Ir. Times*, 1 Nov. 1939.

35 *Times*, 27 Jan. 1940; *Cork Examiner*, 4 Nov. 1939.

36 *Everybody's Weekly*, 9 Dec. 1939.

37 *Ir. Times*, 1 Nov. 1939.

38 *Times*, 29 Jan. 1940.

39 Audited accounts of sweepstake draws, Oireachtas Éireann Library (OÉL).

40 Central Council minutes, half-yearly meeting, 19 Mar. 1940, IRCA.

41 *Irish Red Cross Monthly Bulletin (IRCMB)*, (Dec. 1945), p. 388.

42 *Ir. Press*, 9 Jan. 1941.

43 *IRCMB*, (July 1942), p. 142; (Oct. 1942), p. 204; Phyllis Gaffney, *Healing amid the ruins: The Irish hospital at St Lô* (Dublin, 1999), p. 16.

44 Cabinet minutes, 17 Dec. 1946, Dept of Defence memo., 'Financing of the Irish Red Cross Society', 10 Mar. 1949, NAI, Department of An Taoiseach (DT) S13774/A.

45 Executive Committee minutes, 31 Oct. 1939, IRCA; *Ir. Times*, 24 Nov. 1939.

46 General Purposes Committee minutes, 8 Nov. 1940, IRCA; *Evening Herald*, 5 Dec. 1940.

47 NAI, PRES 1/P1402.

48 General Purposes Committee minutes, 27 June 1941, IRCA.

49 Ibid., 7 Feb. 1941, IRCA.

50 'Functional chart [provisional] – main lines of responsibility – Hospitals Trust [1940] Ltd.', 28 Mar. 1946, in the possession of Mr John Slevin.

51 'Hospitals Trust (1940) Ltd. – Proposed increases in cost of tickets and prizes in future sweepstakes', 17 May 1974, NAI, DT 2005/7/102.

52 'Sweepstakes under the Public Hospitals Acts', 2 Oct. 1945, NAI, DT S13774/A.

53 Ibid.

54 P. Ó Cinnéide to Secretary, Dept of Justice, 4 Feb. 1946, NAI, DT 13774/A.

55 Royal Commission on Betting, Gaming and Lotteries (RCBG&L), 'Memorandum submitted by Home Office: Irish Hospitals Trust Sweepstakes' [c.1949], The National Archives (TNA), HO45/24349.

56 RCBG&L, Minutes of evidence, Sir Harold Scott, TNA, HO45/24349.

57 RCBG&L, Statement of the Director General of the Post Office, TNA, HO45/24349.

58 RCBG&L, Minutes of evidence, Sir Harold Scott, Commissioner, Metropolitan Police, TNA, HO45/24349.

59 RCBG&L, Minutes of evidence, TNA, HO45/24349.

60 *Report of the RCBG&L* (1951), p. 39.

61   Ibid., Appendix II: Expenditure on football pools, p. 149.

62   Roger Munting, *An economic and social history of gambling in Great Britain and the USA* (Manchester, 1996), pp. 59–61.

63   Ibid., pp. 41, 44 and 47; J. A. Kay, *Good cause for gambling: The prospects for a national lottery in the UK* (London, *c*.1992), Table 1, p. 5.

64   *Royal Commission on Gambling: Final Report* (1978), p. 222.

65   *NY Times*, 16 July 1948; *Chicago Daily Tribune*, 9 July 1948.

66   *NY Times*, 15 Jan. 1949; *Chicago Daily Tribune*, 14 Jan. 1949.

67   Andrews memorandum, pp. 44–5.

68   *Washington Post*, 5, 7, 11 June 1961; *Ir. Times*, 22 June 1961.

69   *NY Times*, 21 Oct. 1949; Andrews memorandum, p. 46.

70   Memo. to Mr Purcell, 6 Nov. 1949, NAI, Department of Tourism, Transport and Communications (DTT&C) F12966/32 (vol. 3).

71   Postmaster General to Secretary of State, 6 May 1948, NARA State DF 841D.513/5–648; despatch from US Legation, 22 Jan. 1948, NARA State DF 841D.513/1–2248.

72   I am grateful to Mr John Slevin for showing me one of these Mexican tickets.

73   Despatch from US legation, Dublin, 16 Sept. 1948, NARA, State DF 841D.513/9–1648.

74   Attorney General Stanley Mosk, 'Report on the Irish Sweepstakes', 3 Feb. 1960, California State Library, Documents Section. I am grateful to Mr Liam Wylie for providing me with a copy of this document. Arthur Webb, *The clean sweep: The story of the Irish hospitals sweepstake* (London, 1968), pp. 161–70.

75   United States v. Dunne (1951) F. Supp. 196, US District Court for the Eastern District of Pennsylvania, Lexis-Nexis Reference 4071.

76   *Ir. Times*, 7 Feb. 1961; Anthony Moore, 'Isaac Wunder orders', in *Judicial Studies Institute Journal*, vol. 1, no. 1 (2001), pp. 137–46; Wunder v. Hospitals Trust (1940) Ltd, Supreme Court (Ó Dálaigh J.), 30 Nov. 1970 (16/1970); Wunder v. Hospitals Trust (1940) Ltd, Supreme Court (Ó Dálaigh J.), 16 Dec. 1970 (70/1969); Wunder v. Hospitals Trust (1940) Ltd, High Court (Kenny J.), 12 Nov. 1973 (1973/2926P), UCD Law Library.

77   'Proposal to appoint a Committee to report on the law relating to gambling and lotteries', 4 Apr. 1950, NAI, DT s6831/b/1.

78   'Gaming, lotteries and pools', 9 June 1952, NAI, DT s6831/b/2.

79   'State-controlled lotteries or pools', 11 Dec. 1952, NAI, DT s6831/b/2; *DD*, vol. 151 (25 May 1955), col. 63.

80   'Gaming, lotteries and pools', 9 June 1952, NAI, DT s6831/b/2.

81   'Football and racing pools', 2 Sept. 1952, NAI, DT s6831/b/2.

82   'State-controlled lotteries or pools, supplementary note', 22 Jan. 1953, Joseph McGrath to Sean McKeon [*sic*], 17 Feb. 1953, NAI, DT s6831/b/2.

83   Gaming and Lotteries Act (1956).

84   *DD*, vol. 153 (2 Nov. 1955) cols 454–5; vol. 151 (25 May 1955), cols 66–7.

85   For a more detailed account of the Mater's dispute with the NHS see Daithí Ó Corráin, *Rendering to God and Caesar: The Irish churches and the two states in Ireland, 1949–73* (Manchester, 2006), pp. 136–40.

86   Rev. Michael P. Kelly, *Belfast's Mater Hospital: Why? present position* (Belfast, 1954), p. 10.

87   Mater Infirmorum Hospital Belfast, *Seventy-fourth annual report, 1958*, pp. 30–1.

88   'Mater Misericordiae [*sic*] Hospital, Belfast, and its allied institutions', 12 Mar. 1949, Maurice Moynihan to Private Secretary, Minister for Defence, 14 Sept. 1949, NAI, DT s13774/a.

89 *Ir. Press*, 26 Feb. 1954.

90 Eamon de Valera to Daniel Mageean, 3 July 1952, NAI, DT s6831/B/2.

91 Dept of Taoiseach memo.', 26 Nov. 1954, NAI, DT s6831/c.

92 'Gaming Bill, 1954: Question of permitting pools or lotteries for the benefit of Charities outside the twenty-six counties', 30 Nov. 1954, NAI, DT s6831/c.

93 Thomas J. Coyne to Minister for Finance, 26 Mar. 1955, NAI, DT s6831/c.

94 *Seanad Debates* (*SD*), vol. 45 (14 Dec. 1955), col. 919.

95 Ibid., cols 918–27; (15 Dec. 1955), cols 930–2, 960–1.

96 Ibid., (14 Dec. 1955), cols 920–1; Gaming and Lotteries Act (1956), section 26; *Ir. Ind.*, 4 May 1956.

97 Workers' Union of Ireland (WUI), *Report of the Annual Delegate Conference, 1949*, pp. 3–4, p. 23.

98 Labour Court Recommendation no. 381 (31 Mar. 1950).

99 Ibid.

100 WUI, *Report of the Annual Delegate Conference, 1950*, p. 6.

101 Labour Court Recommendation no. 381 (31 Mar. 1950).

102 WUI, *Report of the Annual Delegate Conference, 1951*, pp. 22–3.

103 Ibid., *1955*, pp. 65–6; *1957*, p. 8; *1958*, p. 69.

104 Ibid., *1951*, p. 23; *1952*, p. 27.

105 Arrangements with Hospitals Trust for sponsored programmes, NAI, DTT&C 20/57 (vol. 6).

106 Brian Cosgrove, *The yew tree at the head of the strand* (Liverpool, 2001), p. 10.

107 Spencer Freeman to T. J. Monaghan, 4 Nov. 1949; 23 Nov. 1949, NAI, DTT&C 20/57 (vol. 4).

108 Draft letter to Spencer Freeman, Dec 1949, NAI, DTT&C 20/57 (vol. 4).

109 T. J. Monaghan to Secretary, Dept of Posts and Telegraphs, 12 Jan. 1952; 27 Feb. 1952, NAI, DTT&C 20/57 (vol. 4).

110 T. J. Monaghan, memo., 9 Feb. 1952; Freeman 'Note of a meeting at Leitrim House on February 7th, 1952'; memo. to Minister for Posts and Telegraphs, 22 Feb. 1952, NAI, DTT&C 20/57 (vol. 4).

111 Memo. to Secretary, Dept of Posts and Transport, 1 Jan. 1953; letter to Spencer Freeman, 12 Jan. 1953, NAI, DTT&C 20/57 (vol. 4).

112 Spencer Freeman to Minister for Posts and Telegraphs, 19 Feb. 1953, Deputy Chief Engineer to Director General, 30 Oct. 1953, NAI, DTT&C 20/57 (vol. 5).

113 Spencer Freeman to Minister for Posts and Telegraphs, 9 Mar. 1955; M. A. Purcell to Private Secretary, Minister for Posts and Telegraphs, 24 Mar. 1955, NAI, DTT&C 20/57 (vol. 5).

114 M. Ó Dochartaigh to Minister for Posts and Telegraphs, 13 Apr. 1955, DTT&C 20/57 (vol. 5).

115 Dept of Posts and Telegraphs memo., 10 Jan. 1957, NAI, DTT&C 20/57 (vol. 6).

116 M. Ó Dochartaigh, memo., 11 Jan. 1957, NAI, DTT&C 20/57 (vol. 6).

117 Letter to Udo Blässer, 8 Feb. 1957, Dept of Posts and Telegraphs to Patrick McGrath, 6 Feb. 1957, NAI, DTT&C 20/57 (vol. 6).

118 Dept of Posts and Telegraphs statement on change of time for Hospitals Trust programme, 3 Apr. 1957; Spencer Freeman to León Ó Broin, 30 May 1957, NAI, DTT&C 20/57 (vol. 6).

119 Memo. from Controller of Programmes, 3 Apr. 1959, NAI, DTT&C 20/57 (vol. 6).

120 Spencer Freeman to Maurice Gorham, 18 Aug. 1959; George McGrath to Director Radio Éireann, 25 Feb. 1960; *Ir. Ind.*, 7 Mar. 1960, NAI, DTT&C 20/57 (vol. 6).

121 This account of the establishment of Radio Teilifís Éireann (RTÉ) is based on Robert J. Savage, *Irish television: The political and social origins* (Cork, 1996).

122 Sean Ormonde to Seán Lemass, 19 Nov. 1957, NAI, DTT&C tw894 (vol. 3); M. Ó Dochartaigh 'Memo.', 23 Oct. 1957, DTT&C tw894 (vol. 4).

123 Joseph McGrath to León Ó Broin, 13 Nov. 1957, NAI, DTT&C tw894 (vol. 4).

124 'Television & sound broadcasting. Memorandum by Hospitals Trust (1940) Limited', 6 Nov. 1957, NAI, DTT&C tw894 (vol. 4).

125 Brian Havel, *Maestro of crystal: The story of Miroslav Havel* (Dublin, 2005), p. 149.

126 Ibid., pp. 147–53.

127 Ibid., pp. 155–68.

128 Ibid., pp. 184–7, 236–40; 'Waterford Glass: A success story', *Irish Echo*, 10 June 1967; *Ir. Press*, 20 Aug. 1984.

129 'Paddy McGrath', in Ivor Kenny (ed.), *In good company: Conversations with Irish leaders* (Dublin, 1987), pp. 84–5.

130 1958 Irish Hospitals Golf Tournament programme.

131 *Ir. Times*, 24 July 1961; 23 July 1962.

132 Reg Green, *The history of the Grand National: A race apart* (London, 1993), p. 276; *Ir. Times*, 15 Nov. 1962.

133 *Ir. Times*, 17 Mar. 1966.

134 Ibid., 20 Jan. 1971.

135 Welcome, *Irish horse-racing*, p. 200; *Ir. Times*, 26 May 1960; *Ir. Press*, 24 Mar. 1961.

136 *Sunday Despatch*, 4 June 1961; *Irish Field*, 13 Jan. 1962; *Ir. Press*, 28 May 1962.

137 *Dublin Evening Mail*, 16 June 1962.

138 *Belfast News-Letter*, 5 June 1962.

139 *Evening Press*, 30 Apr. 1962, 'A series of six articles on the Irish Sweeps Derby, 1962', NAI, Department of Foreign Affairs (DFA) 334/99(1).

140 Sweeney et al., *The Sweeney guide to the Irish Turf*, Table: 'Ireland's top racehorse owners from 1751 to the present day [2001]', pp. 193–4.

141 http://www.pedigreequery.com/nasrullah, www.secretariat.com/secretariat_history.htm (accessed 5 May 2008).

142 Coleman, 'Joseph McGrath' and 'Patrick William McGrath', in *Dictionary of Irish Biography (DIB)*; *Ir. Times*, 9 July 2005.

SEVEN: DECLINE AND CLOSURE, 1961–87

1   Coleman, 'Joseph McGrath' in *Dictionary of Irish Biography (DIB)*; 'Paddy McGrath' in Ivor Kenny (ed.), *In good company: Conversations with Irish leaders* (Dublin, 1987), p. 82.

2   Roger Munting, *An economic and social history of gambling in Great Britain and the USA* (Manchester, 1996), pp. 51–2.

3   Paul A. Fino, *My life in politics and public service* (New York, 1986), p. 154; *LA Times*, 23 Nov. 1966; Munting, *An economic and social history of gambling in Great Britain and the USA*, pp. 72–3.

4   Suzanne Morton, *At odds: Gambling and Canadians, 1919–1969* (Toronto, 2003), p. 5.

5   Joan Vance, *An analysis of the costs and benefits of public lotteries: The Canadian experience* (New York/Ottawa, 1989), p. 66; *Reports of the Joint Committee of the Senate and House of Commons on capital punishment (July 27, 1956), corporal punishment (July 11, 1956), lotteries (July 11, 1956)* (Ottawa, 1956), pp. 64–71.

6   Vance, *An analysis of the costs and benefits of public lotteries*, p. 75.

7   Ibid., pp. 88–92.

8   Munting, *An economic and social history of gambling in Great Britain and the USA*, p. 79.

9   *Ir. Times*, 5 Feb. 1965, 18 Mar. 1967; 'Memo. by the Chancellor of the Exchequer to cabinet re. national lottery', 5 Mar. 1968, The National Archives (TNA), PREM 13/2148; Munting, *An economic and social history of gambling in Great Britain and the USA*, p. 75.

10 Patrick McGrath to Donogh O'Malley, 24 June 1966, National Archives of Ireland (NAI), Department of An Taoiseach (DT) 97/6/637.

11 'Proposals to organise additional sweepstakes under the auspices of Hospitals Trust (1940) Ltd', 10 Nov. 1966, NAI, DT 97/6/637.

12 'Proposals for increase in funds to be raised by Hospitals Sweepstakes', NAI, DT 97/6/637.

13 Patrick McGrath to Donogh O'Malley, 24 June 1966, 'Proposals for increase in funds to be raised by hospitals sweepstakes', Seán Flanagan to Seán Lemass, 18 Aug. 1966, NAI, DT 97/6/637.

14 'Memo. for Government: Proposals for increase in funds to be raised by Hospitals Sweepstakes', 22 Aug. 1966; 'Proposals to organise additional sweepstakes under the auspices of Hospitals Trust (1940) Ltd', 10 Nov. 1966 NAI, DT 97/6/637.

15 'Proposals to organise additional sweepstakes under the auspices of Hospitals Trust (1940) Ltd', 10 Nov. 1966 NAI, DT 97/6/637.

16 N. S. Ó Nualláin to Private Secretary, Minister for Justice, 21 Dec. 1966, NAI, DT 97/6/637.

17 'Memo. for Government: Proposals for increase in funds to be raised by Hospitals Sweepstakes', 22 Aug. 1966, NAI, DT 97/6/637.

18 See various letters from charitable organisations and Federation of Voluntary Charitable Organisations (FVCO) in NAI, DT 99/1/148; *Ir. Press*, 14 Mar. 1967.

19 'Proposals to organise additional sweepstakes under the auspices of Hospitals Trust (1940) Limited', 25 Apr. 1967, Cabinet decision 28 May 1967, NAI, DT 99/1/148.

20 'Hospitals Trust (1940) Ltd. – Proposed increases in cost of tickets and prizes in future sweepstakes', 17 May 1974, NAI, DT 2005/7/102; audited accounts of sweepstake draws, Oireachtas Éireann Library (OÉL).

21 'Hospitals Trust (1940) Ltd. – Proposed increases in cost of tickets and prizes in future sweepstakes', 17 May 1974, NAI, DT 2005/7/102.

22 'Sweeps memo.', 2 July 1974, NAI, DT 2005/7/102.

23 *Ir. Times*, 12 Dec. 1975; *Dáil Debates* (*DD*), vol. 291 (16 June 1976), col. 1138.

24 *Ir. Times*, 22 Mar. 1977, 31 Aug. 1979.

25 Figures calculated from results of draws in Irish daily newspapers.

26 D. Ó Súilleabhain to Private Secretary, Minister for Justice, 5 July 1974, NAI, DT 2005/7/102; audited accounts of sweepstake draws, OÉL.

27 Spencer Freeman, 'Weekly sweepstakes: Application for permission', 6 Jan. 1975, NAI, DT 2005/7/102.

28 DT memo., 17 Sept. 1974, NAI, DT 2005/7/102.

29 Denis Larkin to Liam Cosgrave, 20 Dec. 1974, NAI, DT 2006/133/63.

30 DT memo., 17 Sept. 1974, NAI, DT 2005/7/102.

31 Spencer Freeman, 'Weekly sweepstakes: Application for permission', 6 Jan. 1975, NAI, DT 2005/7/102.

32 F. G. Doherty to Liam Cosgrave, 13 Aug. 1975, NAI, DT 2006/133/63.

33 'Memo. for Government: Proposals by Hospitals Trust (1940) Limited to organise weekly sweepstakes', 22 Oct. 1975, NAI, DT 2006/133/63.

34 Audited accounts of sweepstake draws, OÉL.

35 *Ir. Press*, 16 Jan. 1976; Dept of Justice memo., 1 Mar. 1976, H. S. Ó Dubhda to Private Secretary, Minister for Justice, 3 Mar. 1976, NAI, DT 2006/133/63.

36 Public Hospitals (Amendment) Act (1976).

37 F. G. Doherty to Liam Cosgrave, 16 Mar. 1976, NAI, DT 2006/133/63.

38 J. R. Kennerley to An Taoiseach, 1 Mar. 1976, NAI, DT 2006/133/472.

39 Patrick Cooney to Liam Cosgrave, 12 Mar. 1976, NAI, DT 2006/133/472.

40 V. Mulcahy to Mr McCarthy, 26 Apr. 1976, Mr Kirwan to Secretary, Dept of Taoiseach, 12 May 1976, NAI, DT 2006/133/472.

41 Patrick Cooney to Liam Cosgrave, 12 Mar. 1976, NAI, DT 2006/133/472.

42 Mr Kirwan to Secretary, Dept of Taoiseach, 12 May 1976, NAI, DT 2006/133/472.

43 V. Mulcahy to Mr McCarthy, 26 Apr. 1976, Mr Kirwan to Secretary, Dept of Taoiseach, 12 May 1976, NAI, DT 2006/133/472.

44 Thomas O'Hanlon, 'A good thing in the Irish sweepstakes – for the owners', in *Fortune* (Nov. 1966), pp. 170–3.

45 *Ir. Times*, 6 Oct. 1969.

46 John Horgan, *Irish media: A critical history since 1922* (London / New York, 2001), p. 150; *Hidden history: If you're not in. . .*, RTÉ 1 television, 2 Dec. 2003. Joe MacAnthony, 'Where the sweep millions go', *Sunday Independent*, 21 Jan. 1973.

47 James Stewart-Gordon, 'The odds? 450,000 to one', in *Readers' Digest* [US edition] (Apr.1959), pp. 93–7.

48 Joe MacAnthony, 'Where the sweep millions go', *Sunday Independent* (*Sun. Ind.*), 21 Jan. 1973.

49 Editorial, *Sun. Ind.*, 21 Jan. 1973.

50 Interview with Mr John Slevin, 7 Aug. 2007.

51 *Newsweek*, 12 Feb. 1973, p. 42.

52 Horgan, *Irish media*, p. 150; John Horgan, *Broadcasting and public life: RTÉ news and current affairs, 1926–1997* (Dublin, 2004), p. 151.

53 'Irish Hospitals Sweepstakes: The facts' (I am grateful to Mr John Slevin for showing me a copy of this pamphlet).

54 *If you're not in . . .*

55 *Dáil Debates* (*DD*), vol. 291 (16 June 1976), cols 1110–18 and 1158.

56 Ibid., cols 1142 and 1127–8.

57 Ibid., col. 1140.

58 Ibid., cols 1126–7.

59 *Seanad Debates* (*SD*), vol. 84 (17 June 1976), cols 431–3.

60 Ibid., cols 436 and 439.

61 Ibid., col. 435.

62 Information supplied by Mr Liam Wylie; *Ir. Times*, 14 July 1973.

63 *If you're not in . . .*

64 Horgan, *Broadcasting and public life*, pp. 151–3; Charlie Bird and Kevin Rafter, *This is Charlie Bird* (Dublin, 2006), pp. 37–8; *If you're not in . . .*; *Today Tonight Special: The Sweep*, 22 Jan. 1992.

65 *If you're not in . . .*

66 Information supplied by Mr Liam Wylie.

67 Joe MacAnthony, 'How I exposed the sweepstakes scandals', *Ir. Independent*, 6 Dec. 2003; Stephen Dodd, 'Irish sweepstake scandal remains a lesson to us all', Liam Collins, 'The Sweep dynasty that failed the test of time' and Martin Fitzpatrick, 'Sweepstakes' McGraths ahead of their time', in *Sun. Ind.*, 7 Dec. 2003.

68 Labour Court Recommendation no. 2203 (29 Sept. 1967).

69 *Ir. Times*, 18 Oct. 1967.

70 Ibid., 26 Sept. and 10 Oct. 1967.

71 Workers' Union of Ireland (WUI), *Report of the General Executive Committee, 1968–9*, pp. 76–8.

72 Labour Court Recommendation no. 2556 (22 Mar. 1971).

73 *Ir. Times*, 22 Feb. 1969; interview with Mr John Slevin, 7 Aug. 2007.

74 WUI, *Report of the General Executive Committee, 1968–9*, p. 77.

75 Interview with Mr John Slevin, 7 Aug. 2007.

76 *Ir. Times*, 20 Apr. 1970.

77 Ibid., 22 and 27 Feb. 1969.

78 Ibid., 27 Feb. 1969.

79 Ibid., 14 Sept. 1960.

80 Interview with Mr John Slevin, 7 Aug. 2007.

81 Ibid.

82 *Ir. Times*, 7 June 1972, 11 July 1973 and 4–6 Dec. 1973.

83 Ibid., 26 Jan. 1974.

84 Ibid., 25 July 1973 and 26 Jan. 1974.

85 Ibid., 19 Dec. 1974, 27 Mar. 1975, 8 Oct. 1977; interview with Mr John Slevin, 7 Aug. 2007.

86 Interview with Mr John Slevin, 7 Aug. 2007.

87 *Ir. Times*, 18 Feb. 1975.

88 Ibid., 22 Feb. 1975.

89 Labour Court recommendations no. 4242 (5 Apr. 1977), no. 8393 (27 Oct. 1983), AD-80-3 (23 Nov. 1983).

90 *Ir. Times*, 19 May 1977, 30 May 1977, 31 May 1977, 30 June 1977, 7 July 1977.

91 Ibid., 20 Sept. 1975.

92 Ibid., 10 Feb. 1978.

93 Ibid., 15 June 1979.

94 'Paddy McGrath', in Kenny (ed.), *In good company*, p. 85.

95 *Ir. Times*, 31 Oct. 1980; interview with Mr John Slevin, 7 Aug. 2007.

96 Michael Roche, 'Avenue Investments: Jeffers gambled, McGrath lost', in *Irish Business* (Sept. 1984), p. 28.

97 Frank McDonald, *The destruction of Dublin* (Dublin, 1985), p. 129.

98 *Ir. Times*, 12 Feb. 1980.

99 Roche, 'Avenue Investments', p. 23.

100 *Ir. Times*, 22 Nov. 1960, 14 Nov. 1963.

101 Ibid., 22 Nov. 1967, 31 Mar. 1969.

102 Ibid., 25 June 1977.

103 Ibid., 24 July 1981; Coleman, 'Patrick William McGrath', in *DIB*.

104 *Ir. Times*, 12 Feb. 1980.

105 Ibid., 28 July 1972.

106 Ibid., 23 Mar. 1974.

107 Ibid., 12 July 1990.

108 'Paddy McGrath', in Kenny (ed.), *In good company*, p. 89.

109 Frank Fitzgibbon, 'Why Avenue is hocking the family heirloom', in *Business and Finance* (26 Apr. 1984), pp. 12–13.

110 *Ir. Times*, 15 Aug. 1984; Fitzgibbon, 'Why Avenue is hocking the family heirloom', p. 13.

111 Coleman, 'Patrick William McGrath' in *DIB*; *Ir. Times*, 19 Apr. 1984, 15 Aug. 1984, 12 July 1990.

112 Fitzgibbon, 'Why Avenue is hocking the family heirloom', p. 12.

113 *Ir. Times*, 17 Oct. 1972, 9 Sept. 1980; Fitzgibbon, 'Why Avenue is hocking the family heirloom', p. 12.

114 Roche, 'Avenue Investments', pp. 23–8.

115 *Ir. Times*, 1 Aug. 1987, 8 July 1988, 13 Oct. 2001; Conor Kennedy and Daragh O'Shaughnessy, 'Anti-avoidance – restrictions in tax planning', www.cpaireland.ie/UserFiles/File/Accountancy%20Plus/Taxation/March%202006/Anti-Avoidance.pdf; 'Patrick McGrath and Ors. v. J. E. McDermott (Inspector of Taxes)', in B. H. Giblin and Susan Keegan (eds), *Irish tax reports, vol. III: 1978–87* (Dublin, 1994), pp. 683–705.

116 *Ir. Times*, 26 Apr. 1968.

117 Denis Larkin to Liam Cosgrave, 20 Dec. 1974, NAI, DT 2006/133/63.

118 *DD*, vol. 346 (7 Dec. 1983), col. 1391; *Ir. Times*, 3 Oct. 1984; *DD*, vol. 354 (27 Nov. 1984), col. 699.

119 *Ir. Times*, 2 Aug. 1985, 12 Sept. 1985.

120 Ibid., 14 Sept. 1985.

121 Ibid., 25 Sept. 1985.

122 Ibid., 14 Sept. 1985.

123 Interview with Mr John Slevin, 7 Aug. 2007.

124 *Ir. Times*, 19 Feb. 1986, 27 Mar. 1986, 18 July 1986, 3 Dec. 1986; *DD*, vol. 370 (2 Dec. 1986), cols 1087–8; interview with Mr John Slevin, 7 Aug. 2007.

125 *Ir. Times*, 11 Jan. 1986, 27 Feb. 1987.

126 Ibid., 8 Oct. 1986.

127 Interview with Mr John Slevin, 7 Aug. 2007; *Ir. Times*, 12 Feb. 1987; Irish Hospitals Sweepstakes Trust House Association, submission to Labour Court, 25 May 1987 (I am grateful to Mr John Slevin for a copy of this document).

128 *DD*, vol. 372 (30 Apr. 1987), col. 792.

129 *Ir. Times*, 26 June 1984, 9 Jan. 1987, 1–2 Mar. 1988, 28 July 1988.

130 Irish Hospitals Sweepstakes Trust House Association, submission to Labour Court, 25 May 1987.

131 *Ir. Times*, 4 and 11 Nov. 1987.

132 Ibid., 8 Mar. 1988; interview with Mr John Slevin, 7 Aug. 2007.

133 *Ir. Times*, 14 Feb. 1991.

134 Interview with Mr John Slevin, 7 Aug. 2007.

135 *Ir. Times*, 12 Mar. 1987, 28 July 1988.

136 *DD*, vol. 402 (15 Nov. 1990), col. 1594; Public Hospitals (Amendment) Act (1990).

137 *DD*, vol. 403 (27 Nov. 1990), cols 161–2, *SD*, vol. 126 (5 Dec. 1990), cols 1946–8 and 1972.

138 Ibid., vol. 402 (15 Nov. 1990), col. 1571.

139 *Ir. Times*, 18 June 1992, 11 Mar. 1993.

140 Ibid., 29 July 1993.

141 Interview with Mr John Slevin, 7 Aug. 2007; Hospitals Trust (1940) Ltd (Payments to Former Employees) Act (2000).

142 *DD*, vol. 522 (29 June 2000), col. 1018.

143 Ibid., col. 1016.

144 Ibid., vol. 336 (16 June 1982), cols 455–8.

145 Irish Shipping Limited (Payments to Former Employees) Act (1994).

EIGHT: THE SWEEPSTAKE AND HOSPITAL DEVELOPMENT, 1939–87

1   Hospitals Commission, *Fifth general report, 1939 1940 and 1941* (Dublin, 1943), pp. 6–7.

2   Ibid.; *Seanad Debates (SD)*, vol. 23 (31 Mar. 1943), col. 1772.

3   Hospitals Commission, *Sixth general report, 1942, 1943 and 1944* (Dublin, 1946), p. 8.

4   Sr Mary Bernard Carew to Revd Dr Wall, 27 Apr. 1940, National Archives of Ireland (NAI), Department of An Taoiseach (DT) s12303/a.

5   J. Hurson to M. Ó Muimneacháin, 21 Oct. 1942; 'Hospital development in Dublin: Present position', 11 Nov. 1946, DT s12303/a.

6   Hospitals Commission, *Sixth general report*, pp. 8–9.

7   H. E. Counihan, 'St Laurence's Hospital', in J. D. H. Widdess, *The Richmond, Whitworth & Hardwicke hospitals: St Laurence's, Dublin, 1772–1972* (Dublin, 1972), pp. 148–51; St Laurence's Hospital Act (1943), section 5 (4); John Corcoran, 'Dublin hospitals – voluntary or state', in *Irish Journal of Medical Science (IJMS)* (Feb. 1948), p. 58.

8   Corcoran, 'Dublin hospitals', p. 57; Dublin Fever Hospital Act (1936); Tuberculosis (Establishment of Sanatoria) Act (1945).

9   Assistant Secretary, Dept of Local Govt and Public Health to Secretary, Rotunda Hospital, 23 May 1942, NAI, DH a104/1 (vol. 3). Similar letters were sent to other voluntary hospitals.

10   Hospitals Commission, *Seventh general report, 1945, 1946 and 1947* (1949), p. 4.

11   Ibid., *Sixth general report*, p. 5.

12   Ibid., pp. 6–8.

13   *Ir. Times*, 20 Feb. 1941.

14   Ibid., 30 May 1941.

15   Corcoran, 'Dublin hospitals', p. 56.

16   Dublin Hospitals Bureau, *Report of working, for period 1 June 1942–31 December 1944* (supplement to Hospitals Commission, *Sixth general report*), p. 254.

17   Ibid., *for period 3 June 1941–31 May 1942* (supplement to Hospitals Commission, *Fifth general report*), p. 275.

18   Ibid., *for period 1 June 1942–31 December 1944*, p. 253 and Dublin Hospitals Bureau, *Report of working, for period 1 January 1945–31 December 1947* (supplement to Hospitals Commission, *Seventh general report*), p. 301.

19   Ibid., *for period 3 June 1941–31 May 1942*, p. 276.

20   Ibid.

21   Ibid., *for period 1 June 1942–31 December 1944*, p. 256.

22   Ibid., *for period 1 January 1945–31 December 1947*, pp. 303–4.

23 *Seanad Debates (SD)*, vol. 27 (31 Mar. 1943), col. 1717.

24 Ibid., col. 1719.

25 Ibid., cols 1721–6.

26 Ibid., col. 1727.

27 Ibid., col. 1736.

28 Ibid., col. 1732.

29 Ibid., col. 1744.

30 Ibid., cols 1738 and 1742.

31 Ibid., cols 1762–3 and 1769.

32 See Ruth Barrington, *Health, medicine and politics in Ireland, 1900–1970* (Dublin, 1987), chs 7–8; Greta Jones, *'Captain of all these men to death': The history of tuberculosis in nineteenth and twentieth-century Ireland* (Amsterdam, 2001), chs 7–8.

33 John Horgan, *Noël Browne: Passionate outsider* (Dublin, 2000), pp. 75–6; Barrington, *Health, medicine and politics*, pp. 204–5.

34 Noël Browne, *Against the tide* (Dublin, 1986), p. 115.

35 These calculations are based on the accounts of the Hospitals Trust Fund, published in the seven general reports of the Hospitals Commission.

36 'Hospitals Trust funds and new hospital works' [*c*.Nov. 1944], NAI, Department of Health (DH) A104/6 (vol. 6).

37 'Treatment of tuberculosis', 10 Jan. 1945, NAI, DT s13603A.

38 'Hospitals Trust funds and new hospital works' [*c*.Nov. 1944], NAI, DH A104/6 (vol. 6).

39 *Dáil Debates (DD)*, vol. 95 (31 Jan. 1945), cols 1869–70.

40 Jones, *'Captain of all these men to death'*, pp. 159–60.

41 *DD*, vol. 95 (31 Jan. 1945), col. 1880.

42 Barrington, *Health, medicine and politics*, p. 164.

43 *DD*, vol. 95 (31 Jan. 1945), col. 1884.

44 Tuberculosis (Establishment of Sanatoria) Act (1945), section 5.

45 *DD*, vol. 95 (31 Jan. 1945), col. 1948, (7 Feb. 1945), col. 2384.

46 Ibid., (1 Feb. 1945), cols 2102–3.

47 Ibid., (31 Jan. 1945), col. 1939.

48 Barrington, *Health, medicine and politics*, pp. 156–61.

49 *Report of the Departmental Committee on the Health Services, 1945*, p. 78, Royal College of Surgeons in Ireland, James Deeny papers.

50 Ibid., pp. 84 and 5–6.

51 *First Report of the Department of Health, 1945–9*, p. 65.

52 *DD*, vol. 111 (6 July 1948), cols 2273–5.

53 Ibid., col. 2273.

54 Horgan, *Noël Browne*, pp. 75–6.

55 Ibid., p. 82.

56 *DD*, vol. 111 (6 July 1948), col. 2311.

57 Ibid., (6 July 1948), col. 2273.

58 Ibid., vol. 117 (6 July 1949), cols 229 and 314.

59 Ibid., vol. 110 (12 May 1948), cols 1379–80.

60 J. J. McElligott to P. Ó Cinnéide, 31 July 1948 and 23 Mar. 1949, NAI, DH H34/8c.

61 P. Ó Cinnéide to J. J. McElligott, 11 Apr. 1949; J. J. McElligott to P. Ó Cinnéide, 30 Sept. 1949, NAI, DH H34/8c.

62 *Report of the Department of Health, 1951–2*, Appendix 14: Accounts of the Hospitals Trust Fund for the years 1947 to 1951, pp. 95–127.

63 J. J. McElligott to P. Ó Cinnéide, 25 Apr. 1949, NAI, DH H34/8c.

64 'Hospitals construction programme, 1949–55', 1 Dec. 1949, NAI, DH H34/8A (vol. III).

65 'Memorandum for government: The financing of the short-term hospital building programme', 11 Sept. 1951, NAI, DT S12303A; P. Ó Cinnéide to Secretary, Dept of Finance, 19 Dec. 1952, NAI, DH H34/8A (vol. III); *Report of the Department of Health, 1950–1*, p. 62.

66 Ryan replaced Browne when the inter-party government was defeated by Fianna Fáil in the 1951 General Election.

67 'Memo. for government: The financing of the short-term hospital building programme', 11 Sept. 1951, M. Ó Muimhneacháin to Private Secretary, Minister for Health, 22 Apr. 1952, NAI, DT S12303A.

68 Central Statistics Office (hereafter CSO), *Statistical Abstract of Ireland, 1958*, Table 171, p. 204; P. Ó Cinnéide to Secretary, Dept Finance, 14 Oct. 1953, NAI, DT S12303A.

69 'Hospitals Trust Fund – disbursement in connection with the building programme', 14 Mar. 1952, NAI, DH H34/8A (vol. III).

70 *Report of the Department of Health, 1952–3*, p. 41.

71 *Ibid., 1955–6*, pp. 62–4; *1956–7*, p. 56.

72 P. Ó Cinnéide to Secretary, Dept of Finance, 17 May 1954, NAI, DH H34/8A (vol. III).

73 Maurice Moynihan to Private Secretary, Minister for Health, 22 July 1953, NAI, DH H34/8A (vol. III); 'Memo. for the cabinet committee on the provision of employment', 31 Dec. 1953; M. Ó Muineacháin to Private Secretary, Minister for Health, 8 Jan. 1954, NAI, DT S12303A.

74 P. Ó Cinnéide to Secretary, Dept of Finance, 17 May 1954, NAI, DH H34/8A (vol. III).

75 P. Ó Cinnéide to Mr Brady, 14 Dec. 1954, NAI, DH H34/8A (vol. III).

76 Ibid., 28 Jan. 1955, NAI, DH H34/8A (vol. III).

77 Gerard Sweetman to T. F. O'Higgins, 4 Jan. 1956, NAI, DH H34/8A (vol. III).

78 'Position in regard to the Hospitals Trust Fund', 26 Mar. 1958, NAI, DT S12303/B/2.

79 *Statistical Abstract of Ireland (SAI), 1958*, Tables 171 and 172, p. 204.

80 I am grateful to Professor Ciarán Ó hÓgartaigh (UCD) for preparing this figures.

81 M. Bhreathnach to Secretary, Dept of Health, 16 Feb. 1956, NAI, DH H34/8A (vol. III); memo to Mr Brady, 16 Aug. 1956, T. F. O'Higgins to Gerard Sweetman, 6 Dec. 1956, NAI, DH H34/8A (vol. IV).

82 P. Ó Cinnéide to Minister for Health, 3 July 1956, NAI, DH H34/8A (vol. III).

83 'Position in regard to the Hospitals Trust Fund', 26 Mar. 1958, NAI, DT S12303/B/2; *Report of the Department of Health, 1957–8*, p. 60.

84 P. Ó Cinnéide to Mr Brady, 14 Feb. 1957, NAI, DH H34/8A (vol. IV).

85 T. K. Whitaker to Minister for Health, 3 Aug. 1957, NAI, DH H34/8A (vol. IV).

86 'Estimates concerning disbursements from Hospitals Trust Fund and possibilities in relation to future hospital building activity', 21 Nov. 1959, NAI, DH H34/8A (vol. IV).

87 *SAI, 1967*, Table 187, p. 239.

88 Minister for Health to Minister for Finance, Nov. 1962, NAI, DH H34/8A (vol. IV).

89 E. de Barra to Dublin Voluntary Hospitals, 23 Aug. 1945, NAI, DH A/104/5 (vol. V).

90 P. Ó Cinnéide to Secretary, Hospitals Commission, 5 Oct. 1948, NAI, DH A104/6 (vol. VI).

91 *DD*, vol. 122 (11 July 1950), col. 1222.

92 Barrington, *Health, medicine and politics*, pp. 204–5.

93　E. de Barra to Secretary, Dept of Health, 14 Nov. 1951, NAI, DH A104/9 (vol. VIII).

94　Lord Wicklow to Secretary, Hospitals Commission, 20 Sept. 1951, NAI, DH A104/9 (vol. VIII).

95　T. G. Moorhead to Michael Doran, 15 Jan. 1952, NAI, DH A104/9 (vol. VIII).

96　Sir Patrick Dun's Hospital Act (1954).

97　Memo. to Mr Dowling, 22 Nov. 1951, NAI, DH A104/9 (vol. VIII).

98　P. MacCormaic to Secretary, Dept of Health, 29 Feb. 1952, NAI, DH A104/9 (vol. VIII).

99　Ibid., 22 Dec. 1952, NAI, DH A104/10 (vol. X).

100　Ibid., 16 Dec. 1954, NAI, DH A104/14; 'Grants towards deficits', *c.*Oct. 1956, NAI, DH, H34/8A (vol. IV).

101　E. de Barra to Secretary, Dept of Health, 14 Nov. 1951, NAI, DH A104/9 (vol. VIII).

102　Memo. to Secretary, Dept of Health, 6 Dec. 1947, NAI, DH A104/5 (vol. V).

103　O. P. Hargadon, 'Irish hospital finances', in *Administration*, vol. 4, no. 3 (autumn 1956), pp. 25–6.

104　Barrington, *Health, medicine and politics*, pp. 237 and 246.

105　T. F. O'Higgins to Gerard Sweetman, 3 Jan. 1957, NAI, DH H34/8A (vol. IV).

106　Minister for Health to Minister for Finance, Nov. 1962, NAI, DH H34/8A (vol. IV).

107　*Church of Ireland Gazette*, 1 June 1951.

108　Adelaide Hospital Financial Position, 1953, NAI, DT S15491.

109　J. M. Barry, *Victoria Hospital Cork: A history, 1874–1986* (Midleton, 1992), pp. 216 and 222.

110　J. A. Robins, 'The Irish hospital', in *Administration*, vol. 8, no. 2 (summer 1960), p. 161.

111　James Deeny, *To cure and care: Memoirs of a chief medical officer* (Dublin, 1989), p. 143.

112　Ibid., pp. 167–8.

113　Department of Health, *The health services and their further development* (Jan. 1966); Barrington, *Health, medicine and politics*, pp. 261–2.

114　Peter Gatenby, 'The beginning of the federated Dublin voluntary hospitals', in David FitzPatrick (ed.), *The Feds: An account of the Federated Dublin Voluntary Hospitals, 1961–2005* (Dublin, 2006), pp. 19–24.

115　*Outline of the future hospital system: Report of the Consultative Council on the General Hospital Services* [FitzGerald Report] (1968), pp. 17–20.

116　Ibid., pp. 22–32.

117　Ibid., pp. 41–6.

118　Ibid., pp. 116–18.

119　'Publication of report of consultative committee on the general hospital services', 21 June 1968, NAI, DT 99/1/118.

120　NAI, DT 2003/16/112; see also James Bennett to Jack Lynch, 21 Apr. 1969, DT 99/1/118; John Kilmartin to various TDs, 9 Sept. 1970 and J. Taaffe to Jack Lynch, 6 Oct. 1970, DT 2002/8/132.

121　Barrington, *Health, medicine and politics*, p. 269.

122　'Proposed statement about minimum rights attaching to the proprietorship of voluntary hospitals', 27 May 1971, NAI, DT 2002/8/132.

123　Barrington, *Health, medicine and politics*, pp. 271–4.

124　NAI, DT 2005/7/76.

125　*SAI, 1981*, Table 178, p. 209.

126　*Ir. Times*, 7 Dec. 1972.

127 Ian Howie, 'The emergence of a hospital system to meet the challenges of 2000 and beyond', in FitzPatrick (ed.) *The Feds*, p. 35.

128 Davis Coakley, 'From foundling hospital to university teaching hospital: The development of St James's Hospital', in ibid., pp. 16–17.

129 *Ir. Times*, 30 Nov. 1987.

130 Hilary M. C. V. Hoey and Meadhbh O'Leary, 'The National Children's Hospital', in FitzPatrick, *The Feds*, p. 124.

131 Fergus O'Ferrall, 'The formation of the Adelaide and Meath Hospital, Dublin: Incorporating the National Children's Hospital' and David McConnell, 'The Adelaide Hospital – the last Protestant general teaching hospital in the Republic of Ireland', in ibid., pp. 41–57 and 67–76.

CONCLUSION

1   *Dáil Debates*, vol. 522 (29 June 2000), col. 1019.

Bibliography

—

PRIMARY SOURCES

REPUBLIC OF IRELAND

Dublin

An Comhairle Leabharlanna/The Library Council
Hospital Library Council papers

Companies Registration Office
Hospitals Trust (1940) Ltd file

Irish Labour History Museum
Irish Women Workers' Union archives

Irish Red Cross
Irish Red Cross archives

Labour Court
Recommendations
    No. 381 (1950)
    No. 2203 (1967)
    No. 2556 (1971)
    No. 4242 (1977)
    No. 8393 (1983)
    AD 80–3 (1983)

Military Archives
G2 files

National Archives of Ireland
Department of Finance
Department of Foreign Affairs
Department of Health
Department of Justice
Department of An Taoiseach

Department of Transport, Tourism and Communications
Dissolved Companies files
Office of the Attorney General
Office of the Secretary to the President

National Library of Ireland
Hospitals Trust cypher [Lot 559 Mealys' independence sale, Apr. 2008]
Hospitals Trust newspaper scrapbooks [uncatalogued]
Joseph McGarrity papers
Piaras Béaslaí papers

National Maternity Hospital, Holles Street
Annual reports
Minute books

Oireachtas Éireann Library
Audited accounts of sweepstakes draws, 1930–87

Royal College of Physicians of Ireland
Diaries of Dr Kathleen Lynn [excerpts provided by Dr Margaret Ó hÓgarthaigh]
Records of Sir Patrick Dun's Hospital
Records of St Ultan's Hospital

Royal College of Surgeons in Ireland, Mercer Library
Dr James Deeny papers

Office of General Secretary of SIPTU, Liberty Hall
Federated/Workers' Union of Ireland, *Reports of Annual Delegate Conference and General Executive Committee*

University College Dublin, Archives Department
Maurice 'Moss' Twomey papers
Michael Hayes papers
Michael MacWhite papers

University College Dublin, Law Library
Wunder *v.* Hospitals Trust (1940) Ltd, unreported judgements of the Irish High and Supreme Courts

Private Collections

Professor John Horgan
Memorandum of Joseph Andrews

Mr John Slevin
Miscellaneous documents re. Hospitals Trust (1940) Ltd

NORTHERN IRELAND

Armagh

Cardinal Tomás Ó Fiaich Memorial Library and Archive
Cardinal MacRory papers

Belfast

Queen's University Special Collections: Cardinal Cahal B. Daly Library
Mater Infirmorum Hospital Belfast, *Seventy-fourth annual report* (1958)
Rev. Michael P. Kelly, *Belfast's Mater Hospital: Why? Present position* (Belfast, 1954)

CANADA

Ottawa

National Archives of Canada
Archives of the Canadian Federal Government
        Department of External Affairs
        Department of Justice

Vancouver

Vancouver Public Library
Newspaper clippings collection

GREAT BRITAIN

London

British Library
Irish lottery and sweepstake tickets, collected and arranged by C. L'Estrange Ewen

The National Archives, Kew
Colonial Office
Dominions Office
Home Office
Metropolitan Police Office
Prime Minister's Office
Treasury Solicitor

Reading

BBC Written Archive
J. B. Clark, BBC internal circulating memo. on Irish Free State Broadcasting Service, 23 Nov. 1937 [copy supplied by Dr Peter Martin]

UNITED STATES OF AMERICA

California

California State Library
Report on the Irish Sweepstakes, Attorney General Stanley Mosk, Feb. 3, 1960 [copy supplied by Mr Liam Wylie]

New York

The Tamiment Library, New York University
Seán Prendeville Collection

National Archives and Records Administration, North East Regional Archives
Criminal Cases, Southern District of New York

Rockefeller Archive Center, Sleepy Hollow
Rockefeller Foundation archives

Philadelphia

Falvey Memorial Library, Villanova University
Joseph McGarrity papers

Washington DC
Federal Bureau of Investigation
File no. 61–555: 'Irish activities in the United States', Apr.–Sept. 1939 [Copy supplied by Dr Brian Hanley]
File no. 61–7606: 'Irish Republican Army' [Copy supplied by Mr Ed Morrison, Philadelphia]

National Archives and Records Administration, Washington DC
Post Office Department
State Department

FILM AND SOUND SOURCES

RTÉ Television Archives
Today Tonight special: The Sweep, 22 Jan. 1992
Hidden history: If you're not in. . . , 2 Dec. 2003

Library of Congress Motion Picture Collection
VBM 0204: *Captain and the kids: The winning ticket* (1934)
VBF 5523: *The Flintstones: The sweepstake ticket* (1960)

INTERVIEWS

Mr Alan Dukes, 11 Dec. 2007
Professor J. Kevin Kealy, Dublin, 5 Feb. 2007
Mr John Slevin, Dublin, 7 Aug. 2007

PRINTED SOURCES

OFFICIAL PUBLICATIONS

Ireland

Central Statistics Office. *Statistical abstract of Ireland/Ireland: Statistical abstract*
Dáil Éireann. *Report of the special committee on the Public Charitable Hospitals (Temporary Provisions) Bill, 1923* (1923)
Dáil and Seanad Debates
Department of Health. *Annual reports, 1945–58*
_____ *Outline proposals for the improvement of the health services* (1947)
_____ *The health services and their further development* (1966)
_____ *Outline of the future hospital system. Report of the consultative council on the general hospital services* (1968)
Department of Local Government and Public Health. *Annual reports*
_____ *General reports of the Hospitals Commission*
_____ *Tuberculosis* [white paper] (*c.*1946)
Iris Oifigiúil
Report of the Commission of Inquiry into the Civil Service (1936)
Reports of the Committee of Reference presented to the Minister for Justice

Great Britain

Parliamentary debates: House of Commons and *House of Lords (Hansard)*
Report of the Joint Select Committee on lotteries and indecent advertisements (1908)
Minutes of evidence taken before the Royal Commission on Lotteries and Betting (1932–3)

Royal Commission on Lotteries and Betting, 1932–3: Final Report (1933)
Report of the Royal Commission on Betting, Lotteries and Gaming, 1949–51 (1951)
Royal Commission on Gambling: Final Report (1978)

Canada

Debates of the House of Commons and Senate of the Dominion of Canada
Reports of the Joint Committee of the Senate and House of Commons on capital punishment (July 27, 1956), corporal punishment (July 11, 1956), lotteries (July 31, 1956) (1956)

United States of America

Congressional Record
Foreign Relations of the United States

MISCELLANEOUS PRINTED SOURCES

Medical Research Council of Ireland. *Annual reports*
Hospital Library Council of Ireland, 1937–58 [National Library of Ireland]

PERIODICALS

Catholic Bulletin
Church of Ireland Gazette
Dublin Opinion
Irish Journal of Medical Science
Irish Radio News
Irish Red Cross Monthly Bulletin
Newsweek
Stubbs' Weekly Gazette (Irish Free State and Northern Ireland)
Watchword

NEWSPAPERS

IRELAND

Freeman's Journal
Irish Catholic
Irish Field
Irish Independent
Irish Press
Irish Times
Sunday Independent

GREAT BRITAIN

Daily Mail
The Times

UNITED STATES OF AMERICA

Irish Echo
New York Times
Washington Post

SECONDARY SOURCES

ARTICLES

Barry, Rev. David. 'The moral aspect of sweepstakes – from a Catholic and a Protestant viewpoint', in *Irish Ecclesiastical Record*, 5th series, vol. xxxviii (Sept. 1931), pp. 300–11

Brown, Stephen J. 'Librarians at Cambridge, 22–27 Sept. 1930', in *Studies*, xix, no. 76 (Dec. 1930), pp. 671–6

'C. Hayes, Inspector of Taxes, v. R. J. Duggan', in *Reports of Irish tax cases, vol. 1: 1923–1932* (Dublin: Stationery Office, 1932), pp. 269–81

Coleman, Marie. 'The origins of the Irish Hospitals Sweepstake', in *Irish Economic and Social History*, vol. xxix (2002), pp. 40–55

_____ 'The development of the Irish hospital library service', unpublished paper delivered to the Irish Economic and Social History Society Conference, 18 Nov. 2006

Corcoran, John. 'Dublin hospitals – voluntary or state', in *Irish Journal of Medical Science* (Feb. 1948), pp. 49–64

Counihan, H. E. 'St Laurence's Hospital', in J. D. H. Widdess, *The Richmond, Whitworth & Hardwicke Hospitals: St Laurence's, Dublin, 1772–1972* (Dublin, 1972), pp. 148–54

Daly, Mary E. ' "An atmosphere of sturdy independence": The state and Dublin hospitals in the 1930s', in Greta Jones and Elizabeth Malcolm (eds), *Medicine, disease and the state in Ireland, 1650–1940* (Cork, 1999), pp. 234–52

Egan, Rory. 'Sweeping under the carpet', *Magill* (Apr. 2006), pp. 30–2

Elaine.'An "Irish sweepstakes" party for Saint Patrick's Day', in *Good Housekeeping*, vol. xcviii, no. 3 (Mar. 1934), p. 94

Fitzgibbon, Frank. 'Why Avenue is hocking the family heirloom', in *Business and Finance*, vol. 20, no. 33 (26 Apr. 1984), pp. 12–13

Gorsky, Martin, John Mohan and Martin Powell. 'The financial health of voluntary hospitals in interwar Britain', *Economic History Review*, vol. lv, no. 3 (2002), pp. 533–55

Gorsky, Martin and John Mohan. 'London's voluntary hospitals in the interwar period: Growth, transformation or crisis?', in *Nonprofit and Voluntary Sector Quarterly*, vol. 30, no. 2 (June 2001), pp. 247–75

Hargadon, O. P. 'Irish Hospital finances', in *Administration*, vol. 4, no. 3 (autumn 1956), pp. 13–36

Jones, Greta. 'The Rockefeller Foundation and medical education in Ireland in the 1920s', in *Irish Historical Studies*, vol. XXX, no. 120 (Nov. 1997), pp. 564–80

Kealy, Alacoque. 'Irish Radio Data, 1926–1980', Radio Telefís Éireann Occasional papers series, no. 1 (May 1981)

Kennedy, Conor and Daragh O'Shaughnessy. 'Anti-avoidance – restrictions in tax planning' (Mar.2006)
www.cpaireland.ie/UserFiles/File/Accountancy%20Plus/Taxation/March%202006/Anti-Avoidance.pdf

MacAnthony, Joe. 'Where the sweep millions go', *Sunday Independent*, 21 Jan. 1973

McCarthy, John J. 'The Irish Sweeps', in *Harper's Monthly Magazine*, vol. 169 (June 1934), pp. 49–59

McCarthy, Michael. 'The Shannon scheme strike', in *Old Limerick Journal*, 5 (Dec. 1980), pp. 21–6

McDonald, Fred and Bob Considine. 'Not a clean sweep: the inside workings of the Irish lottery', in *Collier's Magazine* (4 June 1938), pp. 16–17 and 55–7.

Moore, Anthony. 'Isaac Wunder orders', in *Judicial Studies Institute Journal*, vol. 1, no. 1 (2001), pp. 137–46

Moore, Henry. 'Future hospital policy in Dublin', in *Irish Journal of Medical Science* (June 1936), pp. 241–66

Ó Gallchobhair, Eamonn. 'Music – Free State broadcasting II', in *Ireland Today*, vol. 2, no. 8 (Aug. 1937), pp. 64–72

O'Hanlon, Thomas. 'A good thing in the Irish sweepstakes – for the owners', in *Fortune* (Nov. 1966), pp. 170–3

—— 'Drew Pearson – the sweep's US link man', in *Profile* (July 1973), pp. 20–1 [This issue of *Profile* was subsequently withdrawn; therefore, most extant issues for July 1973 do not carry this article]

Panella, Nancy Mary. 'The patients' library movement: An overview of early efforts in the United States to establish organized libraries for hospital patients', in *Bulletin of the Medical Library Association*, vol. 84, no. 1 (Jan. 1996), pp. 52–61

'Patrick McGrath and Ors. v. J. E. McDermott (Inspector of Taxes)', in B. H. Giblin and Susan Keegan (eds), *Irish tax reports, vol. III: 1978–1987* (Dublin, 1994), pp. 683–705

Robins, J. A. 'The Irish hospital', in *Administration*, vol. 8, no. 2 (summer 1960), pp. 145–65

Roche, Michael. 'Avenue Investments: Jeffers gambled, McGrath lost', in *Irish Business* (Sept. 1984), pp. 23–8

Smith, Timothy B. 'The social transformation of hospitals and the rise of medical insurance in France, 1914–1943', in *The Historical Journal*, vol. 41, no. 4 (1998), pp. 1,055–87

Stanhope v. *Hospitals Trust Ltd.* (no. 2) [S.C., I.F.S.] [1936] Ir. Jur. Rep. 25, http://www.justis.com/j-net

Stewart-Gordon, James. 'The odds? 450,000 to one' in *Readers' Digest* (American edition) (Apr. 1959), pp. 93–7

Tarpey, Marie V. 'Joseph McGarrity, fighter for Irish freedom', in *Studia Hibernica*, no. 11 (1971), pp. 164–80

Tierney, Mark. 'The Irish Hospitals Sweepstake and Barrington's Hospital: 1931–1937', in *The Old Limerick Journal*, no. 24 (winter 1988), pp. 114–19

BOOKS

Barrington, Ruth. *Health, medicine and politics in Ireland, 1900–1970* (Dublin, 1987)

Barry, J. M. *The Victoria Hospital, Cork* (Cork, 1992)

Becker, Annette, John Olley and Wilfried Wang (eds). *20th century architecture: Ireland* (Munich/New York, 1997)

Bird, Charlie and Kevin Rafter. *This is Charlie Bird* (Dublin, 2006)

Browne, Noël. *Against the tide* (Dublin, 1986)

Browne, O'Donel T. D. *The Rotunda Hospital, 1745–1945* (Edinburgh, 1947)

Burke, Helen. *The Royal Hospital Donnybrook: A heritage of caring, 1743–1993* (Dublin, 1993)

Coakley, Davis. *Baggot Street: A short history of the Royal City of Dublin Hospital* (Dublin, 1995)

Cosgrove, Brian. *The Yew tree at the head of the strand* (Liverpool, 2005)

Cousins, Mel. *The birth of social welfare in Ireland, 1922–1952* (Dublin, 2003)

Cronin, Seán. *Washington's Irish policy, 1916–1986: Independence, partition, neutrality* (Dublin, 1997)

Crookes, Gearóid. *Dublin's 'Eye and Ear': The making of a monument* (Dublin, 1993)

Daly, Mary E. *Women and work in Ireland* (Dundalk, 1997)

D'Arcy, Fergus. *Horses, lords and racing men* (Kildare, 1991)

Deeny, James. *To cure and care* (Dublin, 1989)

Delaney, Enda. *Demography, state and society: Irish migration to Britain, 1921–1971* (Liverpool, 2000)

Earner-Byrne, Lindsey. *Mother and child: Maternity and child welfare in Dublin, 1922–1960* (Manchester, 2007)

Ewen, Cecil L'Estrange. *Lotteries and sweepstakes* (London, 1932)

Ezell, John Samuel. *Fortune's merry wheel: The lottery in America* (Cambridge, Mass., 1960)

Farmar, Tony. *A history of Craig Gardner & Co: The first hundred years* (Dublin, 1988)

_____ *Holles Street, 1894–1994: The National Maternity Hospital, a centenary history* (Dublin, 1994)

Feeney, J. K. *The Coombe Lying-in Hospital* (Dublin, c.1983)

Feeney, Tom. *Seán MacEntee: A political life* (Dublin, 2008)

Fennelly, Teddy. *Fitz – and the famous flight* (Portlaoise, 1997)

Fino, Paul A. *My life in politics and public service* (New York, 1986)

FitzPatrick, David (ed.). *The Feds: An account of the Federated Dublin Voluntary Hospitals, 1961–2005* (Dublin, 2006)

Fleetwood, John F. *The history of medicine in Ireland* (Dublin, 1983)

Foxrock Local History Club and Dún Laoghaire–Rathdown County Council. *The story of Cabinteely House* (Dublin, 2000)

Freeman, Spencer. *You can get to the top* (Dublin, 1972)

Gaffney, Phyllis. *Healing amid the ruins: The Irish hospital at St Lô* (Dublin, 1999)

Gatenby, Peter. *Dublin's Meath Hospital, 1753–1996* (Dublin, 1996)

Gorham, Maurice. *Forty years of Irish broadcasting* (Dublin, 1967)

Green, Reg. *The history of the Grand National: A race apart* (London, 1993)

Havel, Brian. *Maestro of crystal: The story of Miroslav Havel* (Dublin, 2005)

Horgan, John. *Seán Lemass: The enigmatic patriot* (Dublin, 1997)

_____ *Noël Browne: Passionate outsider* (Dublin, 2000)

_____ *Irish media: A critical history since 1922* (London / New York, 2001)

_____ *Broadcasting and public life: RTÉ news and current affairs, 1926–1997* (Dublin, 2004)

Hospital Library Council, *Special report to mark the 21st anniversary of the Hospital Library Service* (Oct. 1958)

Hospitals Trust. *Irish Hospitals: Facts, figures and photographs* (Dublin, 1938)

_____ *Irish hospitals, 1956–1971* (Dublin, c.1971)

_____ *Irish Hospitals Sweeps charitable achievements* (*n/d*)

_____ *Sweepstake draw programmes*

Hull, Mark M. *Irish secrets: German espionage in wartime Ireland, 1939–1945* (Dublin, 2003)

Hurley, Doran. *Herself, Mrs Patrick Crowley* (London, 1939)

Hutchinson Cockburn, J. *The Christian outlook on lotteries, betting and gambling* (London, 1932)

Jones, Greta. '*Captain of all these men to death': The history of tuberculosis in nineteenth and twentieth century Ireland* (Amsterdam, 2001)

Jones, Mary. *These obstreperous lassies: A history of the Irish Women Workers' Union* (Dublin, 1988)

Kay, J. A. *Good cause for gambling: The prospects for a national lottery in the UK* (London, c.1992)

Kenny, Ivor (ed.). *In good company: Conversations with Irish leaders* (Dublin, 1987)

Lyons, J. B. *The quality of Mercer's: The story of Mercer's Hospital, 1734–1991* (Sandycove, 1991)

Martin, Peter. *Censorship in the two Irelands, 1922–1939* (Dublin, 2006)

Maugham, Somerset. *Sheppey* (London, 1933)

McDonald, Frank. *The destruction of Dublin* (Dublin, 1985)

McMahon, Deirdre. *Republicans and imperialists: Anglo-Irish relations in the 1930s* (London & New Haven, 1984)

Mitchell, David. *A peculiar place: The Adelaide Hospital Dublin, 1839–1989* (Dublin, 1989)

Morton, Suzanne. *At odds: Gambling and Canadians, 1919–1969* (Toronto, 2003)

Munting, Roger. *An economic and social history of gambling in Great Britain and the USA* (Manchester, 1996)

Ó Corráin, Daithí. *Rendering to God and Caesar: The Irish churches and the two states in Ireland, 1949–73* (Manchester, 2006)

Ó Drisceoil, Donal. *Censorship in Ireland, 1939–1945* (Cork, 1996)

O'Dwyer, Frederick. *Lost Dublin* (Dublin, 1981)

Ó hÓgartaigh, Margaret. *Kathleen Lynn: Irishwoman, patriot, doctor* (Dublin, 2006)

O'Sheehan, J. and E. de Barra. *Ireland's hospitals, 1930–1955* (Dublin, c.1955)

Perrier Manda, Veronique and Chris Vander Doelen. *Chasing lightning: Gambling in Canada* (Toronto, 1999)

Pilat, Oliver. *Drew Pearson: An unauthorized biography* (New York, 1973)

Pine, Richard. *2RN and the origins of Irish radio* (Dublin, 2001)

Regan, John M. *The Irish counter-revolution, 1921–1936* (Dublin, 1999)

Rothery, Sean. *Ireland and the new architecture* (Dublin, 1991)

Savage, Robert J. *Irish television: The political and social origins* (Cork, 1996)

Scala, Mim. *Diary of a teddy boy* (Dublin, 2000)

Smith, Brian. *The horse in Ireland* (Dublin, 1991)

Solomons, Bethel. *One doctor in his time* (London, 1956)

Sweeney, Tony, Annie Sweeney and Francis Hyland. *The Sweeney guide to the Irish Turf from 1501 to 2001* (Dublin, 2002)

Swinson, Arthur. *The great air race: England – Australia, 1934* (London, 1968)

Trepannier, Leon. *Sweepstakes: Why they must be legalized for us* (Montréal, 1936)

Vance, Joan. *An analysis of the costs and benefits of public lotteries: the Canadian experience* (New York/Ontario, 1989)

Waller, Rev. B. C. *Sweepstakes: Some hard facts* (Dublin, 1932)

Webb, Arthur. *The clean sweep: The story of the Irish Hospitals Sweepstake* (London, 1968)

Welcome, John. *Irish horse-racing: An illustrated history* (Dublin, 1982)

REFERENCE

American National Biography (Oxford and New York, 1999)

Hickey, D. J. and J. E. Doherty. *A new dictionary of Irish history from 1800* (Dublin, 2005)

Rockett, Kevin (ed.). *The Irish filmography: Fiction films, 1896–1996* (Dublin, 1996)

Royal Irish Academy. *Dictionary of Irish biography* (Cambridge: forthcoming)

UNPUBLISHED THESES

Bradley, Laurence-Marie Gemma. 'John Keating, 1889–1977: His life and work', MA, UCD (1991), 2 vols

Casey, Marion R. 'Ireland, New York and the Irish image in American popular culture, 1890–1960', PhD, New York University (1998)

HOSPITAL ANNUAL REPORTS

Adelaide Hospital
Incorporated Dental Hospital
National Children's Hospital

INTERNET SOURCES

www.irishstatutebook.ie
www.justis.com
www.movietone.com
www.oireachtas.ie
www.oxforddnb.com
www.pedrigeequery.com
www.tcd.ie/irishfilm

Index

___

Abbreviations

HT   Hospitals Trust Limited

HTF   Hospitals Trust Fund

IHS   Irish Hospitals Sweepstakes

USA   United States of America

Abbey Theatre 44

Abbeyleix 78

accident, acute and emergency services 66, 78, 201, 222

Act of Union (1801) 4

Adelaide Hospital 10, 17, 18, 52, 53, 87, 217, 220, 222

Aer Lingus 164, 168

agents and distributors 46, 116–18, 122, 140–1, 176, 180, 182; Andrews as source on 118–21, 122, 123, 125–6, 130, 180; in Britain 30, 91, 97, 104, 106, 117, 122; in Canada 116, 159, 179, 180, 183; Connie Neenan 117, 120, 124–7, 158, 169; Drew Pearson 127–8, 183; Gerard Coughlan 129–30; Joseph McGarrity 118, 120, 123–7, 158, 180; in USA 116–21, 126, 132–7, 138, 140, 141, 158–9, 179; *see also* commissions on sale of tickets

Aintree Grand National 6, 24, 156; *see also* IHS

Aintree racecourse 151, 170, 173

Ajax Trading Company 118

Allen, Denis 57, 64

Allis, Peter 170

Altman's Department Store (New York) 169

America 156

America, north 2, 31, 112, 172–3, 181; market for IHS 42, 103, 104, 112, 116, 117

American Travel Exchange (ATE) 118, 130

American Triple Crown 171

An Post 191

An Post National Lottery Company 191

Andrews, Joseph 50, 118, 119–23, 125, 126, 129, 130, 133, 180

Annie doesn't live here any more (film) 141

Apicella, Antonio 28, 29

Aquitania 7, 134

Art Union Act (UK 1846) 5

Ascot racecourse 171

Associated Hospitals Sweepstake Committee 18, 34, 53, 59, 84, 136, 146–8, 150, 180, 181, 205

Athlone 114; radio transmitter 38, 39, 42, 43, 44, 166, 167

Atholl, John Stewart-Murray, 8th Duke of 108, 109–10

Attorney General: Ireland 7, 8, 123; Britain 90; California 158

audits and auditors 16, 18, 27, 33, 96, 126, 181, 182

Australia 45, 145

Avair 189, 190

Avenue Investments 188, 189, 190

Aynsley China 189, 190

Bačik, Charles 169

Baggot Street Hospital *see* Royal City of Dublin Hospital

Baldoyle racecourse 152

Ballina 78

Ballinasloe 69, 78

Ballyowen TB sanatorium 210

Ballsbridge 34, 148, 149, 172, 185, 187, 192–3, 194

Baltimore (USA) 134

Bank of America 158

Bank of England 97

Bank of India 97

Bank of Ireland 97, 190

banks 91, 92, 97, 133, 138, 158–9, 190; Britain 91, 97, 138; USA 138, 158–9

Barclays Bank 97

Barniville, H. 13

Barrington, Ruth 3, 62, 207, 214

Barrington's Hospital, Limerick 52, 53, 56, 69

BBC 39, 41, 156, 171

BBC Northern Ireland 43

Beaumont Hospital 222

Beaverbrook, Max Aitken, 1st Baron 146
bed bureau 79–81, 82, 148, 200–1
beds 55, 58, 65, 68, 70, 73, 74, 81, 197, 199, 200–1,
    214, 215
Belfast 22, 151, 161, 162, 163
Bellanca 45, 46
Belmont Stakes 171
Belmullet 78
Bennett, Louie 35
Benson, Martin 130, 149
betting 99, 100, 154, 156, 161
Betting and Lotteries Act (Great Britain, 1934)
    6, 23, 40, 44, 100–2, 104, 105, 112, 151, 155
Beveridge plan 203, 204
Beveridge, Sir William 204
Bird, Charlie 183
Black, A. & C. 20
Blackrock, Co. Dublin 47
Blackrock College 41
Blackwell, Sir Ernley 98
Bloodstock Breeders' and Horse Owners'
    Association 150, 171
Board of Trade 146
Boards of Health 59
Boden, Eric 119, 125
Boland, Gerald 41, 161
Bon Secours Hospital, Glasnevin 161
bookmakers 130, 149; Britain 91; USA 111
Bord Fáilte 167, 168, 170
Boston 120, 128, 143
Brennan, Joseph 203
Brennanstown estate 32
Bretherton, Cyril 20
bribery 33, 184
Brigid, Sister 73
Britain 4; Chancellor of the Exchequer 156, 173;
    Conservative Party 89, 91, 107, 156; currency
    regulations 122; depression 94; Director of
    Public Prosecutions 97; Dominions Office
    97, 105, 106; donations to hospitals 56, 95–6,
    107; football pools 89, 156, 168, 173, 174, 177,
    178; greyhound racing 89, 99, 100, 101;
    Home Office 7, 90, 97, 99, 101, 106, 108, 155;
    Home Secretary 89–90, 92, 93, 95, 96–7, 98,
    100, 107; hospital lotteries 89, 95–6, 100,
    107–10, 173; hospitals 58, 74–6, 85, 95–6,
    108–9, 162, 203; House of Commons 21, 89,
    91, 92, 93, 107; House of Lords 89; IRA
    bombing campaign in 124; Irish exports to
    94, 101, 108; and Irish government 7, 95, 97,
    105, 106, 177; land annuities 94–5; Ministry

of Aircraft Production 146; National
    Health Service 162, 163; parliament 41, 104,
    107–8; Protestant churches in 109; racing
    100, 144, 149, 170–1; Select Committee on
    Lotteries (1908) 107; Trade Commissioner
    in Dublin 94, 102, 106; Transport and
    General Workers' Union 91; Treasury 95;
    US Embassy in 45; welfare state 204; *see also*
    agents and distributors; prizes and
    prizewinners; tickets
Britain and IHS: action against 96–8, 99, 139;
    banks and 91, 97, 13; censorship 102;
    Customs and Excise 91, 97, 122; insider
    dealing 131; intelligence 121–2, 123, 126; and
    Irish in Britain 2, 91, 95, 166; Irish
    broadcasts to 38, 41, 43, 166, 168; and Irish
    government 7, 95, 97, 105, 106, 177; judiciary
    and courts 97–8; market for IHS 91, 112, 113,
    152–3, 155; money to Ireland 92, 94–6, 99,
    101, 108, 155, 225; police 97, 99, 105, 107–9,
    155; postal service 5, 21, 91, 92, 96, 97, 104,
    144, 155; press 40, 44, 60, 96, 101–2, 104, 145;
    promoters 93, 95, 97, 103–4; prosecutions
    97–8, 104–5, 109, 151, 155; publicity in 41,
    101–2, 104, 166–7, 168, 224
Britain, lotteries and gambling in 4, 5, 89–90, 91,
    93–101, 107, 109–10, 156, 173; foreign
    lotteries 96–7, 99, 100; hospital lotteries 89,
    95–6, 100, 107–10; legislation 4–5, 13, 89–90,
    97–100, 107–10, 156, 161, 173; national lottery
    100, 173, 191–2; opposition to 90, 95–6, 100,
    107, 108, 109–10; Royal Commissions on
    98–101, 155–6; small lotteries 89–90, 95–6,
    99, 101, 156; Stock Exchange Derby
    Sweepstake 89, 90; sweepstakes 89–90, 92,
    95, 97, 107–8, 173; *see also* Lotteries Act
    (1823), Art Union Act (1846), Lotteries
    (War Charities) Bill (1918), Betting and
    Lotteries Act (1934)
British Board of Film Censors 102
British Colombia 115
British Hospitals Association 108, 109
British International Association 112
British Library Association 85
Brown, Fr Stephen 85, 86
Brown, Governor Gerald 'Pat' 158, 159
Brown, Walter 112
Browne & Nolan 132
Browne, Dr Noël 3, 203, 204, 207–9, 213–14,
    218–19, 225
Brownstown Stud, Co Kildare 32, 149, 171

Building on Reality (Fine Gael/Labour plan for government 1984) 191

Burgett, Clifford, 126

Cabinteely House 32

Cairo Postal Convention (1934) 105

Calcutta Turf Club, Derby Sweepstake 90, 92, 97

California 119,125, 158, 159

California Pacific International Exposition (1934) 119

Cambridgeshire 24, 170

Campbell, Sir Gordon 95

Canada 2, 5, 111, 144, 145, 173; IHS activity in 128, 168, 180, 181, 225; lotteries 111, 112, 114–15, 172–3, 175,181; market for IHS 42, 103, 104, 112; media reports on IHS 179, 183, 226; *see also* agents and distributors; America, north; prizes and prizewinners; tickets

Canadian Army and Navy Veterans' Sweepstake 112

Canadian Cancer Hospitals Sweepstake 112

Canadian Pacific Railway Steamship Services 104

cancer hospitals 53, 65, 69–70, 218

Capital Gains Tax 190, 192, 193

Cappagh Orthopaedic Hospital 8, 16, 59, 60, 67, 88, 197

Captain and the Kids (cartoon) 141

Carson, Lady Ruby 109

Carson, Sir Edward 109

Cashel 78

Casino and International Sporting Club of Monte Carlo 108

Cassidy, Dr Louis 13

Castlebar 78

Castlerea 79

Castlerosse, Valentine Browne, Viscount 92

Catholic Bulletin 14

Catholic Truth Society of Ireland 41

Cearnaigh, Peadar 6

censorship, 102, 149

Central Bank of India 97

Central Racing Advisory Committee 150

Central Remedial Clinic 174, 191

Cesarewitch 6, 24

Charing Cross Hospital (London) 95

Cheltenham Irish Sweeps Hurdle (1969) 175

Cheshire 105

Chicago 125

children's hospitals 10, 65, 67, 77, 79, 88, 207

Church of Ireland Gazette 217

Churchill, Sir Winston 171

City Home and Hospital, Limerick 69

civil servants 49, 63, 122, 148, 154–5, 179, 204, 210, 225

Civil War 20, 35

Clan na Gael 120, 123, 124, 125

Clandillon, Seamus 38

Clann na Poblachta 203

Clann na Talmhan 206

Clare, Co. 38

Clarke, Harry, Studios 25, 26

Clifden 69, 78

clinics 207

Clynes, J. R. 90, 96

Coalition government (Fine Gael/Labour 1973–7) 176, 182, 186, 191, 221

Coast Guard, US 156

Cobh 156

Collier's 49, 140, 141, 179

Collins, Michael 20

Collins, Patrick 122, 123

Comhairle na nOispidéal 221

Commissions on sale of tickets 22, 96, 122, 123, 125, 137, 138, 155, 174, 175, 340; USA 119, 126, 134, 137, 141

Committee of Reference 53–4, 56, 57–60, 61, 64

community health centres 220

Comptroller and Auditor General 62, 182

Connaught Rangers 91

Conservative Party 89, 91, 107, 156

Considine, Bob 140

Constantino, Matteo 28

consultants, hospital 220, 221

Consultative Council on the General Hospital Services 220

convalescent homes 65

Coombe Hospital Linen Guild 11

Coombe Maternity Hospital 6, 13, 52, 55, 67, 212, 214, 218

Cooney, Dr Andy 64, 71, 80

Cooney, Patrick 178, 182

Copenhagen Plan (1948) 167

Córas na Poblachta 121

Córas Tráchtála Teoranta (CTT–Irish Export Board) 168

Corish, Brendan 221, 222

Cork city 4, 6, 33, 57, 114, 122, 209; hospitals 53, 68, 210; North Infirmary 68, 197; Regional Hospital project 68, 212, 213, 218, 220, 222; sanatorium 205, 210; Victoria Hospital 53, 217, 218

Cork, Co. 124, 221
Cork Street Fever Hospital 198, 202
Cosgrave, Liam 176, 186
Cosgrave, W. T. 16, 20, 129, 206
Cospóir, the National Sports Council 191
Costello, Declan 161
Costello, John A. 163
Coughlan, Gerard 129–30
counterfeit tickets, USA 128–9, 135, 138
county homes 62, 212
county hospitals 62, 68, 78, 220, 221
County Infirmary, Limerick 69
Cox & Kings 97
Cox, Arthur 164
Craig Gardner & Company (accountants) 20,
    27, 132–3, 193
Craig, James (TD) 13
Craig, James, 1st Viscount Craigavon 21
Criminal Investigation Department 20
Croker, Richard 32
Cronin, Felix 57
Crowley, Karl A. 134
Crumlin 79, 210
Cuba 129, 144
Cudahy, John 135–6, 137
Cumann na nGaedheal 12, 13, 32, 57, 225
Curragh racecourse 121
Curragh Nursery Handicap 153
customs 97, 109
Czechoslovakia 169

Dáil Éireann 20, 62–3, 83; and HT employees
    145, 195, 224; IHS legislation 12–13, 15–16,
    17–18, 182–3
Daily Express 90, 91
Daily Mail 96, 102
Dalton, Charles 31, 117, 190
D'Alton, John Francis, Catholic Archbishop of
    Armagh 163
Dalton, Owen 190
Daly, Dr de Burgh 50
Daly, Mary 3
Danfay Distributors 189
D'Arcy, Fergus 171
Davison, Sir William 91, 101, 107–8, 109
Dawe, A. P. 22, 114–15
de Gallagh, Count Gerald O'Kelly 96
de Valera, Eamon 83, 95, 101, 105, 108, 124, 136,
    163
Deeny, James 218, 219
Dental Hospital 9, 10, 22

dental hospitals 17
Department of Agriculture 177
Department of An Taoiseach 179
Department of Defence 57, 161
Department of Education 59, 221
Department of Enterprise and Employment 195
Department of External Affairs 92, 136, 142, 158,
    159
Department of Finance 62, 122, 174, 177, 191, 207,
    208–9, 211, 212, 219
Department of Foreign Affairs 177
Department of Health 88, 174, 177, 193, 194,
    203–4, 207–11, 212, 215, 217, 221, 222, 225
Department of Home Affairs (later Justice) 6,
    13, 16, 114
Department of Industry and Commerce 20, 41,
    48
Department of Justice 7, 8, 62, 161, 163, 174, 176,
    178; against expansion of IHS 154, 161, 174,
    175, 176–7, 197; facilitating IHS 51, 83, 154,
    163, 182; and illegality of IHS 154, 177, 181,
    183; role of Minister under 1929 Public
    Hospitals Act 17, 18–19, 46, 53, 62; share of
    profits for promoters and HTF 32, 59, 154–5,
    174, 175
Department of Labour 186
Department of Local Government (from 1947)
    179
Department of Local Government and Public
    Health (Health from 1947) bed bureau
    79–80, 81, 82; hospital legislation 198–9, 202,
    204, 205, 206, 208; hospital library grant
    85–6, 87; medical research 83; and
    promoters' expenses 146–8; sweepstakes
    legislation 19, 3–4, 56, 60–3, 67, 198–9; and
    voluntary hospital deficits 73–4, 75, 76, 199
Department of Posts and Telegraphs 39–44,
    165–8, 224, 225; *see also* postal service
Department of the President of the Executive
    Council 48
depression (1930s) 91, 94, 111, 112, 115, 142
Derby, Frederick Stanley, 16th Earl of 108
Detroit 137
Devlin, Michael 118
dispensaries 207, 210, 218
district hospitals 68, 69, 78, 79, 212, 220, 221
Dodder Investments (later Avenue
    Investments) 188
Doherty, Frank 163
Donegal Carpets 32
Donegal, Co. 68

Donnellan, Michael 206
Donnelly, Horace 131, 134
Doolin, William 81
Doran, Michael 57, 64
Douglas Stuart (bookmakers) 130, 149
Down, Co. 6
Dr Steevens' Hospital 52, 220, 222
Drumcondra 21, 118
Dublin 10, 25, 44, 152, 168–9, 170, 183, 195;
    employment in 36, 37; fear of becoming
    notorious for gambling 15, 29; McGrath
    estate in 32, 188, 190; port 183
Dublin Board of Assistance 81
Dublin Chamber of Commerce 132
Dublin, Co. 32
Dublin Corporation 56, 79, 208, 209, 214, 216,
    217
Dublin County Borough 216
Dublin County Council 179
Dublin Fever Hospital Act (1936) 198
Dublin Fever Hospital, Cherry Orchard 218
Dublin General Hospital, Beaumont 222
Dublin Hospitals Bureau *see* bed bureau
Dublin Methodist Council 14
Dublin Opinion 23
Dublin Regional Sanatorium (now James
    Connolly Hospital) 219, 221
Dublin of the Welcomes (documentary) 102
Dublin Trades Union Council 35, 36, 37
Duggan family 2, 146, 179, 180, 188, 189–90
Duggan, Joseph 116
Duggan, Patrick 146, 153
Duggan, Richard 5–7, 8, 12, 15, 17, 20, 22, 31, 116,
    139, 146, 149, 169, 225
Duggan, Richard (junior) 146
Dukes, Alan 191, 192
Dulanty, J. W. 92, 102, 105
Dunne, Jeremiah 159–60

Easter Rising (1916) 20, 31
Edwards, Lionel 25
Electricity Supply Board 164
Elm Park 211, 212, 221, 222
Elverys 132
embassies, Irish 134, 225
Emergency, The 77, 87
Employer–Labour Conference (ELC) 186
employment 36, 37, 189, 212; in HT 16, 34–7, 154,
    164, 200, 224
Ennis 78
Ennistymon 78

Epsom Derby 6–7, 24, 25, 89, 90, 107, 170
Epsom racecourse 25
Ergas 189
Eucharistic Congress (Dublin 1932) 27, 34
Europe 13, 25, 42, 43, 76, 93, 144, 167, 168, 173, 180
European Economic Community (EEC) 180
European Union 173
Everett, James 36, 37, 145, 147, 148
Expo '67 (Montréal) 173
Exports 94, 101, 108, 114, 115, 142
eye and ear hospitals 6, 53, 95

Fannin Holdings 189, 190
Farley, Jim 133–4, 139
Farmers' Party 14
Farren, Thomas 18
Federal Bureau of Investigation (FBI) 120, 125,
    157
Federated Dublin Voluntary hospitals 220
Federated Workers' Union of Ireland (FWUI)
    see Workers' Union of Ireland (WUI)
Federation of Voluntary Charitable
    Organisations (FVCO) 174, 176, 177, 221
Ferguson, Christy 165
Ferrier Pollock (clothing distributor) 190
fever hospitals 65, 78, 79, 207, 218
Fianna Fáil 18, 57, 60, 61, 64, 94–5, 125, 150; 1932
    election 32, 60, 95, 96; and HT 32, 63, 182,
    193, 195; and HTF funds 174, 208; and
    hospitals 60, 82, 208, 212, 219, 225
Fields, Gracie 27
Fine Gael 163, 191, 211, 221; and sweepstakes 39,
    147, 176, 186; and voluntary hospitals 63, 206
Fino, Paul A. 173
FitzGerald, Professor Patrick 220–1
FitzGerald Report 220
Fitzgerald-Kenney, James 17, 53, 63
Fitzmaurice, Colonel James 45
Fitzpatrick, Bernard 169
Flanagan, Seán 174
Flannery, Frank 191
Fleming, P. J. 31, 50, 117, 118, 119, 136
Flintstones (cartoon) 141
Foot, Isaac 107
foot and mouth disease 149
football pools 89, 156, 168, 173, 174, 177, 178
Foran, Thomas 203
foreign currency 154, 224
Fortune 179
Forum Picture House (London) 91
France 20, 76, 96, 104, 107, 152, 166

fraud 15, 18, 19, 50–1, 99, 123, 126, 128–31, 135, 138, 140–1 155, 180, 182
Freeman, Captain Spencer 2, 20–1, 40, 96, 108, 130, 146, 153, 166, 188, 189, 225
Freeman family 2, 179, 180, 188, 189–90
Freeman, Sidney 2, 20–1, 130–1, 149, 180, 188, 189

Gaelic Athletic Association (GAA) 174
Gael Linn 161, 174, 176
Gaelic League 38
Galway 68, 205, 210, 218, 220
Galway Central Hospital 68
Galway, Co. 69
Galway Regional Hospital 210
Galway Regional Sanatorium 210
gambling 30, 161; opposition to 13–15, 17, 29, 52–3, 154, 177, 178, 217; *see also* Britain; lotteries; Protestantism; USA
Gaming and Lotteries Act (1956) 161–4, 174, 176, 179
gaming machines 161
Garda Síochána 21, 26, 30, 121, 129, 161, 162
Geffen, Philip 129
general elections *1923* 16; *1931* (Britain) 107–8; *1932* 60, 95; *1933* 57
general hospitals 65–6, 69, 70, 80, 197, 199, 201, 203, 207, 211–12, 220, 221
General Post Office 47
general practitioners 13, 200, 201
Geoghegan, James 32, 59
Geoghegan, Justice Hugh 195
Germany 121, 126, 149, 167; East 166
Gilmour, Sir John 100
Glencairn Gallops 32, 171
Globe Investments 190
Glynn, Henry 50
Glynn, Sir Joseph 136, 146
Gogarty, Oliver St John 85
Good Housekeeping 138
Gordon, Harry Pirie 101
Gorey 79
Gorey, Denis 14
Gorham, Maurice 38
Görtz, Herman 121, 123
Government (Irish) 122, 122–3, 133, 157, 178–9, 211; and bed bureau 79–81, 82, 148, 200–1; and Britain 7, 95, 97, 105, 106, 177; and health service 83, 85–6, 203–4, 207, 214, 224, 226; and hospitals 59, 60–1, 63, 83, 163, 197, 198–9, 200, 202, 203, 222, 224, 225; and hospital building programme 197, 202, 204–13, 218–19; and

hospital deficits 209, 210–11, 214–16, 222; and hospital funding for 11, 17, 55, 210, 217, 219, 224; and HT 16, 17, 39, 41–3, 46–9, 51, 114, 117, 122, 146–8, 152, 154–5, 157, 159, 173–9, 179, 180–3, 186, 193–6, 203, 211, 219, 224–6; and HTF 53–4, 56, 61–3, 73, 76, 147–8, 174, 178, 204–13, 216, 217, 219, 222, 225; and labour force 186, 210, 212, 219; and lotteries 160, 163, 174–5, 176, 177, 178, 179, 226; and US government 49, 135–6, 137, 157, 158; *see also* Departments; McGrath, Joseph
Graham, J. C. 27
Grand National *see* Aintree
Gregg, Dr J. A. F., Church of Ireland Archbishop of Dublin 14, 52
Gresham Hotel 40
greyhound racing 89, 99, 100, 101, 176, 177
Griffin, Joseph 153, 169
Griffin, Noel 169, 189
Grindlay & Company 97
Guinness brewery 164

Hammond, Aubrey 25
Hanna, Justice Henry 50
Harcourt Street Hospital 59; *see also* National Children's Hospital
Hardwicke Hospital 55, 198
Harney, Mary 195
Harold's Cross Hospice 214
Harper's Magazine 138, 141
Harriman, Grace 143
Hastings, Selina 22
Haughey, Charles 195
Havel, Miroslav 169
Health Act (1953) 216
Health Act (1970) 221
health insurance 5, 15, 76, 200, 216
health service 177, 181, 182, 194, 204, 207, 220; *see also* hospitals
Health services and their further development, The (white paper 1966) 220
Heilgers, Captain F. F. A. 100
Heney, Michael 183
Hibernian Insurance 189, 190
Hickey, E. W. 134
Hidden History series (RTÉ) 184
Higgins, Michael D. 191
High Court 7, 28, 50, 160, 190, 195
Historical Society, TCD 191, 200
Hogan, Patrick 38
Holland 98

Holles Street Skin and Cancer Hospital 6, 7
Hollywood 44
Hoover, Herbert 131, 142
Hoover, J. Edgar 120
Horgan, John 3, 183
hospital building: building costs 209–10, 214,
    219; and hospital deficits 70, 73–4, 77, 205,
    208–9, 211–14, 216–17, 218; Noël Browne
    204, 207–9, 213, 218–19, 225; plans 198, 202,
    205, 207, 210, 211–12; pre-war 10, 17, 54–5, 57,
    58–9, 65, 67, 68–9, 70, 73–4, 77–9, 204;
    progress of 197, 202, 204, 207–13, 216–17,
    218–19, 226; state funding for 209, 210–12,
    218–19; sweepstake funding for 54, 154, 174,
    194, 204–13, 216–17, 218, 219, 224, 225, 226;
    TB sanatoria 198, 205, 206, 208, 210, 218–19
hospital deficits 70, 71, 75, 76, 199, 213, 214,
    215–16, 218; and hospital building
    programme 70, 73–4, 77, 205, 208–9, 211–14,
    216–17, 218; hospital expenditure 71–4, 75,
    76–7, 199–200, 213, 215–16; and Hospitals
    Commission 70–2, 75–7, 199, 202, 213, 215;
    local authority contribution towards 200,
    206, 207, 213, 216; solutions suggested 76,
    200, 203, 205, 216; state contribution
    towards 209, 210–11, 214–16, 222; sweepstake
    funding 16, 70–3, 75–7, 203, 205, 208, 209,
    210, 211, 212–17, 218, 219, 222; in UK
    hospitals 74–5
Hospital Library Council 86, 87, 88
hospital library service 62, 84–8
Hospital Sunday Fund 10, 55, 217
hospitals 9, 57, 58, 60, 66, 70, 71, 73, 80, 87,
    200–1; accident, acute and emergency
    services 66, 78, 201, 222; amalgamations and
    mergers 10, 11, 54, 61, 63, 65–7, 77, 79, 197,
    202, 220, 221; budgets 72, 75, 76–7; claims for
    sweepstake funding 57, 58–9, 60, 64;
    consultants, appointment of 220, 221;
    contributory schemes 76, 200; co-operation
    and co-ordination between 54, 58, 60, 78,
    80, 220; duplication of services 55, 58, 63, 78;
    expenditure 8, 54, 71, 72–3, 74, 215–16, 224;
    federation 65, 220; governors 55, 57, 64, 74,
    198, 214, 217; inspections of 53, 57, 61, 64, 65,
    75; legislation 198–9, 202, 204, 205, 206, 208,
    216, 221; management and administration
    72, 216, 220, 221; medical staff 58, 66, 81, 198;
    rationalisation 10, 11, 65, 67, 197, 198, 203;
    reform 60, 61, 63, 72, 207, 220;
    regionalisation 207, 220; repair and

maintenance 55, 70, 74, 205–6, 212, 219;
    salaries and wages 73, 200, 214, 215–16;
    specialists 58, 66, 67, 81, 221; staff 73, 200;
    teaching 8, 11, 66, 67, 81, 84, 198; *see also*
    Britain; government; hospital building;
    hospital deficits; children's; county; dental,
    district; eye and ear; fever; general; local
    authority; maternity; mental; orthopaedic;
    psychiatric; private; public; regional and
    voluntary hospitals; names of individual
    hospitals
Hospitals Commission 61, 83–4, 86; and bed
    bureau 79–83, 201; functions of 61–2, 64;
    and hospital deficits 70–2, 75–7, 199, 202,
    213, 215; hospital inspections 61, 64, 65, 75;
    reports of 64–70, 71, 77–9, 83, 197, 199,
    201–3, 207, 218, 220, 224–5
Hospitals Trust Board 62, 147, 193, 206
Hospitals Trust Fund 34, 61–2, 210; 65, 72, 76–7,
    83, 103, 140, 144, 174–8, 192,194, 200, 205–6,
    209, 210–13, 216–17, 218–20, 222;
    investments 72, 208–9, 213; organisation of
    61–2, 67, 72, 76, 146–8, 175, 204, 206, 212, 213;
    spending capital 204, 205–6, 207–9, 210, 211,
    212, 213, 218, 219, 225; *see also* Committee of
    Reference; government; hospital building;
    hospital deficits; hospitals; Hospitals
    Commission; local authority hospitals;
    sweepstakes fund for hospitals; voluntary
    hospitals
Hospitals Trust Limited 20, 29, 30, 31, 32, 33, 34,
    148, 164, 174, 182, 224–6; administration and
    management 172, 174, 175, 186, 187; benefits
    to Irish state 16, 46, 114, 154, 193, 203, 219,
    224, 225; broadcasting 2, 37–40, 43–4, 165–8,
    224, 225; buildings 21, 25, 26, 32, 33–4, 148,
    149, 172, 185, 187, 192–3, 194; and charitable
    organisations 174, 176, 177, 178; directors 20,
    31–2, 120, 126, 146, 168–70; 172, 177, 179, 180,
    181, 184, 185, 187, 193–4, 200; employees and
    employment 16, 24, 25, 26, 27, 31, 34–7, 55,
    63, 105, 139, 145, 146, 147, 149, 154, 164, 165,
    177, 180, 181, 184, 185, 186, 187, 188, 192–6,
    200, 224, 226; expenses of sweepstakes 15,
    16, 19, 22, 33, 57, 108, 126, 140, 146–9, 154, 174,
    175, 177, 186; fees 19, 22, 32–3, 148, 151, 154,
    175, 182; Foreign Department 31, 33, 48, 50,
    116–17, 119–21, 126, 180, 188; industrial
    relations 164–5, 184–8; and Ireland's image
    abroad 154, 180–1, 182, 183, 200; and Irish
    businesses 132–3, 168–70; irregularities

Hospitals Trust Limited *cont.*
  alleged 120, 122, 123; lack of accountability
  63, 182; liquidation (1940) 145–6, (1987) 192,
  193; private company 182, 193, 194, 225; profits
  154, 168, 174, 175, 177, 179; shareholders 146; *see
  also* Andrews, Joseph; government; Hospitals
  Trust Fund; IHS; McGrath, Joseph; postal
  service; publicity; sweepstakes funds for
  hospitals; World War, Second
Hospitals Trust sponsored programme 37–40,
  43–4, 165–7
House of Industry Hospitals 55, 198
Howard-Bury, Colonel Charles 91
Hughes, Peter 57
Hull (Ontario) Public Maternity Hospital Trust
  Fund 112
Hume Street Cancer Hospital 6, 69
Hurley, Doran 142
Hurricane Charlie (1986) 34, 193
Hurson, James 81
Hutchinson-Cockburn, Rev. J. 96
Hyde, Douglas 152

Illinois 173
imports, from Britain 94
income tax 7, 122; *see also* USA
Income Tax Acts 7
Independent Newspapers 128, 180, 183, 184, 191,
  226
Indiana 138
Indianapolis 129
infectious diseases 205
inflation 8, 73, 175
Inman, Philip 95
International Labour Organisation (ILO) 186
inter-party government (1948–51) 161, 207–9
inter-party government (1954–7) 162, 211
Ireland Today 44
Irish 2,000 Guineas 174
Irish army, military intelligence division (G2)
  121, 122, 123
Irish Business 190
Irish businesses 32; HT 32, 132–3, 168–70;
  manufactured products 19, 25; McGrath
  family 169–70, 171, 181, 184, 188
Irish Catholic 35
Irish Cesarewitch sweepstake 148, 153
Irish Congress of Trade Unions (ICTU) 187
Irish Credit Bank 189
Irish Derby 2, 170–1, 172
Irish Elm 156, 159

Irish Embassy in Washington 134
Irish Friends of Germany 121
Irish Glass Bottle Company 32, 168–9, 188, 190
Irish Hazel 156
Irish High Commission in London 92, 102
'Irish Hospitals' Sweepstakes: the facts' 181
Irish Hospitals Sweepstake Sponsored Programme
  2, 165–7
Irish Hospitals Sweepstakes (IHS) 23, 31, 52, 112,
  144, 224; Aintree Grand National 23–6, 28,
  30, 40, 44, 50, 52, 55, 58, 60, 93, 97, 98, 102–3,
  109, 112, 130–1, 134, 146, 147, 151, 157, 170, 212;
  Cambridgeshire 24, 25–6, 91, 103, 109, 112,
  154, 158, 160, 172, 175, 185; Cesarewitch 25, 26,
  30, 50, 96, 112, 144, 153; closure 188, 191, 192,
  223; draws 18–19, 21–2, 24–7, 34, 40, 91, 102,
  134, 141, 146, 152, 153,188; Epsom Derby 24,
  25, 26, 33, 52, 55, 59, 93, 103, 104, 107, 109, 112,
  130, 134, 137–8; Irish Cesarewitch 148; Irish
  Derby 170–1, 172; Irish Lincolnshire 170;
  proposals to increase number of 161, 173–4,
  175–7, 179, 191; Red Cross sweepstakes
  150–3; Sweeps Hurdle 175, 177, 186, 192;
  tourist attraction 92, 138, 140
Irish Independent 128
Irish International Biochemicals 189
Irish Journal of Medical Science 81
Irish Open Golf Tournament 170
Irish Racing Board 170, 171
Irish Radio News 38, 39
Irish Red Cross Chase 151, 152
Irish Red Cross Hospital, St Lô 152
Irish Red Cross *see* Red Cross
Irish Red Cross Steeplechase (1940) 150–3
Irish Republican Army (IRA) 31, 120, 121, 123,
  124–5, 126
Irish Republican Brotherhood (IRB) 20, 124, 126
Irish Shipping Limited 156, 195–6
Irish state lottery (1780–1801) 4
Irish Swoop 45
Irish Times 6, 14, 82, 193
Irish Tourist Association (ITA) 118
Irish Transport and General Workers' Union
  (ITGWU) 20, 35
Irish Travel 118
Irish Triple Crown 150
Irish Turf Club 171
Irish Union of Distributive Workers and Clerks
  37
Irish Volunteers 20, 124
Irish Wheelchair Association 174

Irish Women Workers' Union (IWWU) 35–6, 37
Isle of Man 22, 29, 190
Italy 28

Jamaica 129
James Connolly Memorial Hospital 219, 221
Jeffers, Alan 188
Jefferson Smurfit Group 188
Jenkins, Roy 173
Jersey 190
Jervis Street Hospital (Charitable Infirmary) 6,
    16, 22, 66, 71, 197, 221, 222
Jessel, Lord 173
John Hinde (postcard company) 189
Johnson, Thomas 15, 19, 33, 63, 225
Johnstown 169
Jones, Edith 85
Jones, Greta 3
journalists 137–8, 139, 179, 180–1, 183, 226
Joynson-Hicks, Sir William 89

Kansas 143
Kansas City, Missouri 128
Kealy, William 117, 118
Keane, Senator Sir John 202–3, 205
Keating, Seán 26
Kelly, Edward 64
Kelly, Helena 121
Kelly, John 119, 126–7, 129
Kelly, Thomas 63
Kelly, Vincent 57
Kenmare 78
Kennedy, Hugh 7
Kennedy, M. J. 63
Kenney, Edward A. 142–3
Kentucky Derby 171
Kernoff, Harry 25
Kerry, Co. 68
Kiernan, T. J. 38, 39, 92
Kildare, Co. 32, 68, 149, 188
Kilkenny 78
Kilkenny, Co. 31
Killarney 78, 79
Kilroy, Michael 64
Knock 185
Korean War 209, 219

Labour Court 165, 184–5, 186, 187, 193, 195
Labour Party 15, 36, 37, 38, 145, 147, 176, 182–3,
    186, 191, 221
Labour Party (Britain) 90, 173

Ladbrokes 22, 28, 91
LaGuardia, Fiorello 142
Lalor, P. J. 182
land annuities 94–5, 106
Lang, Dr Cosmo, Archbishop of Canterbury 108
Laois, Co. 31, 118
Larkin, Denis 176, 191
Larkin, James (Junior) 164
Lee, Thomas 116
Leinster 68
Leinster 5
Leitrim, Co. 68
Lemass, Noel 20
Lemass, Seán 41, 42
Leopardstown Chase (1943) 174
Leopardstown racecourse 151
Letterkenny 78
Liberal Party (Britain) 93, 107
Library Association of Ireland 85, 86
Liechtenstein 7
Limerick 6, 33, 52, 53, 68, 69, 78, 169, 210
Limerick, Co. 39, 68
Limerick Commercial Club 6
Limerick Leader 8
Limerick Regional Hospital 210
Lincoln Sweepstake 40, 118, 186, 187
Listowel 79
Little, P. J. 18
Liverpool 92, 98, 105
Lloyds Bank 91, 97
local authorities 10, 56, 176, 179, 200, 206, 207,
    208–9, 212, 216, 217
local authority hospitals 53–4, 56, 61, 69, 77–9,
    83, 86–7, 194, 204, 206, 207, 212, 220, 221; *see
    also* county hospitals; municipal hospitals;
    St Kevin's Hospital; TB; voluntary
    hospitals
Local Loans Fund 212
London 28, 74, 91, 92, 95, 100, 107, 120, 155, 166
London Metropolitan Police 91, 93, 97, 99, 155
London to Melbourne Air Race (1934) 24, 45
Londonderry, Charles Vane-Tempest-Stewart,
    7th Marquess of 95, 100
Los Angeles 135
Loto-Canada 173
lotteries 4–8, 6, 7, 8; Europe 13, 93; small 161–2,
    174, 176, 178; *see also* Britain; Canada;
    gambling; sweepstakes legislation; USA;
    YP Pools
Lotteries Act (1823) 5, 7, 109, 163
Lotteries (War Charities) Bill (1918) 89

Louisiana 111
Luton 30
Lynn, Dr Kathleen 52, 67, 74

MacAnthony, Joe 3, 131, 180–1, 182, 183, 184, 226
McArdle, J. S. 13, 14, 15
MacBride, Seán 207
McCann, John 208
McCartan, Dr Patrick 124
McCarthy, John 138–9
McDonald, Fred 140–1
MacDonald, Ramsay 95
McDonnell, John 104
McDunphy, Michael 48
McElligott, J. J. 208, 209, 219
MacEntee, Seán 122–3, 208, 212
MacEoin, Seán 161
McGarrity, Joseph 118, 119, 120, 123–4, 125–7, 158, 180
MacGonigal, Maurice 25
McGranery, James 125
McGrath family 2, 125, 169–70, 171, 172, 179–80, 181, 184, 188–90; *see also* under individual names
McGrath, Joseph 44, 84, 109, 183, 190; early career 20–1, 31, 35; and HT 20–1, 27, 31–2, 35–7, 43, 90, 96, 103–4, 106, 145–6, 152, 165, 167, 168, 185 208, 212; and government 32, 43, 46, 48, 49, 106, 205, 207–8; investment in Irish industry 32, 169–70; personal wealth 32, 139, 225; racing 32, 149–50, 170–1; salaries, fees dividends 32, 154;
McGrath, Joseph (Junior) 171, 181, 188, 189, 190
McGrath, Patrick (Paddy) 169–70, 171, 172, 173–4, 175–6, 181, 183, 186, 188–90, 192
McGrath, Séamus 171, 181, 188, 189, 190
McGrath, Tom 187
McLean, James 30
Macmillan, Harold 156
MacNeill, James, Governor General 21
MacNeill, Major General Hugo 121
McQuaid, John Charles 41, 197
MacWhite, Michael 127, 131, 132, 135, 142
Mageean, Daniel, Catholic Bishop of Down and Connor 163
Magennis, William 13
Maguire, Justice Conor 151
Mahaney, Thomas O. 128
Main, David 130
Mallow 78, 221
Man of Aran (film) 27

Manchester 50, 92
Manchester November Handicap 5, 19, 21–2, 24, 30, 40, 57, 59, 91, 92, 93, 96, 97, 103 131, 140
Mangan, Henry 57
Mansion House 21, 33
Martin, Eamon 31, 153
Massachusetts 30, 143, 173
Massachusetts Council for Legalizing Lotteries 143
Mater Hospital Sweepstake (1922) 5–6, 7, 12, 20
Mater Infirmorum Hospital, Belfast 161, 162–3
Mater Misericordiae Hospital, Dublin 5–6, 7, 12, 20, 66, 71, 73, 77, 114, 191, 197, 214, 221
maternity hospitals 55, 65, 67, 68, 69, 207
Mayo, Co. 64, 68
Meath, Co. 32, 68
Meath Hospital 7, 10, 11, 47, 53, 55, 65, 77, 197, 220, 222
medical education 8, 11, 66, 67, 81, 84, 198, 220, 221
Medical Officer of Health for Dublin City 80
medical profession 13, 58, 66, 74, 81, 82, 198, 200, 201, 214, 220, 221, 222
Medical Register 11
medical research 11, 62, 81, 83, 84
Medical Research Council of Ireland (MRCI) 83
Meenan, Patrick 84
Melbourne 24, 45
Memory Computer 189, 190
mental hospitals 207
mentally handicapped, accommodation for 210, 211
Mercantile Bank of India 97
Mercer's Hospital 10, 52, 65, 77, 197, 220, 222
Mercy Hospital, Cork 68
Meredith, James Creed 29, 30
Methodism 14, 134
Metro Goldwyn Mayer (MGM) 44, 102, 128
Mexican National Lottery 157–8
Mexico 128, 157–8
Michelson, Charles 167–8
Midleton 78
Millstreet 78
Milroy, Seán 12, 15
Miss Dorothy (aeroplane, formerly *Irish Swoop*) 45
Mohan, John 74
Mohill 78
Mollison, Jim 45–6
Monaghan 78
Monaghan, Co. 64, 78

Monaghan, T. J. 166
Monte Carlo 108
Mooney's Irish Bar (London) 91
Moore, Professor Henry 73–4, 81, 82, 83, 200, 203
Moorhead, Professor Thomas Gillman 66, 82
Moran, Agnes 119, 125
Moran, Paul 119, 125
Morning Post 91, 101
Morrissey, Dan 39
Morton, John 118
Mosk, Stanley 158–9
Mosse, Samuel 4
mother-and-child scheme 204, 208
motor cycle races, Britain 99
Mountjoy Jail 121
Moynihan, Maurice 49
Mullingar 78
municipal hospitals 80, 81, 82
Murnaghan, Justice James 160
Mutual Club Limited, Vaduz 22

Naas 79
Nagle, Ken 170
Nasrullah (horse) 171
National Children's Hospital, Harcourt Street
    10, 16, 17, 22, 54, 56, 67, 77, 214, 220, 222–3
National Health Insurance Society 76
National Health Service (NHS) (UK) 162, 163
National Hospital Trustees (later Hospitals
    Trust Board) 62
national insurance 216
National Library of Ireland 117
National Lottery (Ireland) 176, 178, 179, 180,
    191–2, 193, 194, 226
National Maternity Hospital, Holles Street 10,
    11, 12, 16, 22, 54, 55, 67, 79
National University of Ireland (NUI) 183
national wage agreements 186, 187
Neenan, Connie 117, 120, 122, 123, 124–5, 126–7,
    158, 169
Nenagh 78
Nesbitt, Timothy 104
neutrality 149
New England 128
New Hampshire 172–3
New Jersey 129, 138, 142, 158, 173
New Orleans 138
New Rochelle 129
New Ross 79
New York 25, 104, 118–19, 120, 124, 125–6, 128, 129,
    130–1, 134–5, 142, 143, 156, 158, 160, 169, 173

New York Curb Exchange 124
New York Lottery 175
New York Times 111, 128, 130, 134, 137, 138, 142
New York Times Magazine 137
New Zealand 27
Newport News, Virginia 156
Newspaper Club 91
newspapers *see* press
Newsweek 181
Ní Ghráda, Máiréad 40
Nolan, Joseph 50
North Infirmary, Cork 68, 197
Northern Ireland 21, 22, 43, 100, 150, 151, 153, 162,
    166
nuns 59, 73, 200
nurses and nursing 56, 73, 74, 83, 200
nursing homes 71, 220

O'Brien, Conor 180
obstetrics 58
O'Carroll, Joseph 64
Ó Ceallaigh, Dr Seumas 64
O'Connell, Dr John 182–3
O'Connor, Christy (Senior) 170
Ó Dálaigh, Cearbhall (Chief Justice) 160–1
Odearest 189
O'Doherty, Liam 57, 64
O'Donoghue, Rita 47
O'Donovan Rossa, Jeremiah 143
O'Donovan Rossa, Sheila 143
O'Duffy, Eoin 21, 121, 129
Ó Gallchobhair, Eamonn 44
O'Hanlon, Rory 193, 194
O'Hanlon, Thomas 179, 183
O'Higgins, Kevin 13, 15, 17, 18
O'Higgins, T. F. 211, 219
Ohio 128, 143
Oireachtas 18, 34, 92, 122, 128, 147, 148, 150, 162,
    181, 194; *see also* Dáil Éireann; Seanad
    Éireann; Senate
O'Kelly, Seán T. 73, 74, 82
O'Kiersey, Michael 125
O'Leary, Michael 186
Olympics, Amsterdam (1928) 129
Olympics, Montréal (1976) 173, 181
O'Mahony, Maisie 121
O'Malley, Desmond 182
O'Malley, Donogh 174, 221
Ó Moráin, Donal 183
O'Nolan, D. J. 15
O'Nolan, Fr John 6, 15

Ontario 114
O'Reilly, Frank 41
O'Reilly, Philip 41
Ormsby, Lambert 15
orthopaedic hospitals 8, 16, 53, 59–60, 67, 88, 197, 210
orthopaedics 58
O'Shannon, Cathal (Senior) 15
O'Sheehan, Jack 31, 141
O'Sullivan, Mr Justice 163
Our Lady's Hospital for Sick Children, Crumlin 210
outpatients 77, 197

paediatrics 58
Paramount film studios 27
Paris 107
Paris-Soir 96
patients: fee-paying 10, 55, 81, 199, 200, 203, 205, 216; free 10, 15, 18, 56, 73, 81, 199, 200, 205
Peamount Sanatorium 16
Pearson, Drew 127–8, 183
Pegler, Westbrook 139
Peig 86
Pennsylvania 128
People's National Party 121
Peters, William 94
petrol rationing 149
Philadelphia 119, 124, 125, 134, 138, 156, 159
Phoenix Plate Sweepstake 148, 152
Pilat, Oliver 127, 183
Pim's 32
Polio Fellowship of Ireland 174
Politics Programme (RTÉ 1978) 183–4
Popeye (cartoon) 141
population statistics 58
Portarlington 118
Portlaoise 78
Postal Conventions, International 46, 105
postal service 20, 6, 7, 8; foreign international postal regulations 46–9, 122, 123, 180; and HT 46–7, 48–9, 51, 149, 157, 224, 225; post office strike (1979) 188; in wartime 144, 149; *see also* Britain; USA
Powerscourt, Mervyn Wingfield, 8th Viscount 17, 32–3, 55, 59, 150
Powerscourt Townhouse shopping centre 190
Powerscourt, Wendy, Viscountess 150
Preakness Stakes 171
premium bonds, Britain 156
Prescott, F. R. 22

press 165, 184, 191; *see also* Britain; Independent Newspapers; *Irish Times*; USA
Price, Clair 138
Price Waterhouse Coopers Group 27
private hospitals 73
private [nursing] homes 71
prizes and prizewinners 18, 23, 24, 48, 141, 144, 188; Britain 21, 22, 28–9, 90–3, 98, 101–3, 104, 109, 152, 153; Canada 22, 30, 31, 112, 113, 114–15, 175; Ireland 153, 175; prize fund 24, 174, 175, 177; sellers prizes 18, 22; unclaimed prizes 193, 194; USA 22, 30–1, 111–14, 128, 133, 137, 138, 141–2, 144, 152, 153, 157, 175
Profile 183
Progressive Democrats 195
Promotions Limited (from 1930 Hospitals Trust Limited) 20
protection money 117
Protestantism 10; attitudes to gambling and sweepstakes 14, 17, 27, 52–3, 95,109, 115; Methodism 14, 134; Protestant voluntary hospitals 1, 8, 18, 52–3, 59, 67, 217–18, 221, 222–3
Provincial Bank 56
Provincial Wholesale Newsagents' Association 102
psychiatric hospitals 62, 78, 79, 87
psychiatric patients, accommodation for 211
public hospitals 65, 68, 71, 87, 220, 221
Public Charitable Hospitals Bill (1923) 12–16, 17, 18–19
Public Charitable Hospitals (Amendment) Acts (1931, 1932) 53, 56, 62
Public Hospitals Act (1933) 60–3, 64, 67, 70, 82, 85, 86; section 2 of 117, 180, 181, 182, 225
Public Hospitals (Amendment) Acts (1939) 146–9, 150, 180
Public Hospitals (Amendment) Act (1940) 82, 148
Public Hospitals (Amendment) Act (1976) 88, 177–9, 182
Public Hospitals (Amendment) Act (1990) 194, 224
publicity (HT) 37–46, 102, 139, 152; advertising 39, 41, 51, 165, 168, 170, 181, 184, 188; in Britain 41, 101–2, 104, 166–7, 168, 224; broadcasting 2, 37–44, 165–8, 224, 225; international exhibitions 118–19; London to Melbourne Air Race 24, 45; newspapers 40, 41, 44; sports sponsorship 170–1; in USA 112, 116, 118–19, 127–8, 131, 133, 134, 136, 168

Quinlan, Patrick 183
Quirke, Captain 29

racecourses: Britain 25, 100, 170, 173; Ireland 121, 151, 152, 153, 174
racehorses 28, 130, 138, 149–50, 151, 171
racing 40 188; Britain 24, 100, 149, 170; Ireland 144, 149–50, 151–3, 170–1, 174; McGrath, Joseph 32, 149–50, 170–1; results 40, 165; USA 111, 171
radio 2, 37–44, 43, 165–8, 224, 225
Radio Éireann / Radio Telifís Éireann (later RTÉ) 2, 38–44, 165–8, 183, 224, 225; *see also* 2RN
Radio Luxembourg 166, 167
Radio Telegraph Convention of Madrid, International 41
radium 69–70
rates 53, 86, 203, 206, 213
Rathdrum 78
Rathmines 56
Rathmines Urban District Council 56
Ray, Betty 185
Readers' Digest 180
Reading, Pennsylvania 128
recession (early 1980s) 189
Red Cross: British 85, 127, 150, 151, 152; Irish 150, 151, 152; Northern Ireland 150; sweepstakes 150–3
regional health boards 220, 221
regional hospitals 68, 220, 221
Rehabilitation Institute 191
Report of the Departmental Committee on the Health Service 207
Revenue Commissioners 7, 122, 123, 190, 192
Rhodesian Sweep 144
Rice, Charles 125
Rice, Eamonn 125
Rice, James 151
Richmond Hospital 55, 66, 77, 197, 198, 222
Ringsend 169
'Ripley's Believe it or Not' column 138
R. J. Goffs (bloodstock sales) 189
Robins, Dr Joseph 218
Robinson & Keefe (architects) 34
Robinson, John J. 34
Robinson, Mary 183
Rockefeller Foundation 11, 78, 83
Romeike & Curtis (press-cutting Agency) 101
Roosevelt, Franklin D. 142
Roscommon 68, 78

Rothermere, Harold Harmsworth, 1st Viscount 96
Rothschild, Lord Nathaniel 156
Rotunda Maternity Hospital 4, 18, 52–3, 54, 67, 73, 79
Rowlatt, Sir Sidney 98
Rowlette, Dr Robert 74, 150, 202, 203
Royal Academy of Medicine in Ireland (RAMI) 83, 84
Royal Aero Club 45
Royal City of Dublin Hospital (Baggot Street) 10, 52, 54, 65, 77, 197, 220, 222
Royal College of Physicians of Ireland (RCPI) 66, 83
Royal College of Surgeons in Ireland (RCSI) 82, 83
Royal Commission on Betting, Lotteries and Gaming (1949–51) 155–6
Royal Commission on Gambling (1978) 156
Royal Commission on Lotteries and Betting (1932–3) 98–101
Royal Eye Hospital (London) 95
Royal Hospital, Donnybrook 53
Royal Victoria Eye Ear Hospital 6, 53
Russell, Seán 125
Ruttledge, Patrick 150
Ryan, Dr James 208, 210, 217

St Andrew's Catholic Club 6
St Anne's Cancer Hospital 69
St Bartholomew's Hospital, London 95, 107
St Catherine's Hospital 4
St James's Hospital (formerly South Dublin Union, St Kevin's) 66, 218, 222
St John's Hospital, Limerick 69
St Joseph's blind institution, Drumcondra 21
St Kevin's Hospital (formerly South Dublin Union, now St James's Hospital) 66, 201, 221, 222
St Laurence's Hospital Act (1943) 198
St Laurence's Hospital (proposed) 198, 211–12, 213, 218, 220, 221, 222
St Leger (English, 1933) 109
St Leger (Irish) 174
St Louis, Missouri 137
St Luke's Cancer Hospital 218
St Mary's Orthopaedic Hospital, Cappagh *see* Cappagh Orthopaedic Hospital
St Mary's Orthopaedic Hospital, Cork 210
St Nicholas's Hospital 4
St Patrick's Cathedral 14

St Patrick's Incurable Hospital, Cork 53
St Paul, Minnesota 138
St Ultan's Infant Hospital 9, 10, 16, 22, 53, 54,
      55–6, 67, 77, 222
St Vincent's Hospital 6, 10, 66, 197, 212, 218, 220,
      221, 222
Samuel, Sir Herbert 93, 98
San Diego exposition (1935–6) 119
sanatoria 53, 69, 198, 205–6, 213, 219; *see also* TB
Saurin, Frank 31, 153, 172
Scala, Emilio 28, 29, 30
Scala, Geofredo 29
School of Physics, TCD 197
Scotland 5, 22, 90, 96, 97, 155
Scott, Michael 198
Scott, Sir Harold 155
Seanad Éireann 147, 164, 176, 183, 186, 202
Senate (later Seanad) 18, 19, 63, 85
Senders Fries Berlin 167
7 Days (RTÉ programme) 179
Shamrock Sweeps 188
Shanks, George 41, 42, 168
Shannon Scheme 20, 35
Shepherd, A. F. 107
Siemens-Schuckert 20
Sinn Féin 20, 31
Sir Patrick Dun's Hospital 9, 10–11, 16, 22, 54,
      56, 65–6, 73, 74, 77, 197, 214, 220, 222
Sisters of Charity 66, 67, 197
Slevin, John 194, 195
Sligo, Co. 68, 78, 79
slum housing 63
Smith Group 189, 190
Smith, Hugh 138
smuggling *see* tickets
Smyth, P. L. 6, 15–16
social welfare 186, 193, 216
Solomons, Dr Bethel 52
South Africa 5, 20, 22, 50, 144
South Charitable Infirmary, Cork 68
South Cork Board of Public Assistance 68
South Dublin Union workhouse hospital (later
      St Kevin's Hospital, St James's Hospital) 66
Southampton 151
Special Commissioners of Income Tax 7
specialist hospitals 65, 67, 70, 80
specialists 58, 66, 67, 81, 221
sponsored radio programme 37–44, 165–7
Sports Federation of Ireland 161
sports sponsorship 170–1
Spring, Dick 191

Squash Ireland 189
SS *Capulin* 134
stamp duty 148, 203, 210, 224
Stanhope, James Robb 50, 180
Stanley, Sir Arthur 108
Stanton, C. Rebel 25
Stefanoff, Bello 137
Stephen, Nora 185
Stevenson, Lincoln 135
Stevenson, Oscar 135
Stoney, Richard Atkinson 66
Stubbs Gazette 130
Sunday Express 92
Sunday Independent 180, 184
Supreme Court 7, 50, 160, 190
Sweeps Hurdle 175, 177, 186, 192
Sweepstakes Annie (film) 141
Sweepstakes funds for hospitals 16, 17–19, 52, 54,
      62, 77–9, 179, 206, 219, 223, 224–6; allocation
      of funds 15, 22, 53–7, 59, 60, 61–4, 67, 73,
      75–6, 200, 202, 204; division of between
      hospitals and promoters 147–8, 152, 177–8,
      180, 182, 184, 192; eligibility conditions
      17–19, 53, 67, 74; hospital claims for 55, 57,
      58–9, 64, 76; for hospital library service 85–8;
      for medical research 62, 83–4; *see also* local
      authority hospitals; voluntary hospitals
Sweepstakes Winner (film) 141
Sweetman, Gerard 211
Swinford 78
Switzer's 189, 190

Talbot motor assembly plant 195
Tallaght 222, 223
Tallaght Hospital 222, 223
taxation 7, 32, 122, 123, 190–1, 194, 203; *see also*
      USA
TB 69, 78, 84, 87, 88, 204, 205–6, 225; eradication
      campaign 208; legislation 198, 205, 206, 208;
      sanatoria and hospitals 69, 78, 205–6, 207,
      210, 219
television broadcasting 3, 167–8, 183–4
Television Commission 168
Temple Street Children's Hospital 67, 214
Thomas, J. H. 95, 105
Thrift, Professor William 15
tickets: counterfeit 128–9, 135, 138; free 18, 96;
      prices 31, 144, 154, 172, 175, 176, 235; sales 15,
      16–17, 18, 39, 51, 172, 176–8, 184; sales in
      Britain 21, 23, 40, 90–5, 96–8, 99–100,
      101–6, 108, 109, 112 144, 151, 152–3, 155–6, 166;

sales in Canada 42, 103, 104, 112, 114–15, 175;
sales in Ireland 153; sales in Northern
Ireland 21; sales in USA 23, 24, 48, 103, 104,
111–13, 115–18, 131–6, 139–40, 157, 158–60;
shares in 28, 29, 30, 31, 130; smuggling 42,
91, 98, 104–5, 116–18, 126, 134–5, 155–6, 180,
183; *see also* agents and distributors
Times, The 101, 108
Tipperary 39, 68
Tobin, Liam 129
Today Tonight Special (RTÉ 1992) 184
Toome (Co. Down) sweepstake 6, 15
Torney, John 22
Toronto 115
Touche Ross (consultants) 191
trade unions 35, 37, 164–5; Britain 91; and HT
35–7, 164–5, 185, 187; and union recognition
164–5, 179, 180, 187; *see also* Irish Transport
and General Workers' Union; Irish Women
Workers Union; Workers' Union of Ireland
Tralee 78
Travel Goods, Portarlington 118
Treaty, Anglo-Irish 20, 31, 124
Trimblestown 32
Trinity College Dublin (TCD) 13, 15, 66, 183,
191, 197, 200
Tuberculosis (Establishment of Sanitoria) Act
(1945) 198, 205, 206, 208
Tullamore 78
2RN (later Radio Éireann) 37–8, 39, 40
Twomey, Moss 124, 125

Ulster Unionist Party 109
unemployment 56, 210, 219
United National Charities Ltd 191
United States of America (USA) 20, 84; Air
Commerce Bureau 45; Congress 136, 142, 143;
consulate in Dublin 111, 112, 120, 121, 126, 130,
132, 135, 137, 157, 159; Democratic Party 125,
142; Embassy in Britain 45; foreign lotteries
111–12, 131, 158; great depression 91, 111, 112,
142; hospitals 58, 85; and IHS 45, 111–13,
116–17, 119–21, 123, 125–31, 134–5, 137–43,
156–9, 160–1, 179, 225; illegal sweepstakes
traffic 119–20, 127–8, 130, 131–7, 139, 156–9;
income tax 120–1, 122, 123; 134, 137, 175;
Irish-American companies as agents 118;
Irish emigration to 91; Irish exports to 114,
115, 142; and Irish government 49, 135–6, 137,
157, 158; Irish in 2, 118, 138, 142; Irish Minister
in Washington 127, 131, 132, 135, 142; Irish
republicans in 120, 123–5, 126; lotteries and
gambling 4, 5, 13, 89, 90, 99, 100, 111–12,
113, 116, 134–7, 142–3, 172–4, 181; market for
tickets 24, 42, 103, 104, 112–13; Money Order
Convention (Ireland/USA) 157; Navy 45;
newspapers and periodicals 49, 127, 131, 133,
134, 137–41, 142, 179, 180–1, 226; Post Office
and 111, 118–20, 127–8, 131–7, 157, 159,; 142,
157; Postmaster General 112, 127, 131, 133–4,
135, 39, 157; publicity in 112, 116, 118–19,
127–8, 131, 133, 134, 136, 168; racing 111, 171;
Republican Party 131; rise in value of dollar
144; Second World War 144, 148, 149, 154;
State Department 135, 158, 159; sweepstake
money as invisible export from Ireland 114,
115, 142; US currency to Ireland 114, 115, 142,
154; US lottery legislation 111, 116, 134–7;
Veterans' Administration 142; Waterford
Glass 169, 188; Western Union 111, 157;
Works Progress Administration 31; *see also*
agents and distributors; America, north;
commissions; prizes and prizewinners;
tickets
United States Daily 127
University College Dublin (UCD) 13, 73, 83,
220, 221
University College Hospital, Galway (formerly
Regional Hospital) 218
unmarried mothers, homes for 62

Vancouver 22, 114, 115
Vernon's Football Pools 178, 179, 191
Viant, S. P. 92
Victoria Hospital, Cork 53, 217, 218
Virginia 4
voluntary hospitals 72, 221, 224; accountability
to state 224; bed bureau 79–82, 200–1;
Britain 74–5, 108, 109; buildings 10, 17, 65;
conflicting interests 58–9, 64–5, 77;
construction 10, 54, 57, 58, 75; donations to
10, 12, 14, 55–6, 217; finances 9, 10, 12, 15, 16,
54, 57, 218; funding 10, 11, 15, 17, 22, 52, 55, 56,
81, 199, 200, 203, 205, 206, 207, 210, 216, 217,
219, 224; and government 59, 60–1, 63, 198–9,
200, 202, 203, 224; Hospitals Commission
224–5; lay controlled 199–200, 214; Northern
Ireland 162; and original purpose of IHS 12,
63, 82, 224; Protestant 1, 8, 18, 52–3, 59, 67,
217–18, 221, 222–3; religious controlled 1, 59,
199, 200, 221; resent use of Sweepstake funds
for public hospitals 61–2, 63, 74, 198–9, 203,

voluntary hospitals *cont.*
206, 224; teaching 8, 66, 81, 198, 220; voluntary principle 11, 59, 60–1, 63, 66–7, 72, 82; *see also* Associated Hospitals Sweepstake Committee; hospital deficits; hospitals; Hospitals Trust Fund; sweepstakes funds for hospitals

Wales 5, 20, 22, 45, 91, 155
Walker, Arnold 114
Wall Street Crash 140
Wallace, Edgar 21
Wallasey 105
Walsh, Andrew 26
Walsh, J. J. 40
Walsh, Louis 164
Walshe, Joseph 136
Waltham Holdings 189, 190
Walton, Herbert 138
War of Independence 31
Ward, Dr Con 62–3, 203, 205–6, 207, 208, 213, 216
Ward, Frank 22
Washington DC 121, 126, 127, 131, 132, 134, 138, 135, 142, 159
Washington Post 138, 141
Waterford 33, 57, 68, 189
Waterford Glass 2, 125, 169–70, 183, 185, 188–9, 190
Watson and Jameson (sail-makers) 189
Webb, Arthur 2
welfare state (UK) 204
Western Union Telegraph Company 111, 130, 157
Westmeath, Co. 78, 114
Westminster 41
White, Dr Harry Vere, Church of Ireland bishop of Limerick 52

White, Dr Vincent 12
Whitworth Hospital 55, 198
Wicklow, Co. 68, 69
Wicklow, William Howard, 8th Earl of 214
Wilmington, North Carolina 156
Winning ticket, The (film) 44, 102, 128
Winnipeg 115
Wireless Telegraphy Act (1926) 42
Witts, John 104
Wong, Anna May 27
Woodbrook Golf club 170
Woodhall, Frederick 98, 105
Woodhall, Thomas 105
Worker's Union of Ireland (WUI, later FWUI) 164; and HT 164–5, 176, 185, 186–7, 194; struggle for recognition by 164–5, 179, 180, 184–7, 191
workhouse hospitals 66
Worksop 22
World War, First 8, 20, 85, 127, 142
World War, Second 121–2, 125; and hospitals 75, 76–7, 147–8, 197, 205, 207; and HT 27, 76, 77, 84, 103, 144–8, 149, 152–4; sweepstakes 25, 144, 150–3, 188; and racing 144, 49–50
World's Fair, New York (1939) 25
Wunder, Isaac 160–1
Wylie, Liam 3, 184

x-rays 69, 73, 74, 75, 197

Yorkshire Penny Bank 97
Youghal 78
YP (Young Philanthropists) Pools (Northern Ireland) 162–4, 174
Yugoslavia 41